Radiographic Imaging for Regional Anesthesia and Pain Management

Radiographic Imaging for Regional Anesthesia and Pain Management

P. Prithvi Raj, MD
Professor of Anesthesiology
Co-Director of Pain Services
Texas Tech University Health
Sciences Center School of Medicine
International Pain Institute
Lubbock, Texas

Leland Lou, MD
Assistant Professor of Anesthesiology
Texas Tech University Health
Sciences Center School of Medicine
International Pain Institute
Lubbock, Texas

Serdar Erdine, MD
Professor of Algology
Medical Faculty of Istanbul
University
Istanbul, Turkey

Peter S. Staats, MD
Associate Professor of Anesthesiology
and Critical Care Medicine
Division of Pain Medicine
John Hopkins University
School of Medicine
Baltimore, Maryland

Meadow Green
Medical Illustrator
Lubbock, Texas

Steven Platten
Computer Specialist
Lubbock, Texas

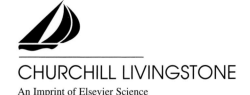

CHURCHILL LIVINGSTONE

An Imprint of Elsevier Science
New York Edinburgh London Philadelphia

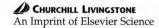

CHURCHILL LIVINGSTONE
An Imprint of Elsevier Science

The Curtis Center
Independence Square West
Philadelphia, Pennsylvania 19106

RADIOGRAPHIC IMAGING FOR REGIONAL ANESTHESIA AND
PAIN MANAGEMENT
ISBN 0–443–06596–9

Distributed in the United Kingdom by Churchill Livingstone, Robert Stevenson House, 1-3 Baxter's Place, Leith Walk, Edinburgh EH1 3AF and by associated companies, branches, and representatives throughout the world.

CHURCHILL LIVINGSTONE and the Sail Boat Design are trademarks of Elsevier Science, registered in the United States of America and/or other jurisdictions.

Notice

Anesthesiology is an ever-changing field. Standard safety precautions must be followed, but as new research and clinical experience broaden our knowledge, changes in treatment and drug therapy may become necessary or appropriate. Readers are advised to check the most current product information provided by the manufacturer of each drug to be administered to verify the recommended dose, the method and duration of administration, and the contraindications. It is the responsibility of the treating physician, relying on experience and knowledge of the patient, to determine the dosages and best treatment for each individual patient. Neither the publisher nor the editor assumes any liability for any injury and/or damage to persons or property arising from this publication.

The Publisher

Library of Congress Cataloging-in-Publication Data

Radiographic imaging for regional anesthesia and pain management / P. Prithvi Raj ... [et al.].
   p. cm.
  ISBN 0–443–06596–9
   1. Conduction anesthesia. 2. Radiography, Medical. 3. Analgesia. 4. Diagnostic
imaging. I. Raj, P. Prithvi.
  RD84 .R33 2003
  617.9′64–dc21

2002067432

Editor-in-Chief: Richard Lampert
Acquisitions Editor: Allan Ross
Developmental Editor: Josh Hawkins
Cover Designer: Ellen Zanolle

EH/MVY

Printed in the United States of America

Last digit is the print number: 9 8 7 6 5 4 3 2 1

To all our family, friends, and colleagues
who have made it possible
for this book to be published

▽ PREFACE

As the practice of pain management expands, so do the responsibilities of monitoring its growth and recognizing the need to sustain its growth. Everyone in the field of pain medicine will agree with us that the basic knowledge of pain mechanisms has grown by leaps and bounds since the 1960s. Similar growth has occurred in pain management teaching facilities, fellowship programs, examination process, books, and journals.

The daily practice of pain medicine is constantly evolving. Although the majority of pain specialists still feel that this field has to be multidisciplinary, this concept is understood differently in the various disciplines. If one asks a psychiatrist or a pharmacologist, he or she would state that chronic pain management is conservative management only with strong emphasis on behavior modification. If one asks an anesthesiology-trained pain physician or a neurosurgeon, they would state that multidisciplinary pain management means interventional techniques with assisted physical therapy and psychotherapy.

Surprisingly, pain patients have taken these conflicting opinions in their own hands and are coming to pain management centers in droves and demanding advanced interventional techniques. This experience has awakened the pain management community. In response, physiatrists, neurologists, orthopedists, and even radiologists are performing interventional techniques in ever-increasing numbers. One may think that this is good for the interventionist, but if considered more seriously, one will realize it is not.

Advanced interventional techniques are not adequately taught in a majority of the training programs. Even the anesthesiologist has less than ideal training in these techniques, as does the neurosurgeon, neurologist, and physiatrist. The teaching of indications and the techniques of performing these procedures is done mainly during weekend courses; some by societies and others by companies interested in selling their own products. Standards of care are often not available. This situation should be corrected immediately. There have to be credible institutions training physicians in proper application of these techniques.

At present, one of the very few texts that describes advanced interventional techniques is *Interventional Pain Management, 2nd edition*, edited by Steven D. Waldman and published by SAUNDERS, Philadelphia.

Although the text and content are authoritative, it does not take the trainee step by step through each procedure. This void needs to be filled. An easy-to-follow, step-by-step training manual for advanced interventional techniques is clearly needed. Special emphasis has to be placed on radiographic imaging as a safe way of doing these procedures. This manual, *Radiographic Imaging for Regional Anesthesia and Pain Management*, was conceived for this purpose. CHURCHILL LIVINGSTONE has been enthusiastic and supportive from the start of this project. One of the editors (PPR) discussed this idea with the other three editors, and here we have it—a unique book on radiographic imaging for interventional techniques.

The editors worked hard at choosing which techniques to describe. They finally came up with 38 techniques amenable to advanced radiographic imaging. Each technique was initially tried on cadavers. This allowed them to decide the correct position of the patient and the fluoroscope. Multiple photographs were taken. The material obtained from this activity led the editors to choose illustrations for line drawing and for radiologic imaging on actual patients. The images were then digitized and labeled by experts in computer technology.

Radiographic Imaging for Regional Anesthesia and Pain Management is the result of long and difficult hours by many people. We hope that our readers will find it easy to read and follow while learning the various procedures. The editors are indebted to many for completing this project. We are grateful to Steven Waldman, Susan Anderson, Miles Day, Gabor Racz, and many others who made it possible to select the best images for this book. We especially thank Marla Hall, Dr. Raj's secretary, who worked tirelessly to complete this project. Our gratitude also goes to Susan Raj, Sterling Brinson, Steven Platten, and Meadow Green for providing invaluable help in getting the book together in good time. Most of all we are thankful to Allan Ross, the publishing editor, for seeing this project through. He was ever so helpful, cheerful, and enthusiastic, which is so rare in the publishing world.

P. Prithvi Raj
Leland Lou
Serdar Erdine
Peter S. Staats

CONTENTS

Topographic Map of the Interventional Technique

Chapter **Head and neck**

6   Trigeminal ganglion
      block and neurolysis
7   Maxillary nerve block
8   Mandibular nerve block
9   Glossopharyngeal nerve block
10   Cervical (C3–C7) nerve root
      block and radiofrequency
      thermocoagulation
11   Sphenopalatine ganglion block
      and neurolysis
12   Stellate ganglion block
13   Atlanto-occipital joint block
14   Atlantoaxial joint block
15   Cervical facets median branch
      block and radiofrequency
      thermocoagulation
16   Cervical epidural nerve block
17   Cervical discogram
18   Brachial plexus block

Chapter **Lumbar/Abdomen**

26   Lumbar sleeve and
      dorsal root ganglion
      block
27   Splanchnic nerve block
28   Celiac plexus block
      and neurolysis
29   Lumbar sympathetic block
      and neurolysis
30   Lumbar facet block and median
      branch blocks
31   Lumbar provocative discography
32   Intradiscal
      electrothermocoagulation
33   Vertebroplasty
34   Psoas and quadratus lumborum
      muscle injection

Chapter **Chest/Thorax**

19   Intercostal nerve block
20   Thoracic sleeve and
      dorsal root ganglion
      block and neurolysis
21   Suprascapular nerve block
22   T2 and T3 sympathetic nerve
      block and neurolysis
23   Thoracic facet block and
      radiofrequency
      thermocoagulation
24   Thoracic epidural block
25   Thoracic discogram

Chapter **Pelvis**

35   Sacral nerve root injection
36   Hypogastric plexus block
      and neurolysis
37   Ganglion of Impar block
38   Sacroiliac joint injection

Chapter **Lower Extremities**

39   Sciatic nerve catheter
      placement and block
40   Piriformis muscle injection

Basic Physics of Radiography

ATOMIC STRUCTURE

Matter is composed of atoms that occupy space. The atoms can be further broken down into elementary components consisting of the electron, proton, and neutron. All known substances, living and nonliving, are from these elemental components. Combinations of these elemental particles determine the atomic structures. The atomic number, based on the number of protons, is used to classify each element.

Protons (positive charge) and neutrons (neutral charge) collectively form the nucleus of the atom. The electrons are often compared to "planets" that orbit the nucleus, or "sun," of the atom (Fig. 1–1). Negative charge from the electrons keeps them orbiting the nucleus in five electron shells labeled K, L, M, N, and O (Fig. 1–2). The K shell is the strongest and requires the most energy to displace an electron from its orbit. If an electron is moved from a higher energy shell to a lower one, energy is released.

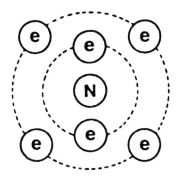

FIGURE 1–1

Atomic structure. A typical atom consists of a nucleus (N), which contains positively charged protons, neutrons (no charge), and negatively charged electrons (e). The electrons orbit around the nucleus. This representation of the carbon atom is not in scale. In actuality, neutrons and protons each constitute 1838 times more mass than electrons.

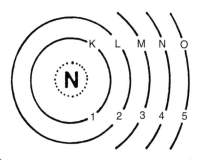

FIGURE 1–2

Electron shell arrangement and binding power. The binding force on the electron shells holding the electrons in orbit around the nucleus weakens as the number of shells increases. The five electron shells shown are labeled K, L, M, N, and O. The K shell possesses the strongest binding power. The electrons in the K shell require the most energy to dislodge from orbit, whereas the electrons in the peripheral shells are easier to displace.

Normally an atom is in a non-ionized state with an equal number of protons and electrons. When this balanced state is disturbed, the displaced orbital electron and the atom from which it originated is called an *ion pair*. This situation can occur with electron bombardment of matter, x-ray bombardment of matter, thermionic emission with electron release, chemically, and many others. If the ionized electron is moved to a higher orbit, this is called *excitation*. In an excited state the displaced electron returns to its original orbit or is replaced by another electron. Often the additional energy needed to ionize the atom is released as photons of electromagnetic energy, heat, or chemical energy.

ELECTROMAGNETIC RADIATION

Electromagnetic energy is arranged in an orderly fashion according to the wavelength. For medical x-rays this range is from approximately 0.1 to 0.5 Å (0.01 to 0.05 nm) (Fig. 1–3). This energy travels in the form of sine

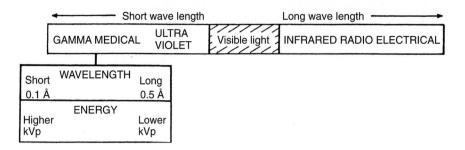

FIGURE 1–3

The relationship of the medical x-ray to the electromagnetic spectrum. In this abbreviated illustration the electromagnetic spectrum runs from gamma radiation (short wavelength) to electrical waves (long wavelength). Within the medical x-ray portion of the spectrum, wavelengths may be short (0.1 Å) or long (0.5 Å). In the medical x-ray range, a short wavelength is produced with high kilovoltage values, whereas a long wavelength is generated by low kilovoltage values.

wave–like oscillations at the speed of light. The oscillations are measured as amplitude, wavelength, and frequency. Amplitude is the height of the wave from the crest to midpoint or trough to midpoint. Wavelength (angstrom) is the distance from one wave to the next. Frequency (hertz) is the measurement of the number of waves passing by a specific point in a given unit of time (Fig. 1–4). X-ray photons are commonly between 0.1 and 0.5 Å and 10^{18} to 10^{21} Hz.

ELECTRICAL ENERGY CONVERSION TO X-RADIATION

Alternating current (AC) is converted into direct current (DC) by an electrical transformer. This direct current is then put into motion (kinetic energy) from cathode to anode in the x-ray tube to produce heat (thermal energy) and x-radiation (radiant energy).

The filament (cathode) of the x-ray tube is heated to incandescence, causing electrons to "boil off" in a process known as *thermionic emission*. The electrons' energy is converted into heat and x-ray energy.

The milliampere setting selects the tube current and determines the heat of the filament. This setting determines the number of released electrons available for interaction. The range of the applied voltage (kilovolt [peak]) determines the wavelength and thus the energy of the x-ray photons. The relation of voltage and amperage to resistance can be expressed by Ohm's law, which states that

$$I = \frac{V}{R}$$

where I = amperage, V = voltage, and R = resistance.

ELECTRON INTERACTION WITH THE ANODE OF THE X-RAY TUBE

More than 99% of the energy is converted to thermal energy (heat). The remaining energy is divided among

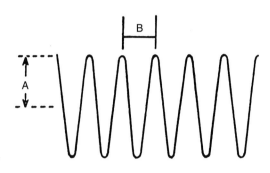

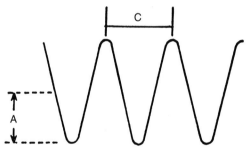

FIGURE 1–4

Sine wave. Electromagnetic energy is transported through space in the form of sine wave–like oscillations. This energy travels at the speed of light, about 186,300 miles per second, and can be schematically illustrated. Components of the sine wave include amplitude, wavelength, and frequency. *Amplitude* refers to the height of the wave from crest to mean value (A). *Wavelength* describes the distance from one crest of the wave to another and represents the distance between two corresponding points on the wave (B and C). *Frequency* is determined by the number of crests or valleys passing through a specific point in a given time. There are more wavelengths in B compared with C. Shorter wavelengths (B) result in increased frequency of the wave.

bremsstrahlung and characteristic radiation. Heat is produced by the energy derived from the movement of the atoms and their quick return to a normal state. The greater the kinetic energy (energy of motion or vibration) produced, the greater the temperature.

Bremsstrahlung radiation is also known as *general radiation*, the *continuous spectrum*, or *white radiation*. Production of bremsstrahlung radiation is from the "braking" action that occurs as the electrons interact with the anode. This process involves electrons that gratingly pass by the heavy nuclei of the metallic atoms in the target material. The attraction between the negatively charged electrons and the positively charged nuclei causes the electrons to be deflected and decelerated from their original path and to lose some of their energies. Since energy cannot be destroyed, the energies lost by the electrons are transformed and emitted as x-ray photons.

The considerable rate of deceleration causes the emission of short wavelength radiation in the form of x-rays. As this braking action varies, so does the intensity of the resultant x-ray energy. In the 80- to 100-kVp ranges, using tungsten anode, these bremsstrahlung rays constitute about 90% of the radiation emitted as x-rays. For example, to produce characteristic radiation with a tungsten target, at least 70 kVp is required for K-shell interaction, because the K-shell electron of tungsten is held with 69.53 effective kilovoltage (see Fig. 1–2). Characteristic radiation produced in the interaction of x-rays with matter is usually referred to as *secondary radiation* and is a form of scatter.

X-RAY INTERACTION WITH MATTER

In diagnostic radiology, there are three types of x-ray energies of importance. Primary x-rays or photons are emitted by the x-ray tube. Scattered x-rays or photons are produced when primary photons collide with electrons in matter. Remnant radiation is the x-rays that pass through the patient and strikes the image detector.

When discussing x-ray interactions with matter, a photoelectric effect and Compton effect are important. The photoelectric effect is the absorption of energy. When the x-ray photon collides with the inner shell electron of an atom, the photon may gives off all of its energy and the collision causes the photoelectric effect along with ionization.

The *Compton effect* refers to the scatter of the ions or radiation as it interfaces with different radiographic densities. If the incoming x-ray photon has increased energy, resulting from increased kilovoltage applied to the x-ray tube, some of that energy is transferred to other atoms with the x-ray photon passing with a decreased energy and slower wavelength. This principle is relevant to the five basic medical radiographic densities: air, fat, water (soft tissue), bone, and metal.

ELECTRICAL CURRENT

There are two basic types of current: alternating and direct. Alternating current of sinusoidal wave shape results from the application of an alternating voltage with its polarity and values reversing direction at regularly occurring intervals, typically 60 times per second (60 Hz) in the United States. Electrical energy in the form of voltage and amperage is usually supplied by commercial power companies and delivered as alternating current, because it is easier to produce and transfer from place to place in this form. Alternating current can be greatly increased or decreased by employing a simple device called a *transformer* (see Transformers).

Direct current may be steady or intermittent. The direction of flow does not change with direct current. To operate many devices, direct current is created from alternating current. This current is easier to put to use but difficult to transmit over great distances.

ELECTRICAL CIRCUITS

In a series circuit, the current passes consecutively through each individual component and can be expressed as $I = i^1 = i^2 = i^3$. With a parallel circuit, current flow is divided among the branches of the circuit and is expressed as $I = i^1 = i^2 = i^3$.

DEFINITIONS

An electrical circuit is used to gather, carry, or direct flowing electron energy. Electrical energy is carried through the circuit by electrical current (electrons in motion). Volts (V) measure the potential difference from start to end of a path. Current (I) or electron flow is measured in amperes (A). There is resistance (opposition) to the electron flow in all circuits, with some absorption and thus loss of energy.

Electrical resistance (R) is measured in ohms (Ω). The term *resistance* is used in reference to a simple direct current. Impedance denotes resistance in alternating current. The resistance of a conductor is directly proportional to the resistivity of the material of which the conductor is formed. Resistance is also directly proportional to the length of the conductor but inversely proportional to the width (cross-sectional area) of the conductor.

Conductors are materials that transport electrons at all levels of energy output. Some materials are able to conduct only when they receive a specific increment of energy; these are known as *semiconductors*. Some materials do not conduct and are thus referred to as *insulators*.

TRANSFORMERS

A transformer does not produce energy—it transforms voltage and current by way of the ratios of their respective windings.

Air-Core Transformer. By placing a coil of wire with current flowing through it, called a *solenoid*, adjacent to a second coil of wire, an air-core transformer is formed. This is the simplest type of transformer.

Open-Core Transformer. To form an open-core transformer, soft iron bars are placed in both the primary and secondary coils. The cores are not electrically connected; they only conduct field lines.

Closed-Core Transformer. A continuous laminated iron bar forming a rectangular annulus is used to support the primary and secondary windings in a closed-core transformer. Again, there are no electrical connections between the coils.

Shell-Core Transformer. A continuous laminated iron bar forming a rectangular figure-8, with the primary and secondary wires wound around the center support, is called a *shell-core transformer*.

Step-Up Transformer. A ratio exists between the primary and secondary currents and is related to the number of turns in the wires in the individual coils. If the number of turns in the wire of the secondary coil exceeds the number of turns in the wire of the primary coil, the transformer becomes a step-up transformer and voltage will be increased.

Step-Down Transformer. If more turns exist in the wire of the primary coil than in that of the secondary coil, the transformer becomes a step-down transformer and voltage will be reduced. The filament circuit uses a step-down transformer.

Autotransformer. An autotransformer is easy to recognize in a circuit schematic. The primary and secondary windings of the autotransformer are connected in series with no electrical insulation between the primary and secondary sides. A large number of contacts (taps) are attached to the different turns of the transformer. Voltage is changed to kilovoltage by a step-up transformer, which operates on the principle of mutual induction to change the voltage ratio.

Three-Phase Transformers. Three-phase transformers are used for three-phase equipment to generate a more homogenous x-ray beam. Three separate circuits are required in an x-ray machine using three-phase power, one for each phase. Each circuit requires its own transformer, rectifiers, line voltage compensator, and so on.

SUMMARY

The production of the x-radiation is dependent on many factors and principles in physics. With advancement of technology, electricity is used to generate x-radiation without the need for radioactive elements in radiographic imaging. These machines can thus be transported easily wherever electricity can be found and x-ray images are needed. General knowledge of the creation of x-radiation and its effects on the matter that it interacts with is important for proper understanding of the use of the radiographic devices. Through knowledge of the safe and appropriate use of x-rays, the physician, patients, and ancillary staff all can minimize their radiation exposure.

FURTHER READING

Cullinan AM, Cullinan JE: Producing Quality Radiographs, 2nd ed. Philadelphia, JB Lippincott, 1994.

CHAPTER 2

Equipment Used for Radiographic Imaging

BASIC COMPONENTS OF AN X-RAY GENERATING SYSTEM

ELECTROMAGNETICS

Electrical charges may be static (at rest) or dynamic (in motion). Electrical current is always surrounded by a magnetic field, which exists only while the current is flowing. The process of electromagnetic induction can produce current from a second wire. Since both coils are not electrically connected, placing a second coil of wire adjacent to the first coil induces an electrical current in the second coil by mutual induction. The force in the second wire loop is directly proportional to the number of turns in the first wire loop.

When the wire of a conductor is coiled, a helix is formed. A helix with current flowing through it is called a *solenoid*. The solenoid, an electromagnet, has a strong magnetic field in its center when current is flowing through the coiled wire.

Rheostats are controls used to add resistance to the circuit to adjust incoming voltage and amperage values. A break in the circuit can be achieved with switches that are used to control the length of time that the current may flow. Fuses or circuit breakers are protective devices that open at present levels of current and thus prevent circuit overloading and damage.

THE X-RAY CIRCUIT

The x-ray circuit is divided into subsections called *primary* (low-voltage) and *secondary* (high-voltage) circuits (Fig. 2–1).

The primary circuit consists of the following:

1. The main switch: Power from an electrical source is turned off and on at this point.
2. A line voltage compensator: This is used to compensate for variations in power supply. It is important to monitor the incoming line voltage. Line voltage compensation is automatic in some units.
3. Fuses or circuit breakers: These are used to prevent equipment overload or tube damage.
4. An autotransformer: This is used to control voltage supplied to the primary of the step-up transformer, to allow for minimal variations in kilovoltage selection.
5. A prereading voltmeter: This indicates the amount of voltage being sent to the primary of the step-up transformer. Kilovoltage is determined by the amount of voltage supplied to the step-up transformer and is present only when the exposure is being made.
6. Timer and exposure switches: Timers are used for manual or automatic exposure control. The timer is situated between the autotransformer and the primary of the step-up transformer.
7. A filament circuit: Thermal energy is created from this circuit to heat the filament of the x-ray tube. High amperage is used to heat the filament for production of thermionic emission. The heating of the filament is then controlled by the rheostats or resistors, which regulate the milliamperage delivered to the filament circuit and resultant heating.
8. A filament ammeter: This is used to measure the filament current.
9. The primary coil of the step-up transformer.

The secondary or high-voltage circuit consists of:

1. The secondary coil of the step-up transformer: This is "center-tapped" to allow a milliampere meter to be installed at ground potential.
2. The milliampere meter: This is used to measure tube current.
3. A milliampere-second (mAs) meter: This is used to measure mAs values at short time intervals.

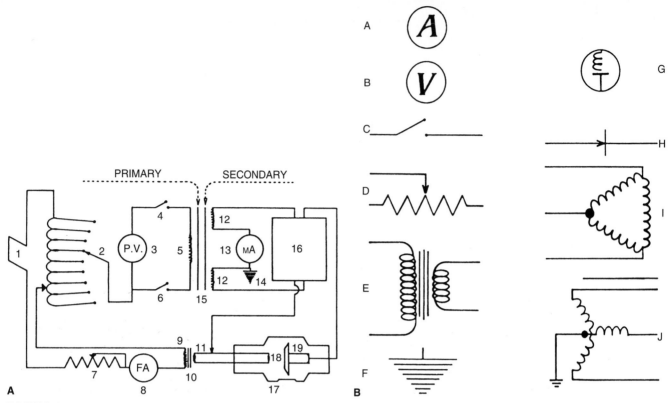

FIGURE 2–1

A, The x-ray–generating circuit is divided into a primary (low-voltage) and secondary (high-voltage) circuit. The primary circuit consists of (1) a main switch, (2) an autotransformer, (3) a prereading voltmeter, (4) fuses or circuit breakers, (5) the primary coil of the step-up transformer, (6) a timer that includes exposure switches, (7) a filament circuit and rheostat, used to vary current to the primary circuit of a step-down transformer to illuminate the filament of the x-ray tube, (8) a filament ammeter, (9) the primary coil of the step-down transformer, (10) the step-down transformer, and (11) the secondary coil of the step-down transformer. The secondary or high-voltage circuit consists of (12) the secondary of the step-up transformer, (13) a milliampere meter, (14) ground, (15) step-up transformer, (16) a rectification system, (17) the x-ray tube, (18) the cathode of the x-ray tube, and (19) the anode of the x-ray tube, including shockproof grounded cables to conduct high voltage from the secondary of the step-up transformer to the tube. Solid-state rectifiers are used to illustrate the rectification segment, since valve tubes (vacuum tubes with illuminated filaments) are no longer in common use. Valve tubes require step-down transformers.

B, Schematic representation of x-ray circuit components. (A) The filament ammeter is usually designated in the circuit by a circular meter containing the symbol A. (B) A voltmeter is similarly indicated by the symbol V. (C) A circuit breaker or a timer is often represented as an open-ended switch. (D) A rheostat is used to vary electrical current to the primary circuit of the step-down transformer. (E) The step-down transformer shown has more turns in the coils of the primary than in the secondary windings. (F) The universal symbol for ground. (G) Vacuum tubes that contain a filament and flat anode can be used for rectification of alternating current to direct current. (H) A solid-state rectifier. Three-phase transformers used for three-phase equipment generate a more homogenous x-ray beam. Three separate circuits are required in an x-ray machine using three-phase power, one for each phase. Each circuit requires its own transformer, rectifiers, line voltage compensator, and so on. In the high-tension transformer the primary coils are wound around separate arms of a core common to all three transformers. (I) A "delta" configuration depicts this arrangement of the coils. (J) The secondary high-tension coils have a common center, each coil radiating outward in a star ("Wye") pattern.

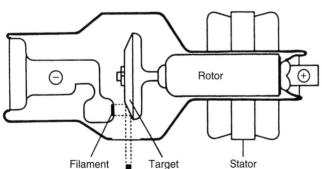

FIGURE 2–2

Basic components of an x-ray tube. A basic component of a radiographic tube is the filament, the source of electrons, at the cathode side of the tube. The cathode, with a high negative potential, includes the focusing cup, which has a negative charge applied to it to "focus" the stream of electrons by the repulsion of like charges. The anode, with a high positive potential, serves as a target for the focused electron stream. A stator rotor system that uses an induction motor rotates the anode at extremely high speed, usually 3000 or 10,000 rpm. A Pyrex envelope houses the cathode and rotating anode and is placed in an oil-filled, lead-lined housing.

4. Rectifiers: The x-ray tube is most efficient when unidirectional high-voltage current is used. Current is made unidirectional for use by the x-ray tube by means of a rectification system which converts alternating current to direct current (DC).

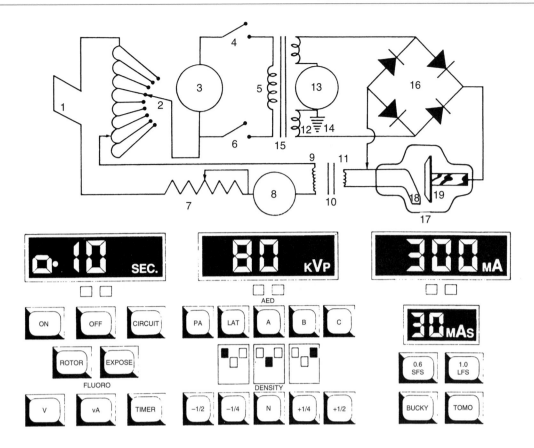

FIGURE 2–3

Operator controls of an x-ray machine. This representation of a control panel is divided into the following segments: kilovoltage and related circuits *(center)*, milliampere settings and focal spot size selection *(right)*, and timer control *(left)*. A representative schematic of the x-ray circuit is shown above the control panel. Depending on the equipment design, these controls can be presented in many configurations. Additional meters such as tube load limits, heat displays, and a direct readout of the fluoroscopic examination time are often found on control panels.

Kilovoltage can be raised or lowered *(center)* as required to adequately penetrate the part being examined. A power "on" and "off" button and a circuit breaker are shown. The rotor control as well as the "expose" button is on the left. At the bottom are fluoroscopic kilovoltage and milliampere stations and a fluoroscopic timer that can be set to limit the length of the fluoroscopic procedure.

The milliampere (mA) readout is shown on the right. Milliamperage can be raised or lowered depending on technical needs. A high milliampere value combined with a short exposure time is sometimes needed to overcome motion. The selection of a moderate milliampere value often permits the use of a small focal spot (SFS) (LFS stands for large focal spot). The focal spots represented in this panel are 0.6 and 1.0 mm in size. Directly above the focal spot selection indicators is a milliampere meter. This device is required when extremely short exposures are used so that an accurate reading of the milliamperes used can be obtained. Below the focal spot size selection are the Bucky "on" and "off" buttons and tomographic selector control.

At the top left of the control panel is the manual timing section. The time of exposure can be raised or lowered by the radiographer, or an AED can be selected. Specific AED sensor indicators for the chest (posteroanterior or lateral) or other Bucky stations are shown. Table Bucky is represented by A, the upright Bucky by B, and the radiographic spot-film component of the fluoroscope by C. The darkened sensors (left, right, or center) indicate the sensors selected for the part under study.

In the lower portion of the AED section on the control panel, density adjustment controls are shown. The center button, labeled N, is intended for use when a normal or preselected density is desired. The (–) control can be adjusted for a ¼ or ½ decrease in density. The (+) control can be adjusted in a similar fashion for an increase in density. When an examination must be repeated, image density should be adjustable by the use of the (–) or (+) setting.

5. Shockproof, grounded cables: These conduct high-voltage current from the secondary of the step-up transformer to the x-ray tube.
6. The x-ray tube.

BASIC COMPONENTS OF AN X-RAY TUBE

The basic component of the x-ray tube starts with the filament. From the source of electrons or cathode side of the tube the electron stream passes through a "focus-ing cup" or area and is directed into the anode. A rotating anode with a high positive potential is often used instead of a stationary anode in a fluoroscope (Fig. 2–2).

This rotating anode allows for quicker dissipation of the heat generated. An extremely high-speed stator motor system is needed to keep the heat produced even and avoid damage to the anode. The x-ray is projected from the x-ray tube into the target area and gathered by the imager to be transformed into a radiographic image.

BASIC OPERATION OF X-RAY TUBE

Once the electrical signal is sent through the circuitry, the filament is energized to "boil off" electrons as a thermionic emission. As the increase of kilovolt (peak) passes through the filament the creation of a higher potential difference results in the emission of electrons beyond the "cloud" of electrons that are found in the vicinity of the filament. The attraction of the electrons into the metal anode (+) surface and the following abrupt stopping of the electrons produce x-radiations and heat. Unfortunately, 99% of this energy is converted into undesired heat and less than 1% is converted into x-radiation.

The variation of the kilovoltage affects the speed of the electrons directed at the anode and generates different wavelengths of the x-rays. For example, a shorter wavelength makes the beam more penetrating. A longer wavelength x-ray is less energetic and less penetrating.

CONTROL PANEL

In clinical practice the control panel is the most common interface of the fluoroscope and the radiographer (Fig. 2–3). From this panel variations in power delivered through the x-ray tube can be controlled for improved images. The milliamperage determines the intensity of the x-ray beam. Kilovoltage determines the speed of the electrons and quality of the x-ray beam. The length of exposure is often measured in seconds and is the most obvious factor in measuring x-ray exposure.

The milliamperage is important in determining the quantity of x-rays produced. In combination with the length of exposure, the milliamperage is important to the quality of the image produced. For a stop-motion situation, the operator may need to combine a high milliamperage with a short exposure time.

Kilovoltage determines the penetrating ability and quality of the x-ray beam. The higher energy release of x-rays results in a greater number of photons to be captured by the imager. This allows for a more detailed and wider range of contrast of the gray scale.

Collimator buttons on the control panel are usually of two varieties: a circular shape and horizontal bars. Ideally the collimators should be used as much as possible to reduce the amount of radiation exposure. For this purpose the radiographer may choose horizontal collimation for facet injections. The circular or "shutter" collimation is best used in techniques that use a "tunnel approach."

The timer is also located on the control panel. There are audible alerts set at 5-minute intervals to remind the fluoroscopist of the actual time of x-radiation exposure. Exposure is best limited by minimizing fluoroscopy time. To simplify the measurement of time, the timer should be reset prior to each new procedure.

Many of the other buttons available for manual control involve the orientation of the fluoroscopic image from left to right, inversion, or rotation. This function is important for the interventional physician in the performance of the procedure. A consistent habit provides continuity and accordingly limits risk and mistakes. For example, left-sided procedures should always be correlated with a left-sided radiographic image to prevent accidentally performing the procedure on the wrong side.

SUMMARY

Although the use of the x-ray machine is often critical for the performance of the interventional procedure, the many manual adjustments discussed are frequently unnecessary. Sensors provide for an automatic mode of adjustment of the milliamperage and kilovolts, enabling ease of use by the physician and the ancillary staff. The most frequent adjustments of the fluoroscopic image are the orientation of the image to minimize physician confusion.

FURTHER READING

Cullinan AM, Cullinan JE: Producing Quality Radiographs, 2nd ed. Philadelphia, JB Lippincott, 1994.

C H A P T E R

3

Radiation Safety

Interventional radiology procedures can require substantial amounts of ionizing radiation and therefore necessitate particularly close attention to radiation management. This chapter reviews radiation units, regulations, and the fundamental principles of radiation management for patients and personnel and examines the procedures and devices designed to reduce patient and staff exposure in interventional radiology.

RADIATION UNITS

The fundamental interactions of x-rays with matter produce ion pairs via photoelectric absorption and Compton scattering.[1] The *coulomb per kilogram* (C/kg) is the unit used to measure the electrical charge produced by x- or gamma-radiation in a standard volume of air by ionization. Previously the *roentgen* unit (about 0.25 mC/kg) was used for this purpose. *Radiation exposure* is the formal term for the process of ion pair production.

The number of ion pairs produced in air does not directly measure the amount of energy deposited in another medium because of the differences in x-ray absorption by different materials.[1] The *gray* (Gy) is used as a measure of the radiation *absorbed dose* (energy deposited per unit mass). A gray is equal to 1 J/kg. The older unit of the rad is equal to 0.01 Gy. These units are of fundamental importance in patient dosimetry.

Ionizing radiations other than x- and gamma rays, such as particles or neutrons, may induce a greater biologic effect for a given absorbed dose. To quantitate this observation, the *sievert* (Sv) is used to measure the *dose equivalent*. The sievert is equal to the number of grays multiplied by a quality factor ranging from 1 to 20 that expresses the degree of biologic insult for equal doses of different types of ionizing radiation. The quality factor for x- and gamma radiation is equal to 1. The older unit of the rem is equal to 0.01 Sv. This unit is most often used in health physics and radiation-monitoring measures for personnel.

RADIATION PROTECTION FUNDAMENTALS

To decrease the absorbed dose to the patient and the staff, the radiation protection principles of time, distance, and shielding must be considered. Radiation dose is directly related to exposure time, so by halving the exposure time, one halves the radiation dose. Personnel who do not need to be in the fluoroscopy suite during all or part of a procedure can reduce their exposure time by simply leaving the area. For other individuals the time is totally controlled by the fluoroscopist. Therefore, to reduce exposure time, the fluoroscopist should never depress the foot switch except while observing the fluoroscopic image.

Because an x-ray beam diverges as it passes through space, radiation intensity decreases as the inverse square of the distance from the radiation source:

$$\frac{I_2}{I_1} = \frac{d_1{}^2}{d_2{}^2}$$

Hence, the distance from a radiation source is doubled; the radiation intensity decreases to one-fourth its original value (Fig. 3–1, *upper graph*). Although this relation holds strictly only for a point source, the distance principle is useful in reducing radiation dose to clinical personnel when the patient is the principal source of scattered radiation. Personnel who do not need to be in the immediate vicinity of the patient should always stay as far away as is reasonable from the portion of the patient that is being imaged.

The attenuation of an x-ray beam (loss of intensity as it passes through matter) is exponential:

$$I = I_0 e^{-\mu x}$$

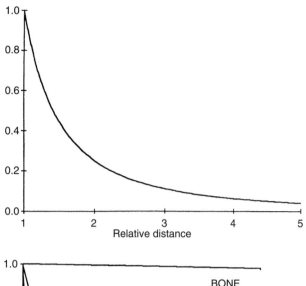

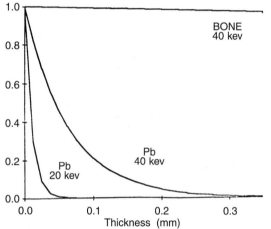

FIGURE 3–1

Upper graph, Reduction of radiation intensity (*y* axis) according to the inverse square of distance law. *Lower graph,* Reduction of radiation intensity with increasing thickness of lead (Pb) and bone at 60 kVp (20 kev) and 120 kVp (40 kev).

where I and I_0 are the initial and transmitted radiation intensity, respectively; μ is the attenuation coefficient of the material (which depends on the atomic number and density of the material and on the energy of the photons); and x is the thickness of the attenuating material. Small amounts of attenuating (shielding) material can greatly reduce the intensity of an x-ray beam. For example, more than 90% reduction of a diagnostic x-ray beam is obtained by using material equivalent to 0.5 mm of lead (the nominal equivalent of a typical lead apron). Examples of exponential attenuation for diagnostic radiology x-ray beams are shown in Figure 3–1 *(lower graph).* Lead aprons should always be worn by anyone in a fluoroscopy suite. Because fluoroscopy is used extensively during some interventional radiology procedures, the continual observation of these fundamental principles is of far greater importance than in other areas of diagnostic radiology.

RADIATION PROTECTION REGULATIONS

Unlike other areas in medicine in which ionizing radiation is used to diagnose or treat disease (e.g., therapeutic radiology, nuclear medicine), x-ray use is not completely regulated at the federal level. No one federal body analogous to the Regulatory Commission exists to supervise the x-rays. Instead regulations concerning equipment are devised by the Center for Devices and Radiology Health within the U.S. Food and Drug Administration (FDA)[2]; the Occupational Safety and Health Administration (OSHA) places limits on the radiation doses of employees in the workplace; and individual states' departments of services place additional regulations on users of x-ray equipment. Although one might expect this decentralization of regulations to be confusing, the state-to-state variation actually is minimal, since most states have patterned their regulations after the recommendations of the National Council on Radiation Protection and Measurements (NCRP). This body has developed an extensive set of regulatory guidelines that have become de facto standards for the safe and proper use of ionizing radiation (summarized in Tables 3–1 and 3–2). Other sources give further details of the general philosophy of radiation protection, as well as specific recommendations for particular situations.[3–9] Two other bodies also publish recommendations for radiation protection: the International Commission on Radiation Protection (ICRP) and the International Commission on Radiological Units and Measurements (ICRU).

The presence of these diverse recommendations is particularly important in interventional radiology, since the maximum quarterly dose to the eyes permitted by OSHA is one third that recommended by other regulatory organizations. These quarterly allowances are

▽ TABLE 3–1 Maximum Permissible Dose Equivalents (mSv)

Area	13 Weeks	Yearly	Cumulative
Total effective dose equivalent	12.5	50	Age × 10
Lens of eye	37.5	150	
Other organs (individually)	125	500	

▽ TABLE 3–2 Maximum Number of Fluoroscopic Procedures in a 3-Month Period Without Exceeding Eye Exposure of 12.5 mSv/Quarter

	Radiation Exposure at Eye Level (mSv/hr)					
Fluoroscopic Time per Procedure (hr)	**10**	**25**	**50**	**100**	**200**	**300**
0.25	50.0	20.0	10.0	5.0	2.5	1.2
0.50	25.0	10.0	5.0	2.5	1.2	0.8
1.00	12.5	5.0	2.5	1.2	0.8	0.4
2.00	6.2	2.5	1.2	0.6	0.3	0.2

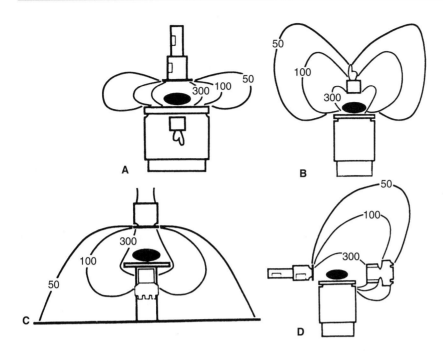

FIGURE 3–2

Scatter radiation from several equipment configurations. Isoexposure lines are given in mR/hr. *A*, Conventional fluoroscopy. *B*, Overhead tube. *C*, Posteroanterior fluoroscopy with C-arm or U-arm. *D*, Cross-table lateral fluoroscopy with C-arm or U-arm. (Courtesy of General Electric Medical Systems Division.)

intended for sporadic exposure, not continuous exposure. Doses should always be kept "*as low as reasonably achievable*" (ALARA).

Concern is often expressed about the absorbed dose to the eye of the fluoroscopist because of the risk of radiation-induced cataracts. This biologic effect appears to have a threshold, in that about 6 Gy of diagnostic x-irradiation over several weeks is necessary to produce cataracts in humans.[3, 10, 11] It may be that absorbed doses of about 15 Gy are necessary to induce cataracts in the diagnostic radiology setting.[6, 10]

STAFF RADIATION DOSE MONITORING

In general, monitoring devices must be worn if it is reasonable likely that a person could receive 25% of the maximum permissible dose in the discharge of his or her duties. This rule most assuredly mandates dose monitoring of the interventional radiologist and anyone else routinely in the fluoroscopy suite during these procedures.

STAFF RADIATION PROTECTION IN FLUOROSCOPY

The radiation exposure of the fluoroscopist is heavily dependent on imaging geometry. Figure 3–2 shows typical isoexposure lines for several imaging configurations; note the tremendous increase in operator exposure with configurations in which the x-ray tube is above the patient. This increase occurs for two reasons: the overall intensity of the scattered radiation beam is approximately 985 greater at the radiation entrance site

on the skin compared to the exit site,[1] and there is less attenuating material (e.g., image intensifier) between the patient and the operator. As a rule of thumb, the maximum operator exposure at a given distance occurs when there is an unobstructed path between an object and the location at which the x-ray beam enters the patient.

In addition to time, distance, and shielding, another important radiation protection parameter is x-ray beam size (Fig. 3–3). The amount of scattered radiation exposure is directly related to beam size. The patient dose and image quality are affected by changes in collimation. Hence, by limiting the beam size to the smallest necessary area, the fluoroscopist can decrease both personnel and patient doses while improving image quality.

RADIATION MANAGEMENT DURING IMAGE RECORDING

Because cine is an extension of fluoroscopy, all of the previous radiation protection considerations apply; however, radiation doses are significantly higher for the patient as well as the staff. Typical patient skin entrance dose rates can range from 200 to 900 mGy/min in fluoroscopy.[12–14]

RADIATION MANAGEMENT IN COMPUTED TOMOGRAPHY

Head and neck entrance doses could range from approximately 3 to 9 mGy for an interventional procedure

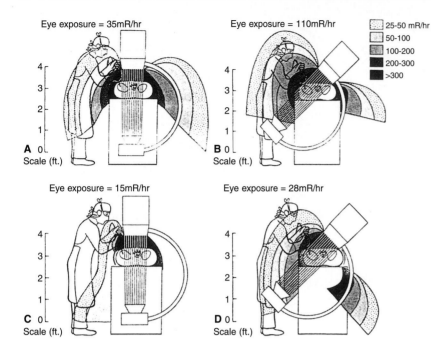

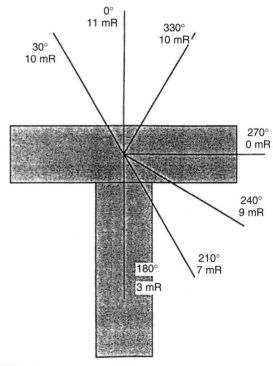

FIGURE 3–3

Scatter radiation reduction with surface shielding (2.8 R/min patient skin entrance exposure). A, Vertical fluoroscopy without shielding. B, Oblique (45-degree) fluoroscopy without shielding. C, Vertical fluoroscopy with a 25 × 15-cm (0.75-mm lead equivalent) surface shield. D, Oblique (45-degree) fluoroscopy with surface shielding in place. (A to D From Young AT, Morin RL, Hunter DW, et al: Surface shield: Device to reduce personnel radiation exposure. Radiology 159:801–803, 1986; with permission of the Radiological Society of North America, Inc.)

involving a table side position for 10 to 20 images. Note that movement to the side of the gantry reduces exposure greatly in comparison to that received when one stands in front of or behind the gantry. In this case, a small step dramatically reduces radiation exposure (Fig. 3–4).

MANAGEMENT OF PATIENT RADIATION DOSE

Interventional procedures exceed all other x-ray imaging procedures in radiation dose. As a rule of thumb, patient skin doses are about 10 times more during interventional procedures than during angiography, and doses from angiographic procedures are about 10 times higher than from conventional gastrointestinal fluoroscopy or CT scanning. Skin entrance doses have been reported in the range of 6 to 18 Gy from certain interventional procedures.[15, 16] In 1994, on the basis of reports of a small number of severely injured patients, the FDA issued a warning to all users of fluoroscopy equipment to beware of doses that can lead to severe skin damage.[31] Acute doses in excess of 2 Gy can lead to erythema and epilation; 6 Gy can cause permanent epilation; 10 Gy can lead to dry desquamation, dermal atrophy, and telangiectasia; and 15 Gy or more can lead to moist desquamation and necrosis. Injury to other organs may also be possible at these dose levels.[15, 17]

In general, reducing radiation doses to the patients also reduces doses to the medical personnel. Several suggestions have been made earlier that reduce both. In addition, using the shortest possible distance between

FIGURE 3–4

Approximate scattered radiation exposures about CT scanner in milliroentgens (mR). Exposures are derived from Reference 18 for a 130-kVp, 50-mA, 10-second, 10-mm scan at a distance of 1 m and a height equal to the isocenter.

the image intensifier and the patient can reduce the dose to the patient's skin. This causes the automatic brightness system of the x-ray generator to drop the radiation output.

SUMMARY

Typical patient entrance dose rates are on the order of 30 mGy/min during fluoroscopy and 500 mGy/min during cine. Staff eye dose rates can range from approximately 0.1 to 1 mGy/hr during fluoroscopy and from approximately 1 to 25 mGy/hr during cine. In general, staff doses are markedly decreased for interventional procedures that use CT, with the greatest reduction if staff members step to the side of the gantry or leave the room during the slice acquisition.

REFERENCES

1. Curry TS, Dowdey JE, Murry RC: Christensen's Introduction to the Physics of Diagnostic Radiology. Philadelphia, Lea & Febiger, 1984.
2. Code of Federal Regulations, Title 21, Parts 1000–1050. U.S. Government, 1985. Revision of the Radiation Control for Health and Safety Act of 1968.
3. National Council of Radiation Protection and Measurements: Recommendations on Limits for Exposure to Ionizing Radiation. NCRP Report No. 91. Washington, DC, 1987.
4. National Council on Radiation Protection and Measurements: Medical X-ray, Electron Beam, and Gamma Ray Protection for Energies Tip to 50 Mev. NCRP Report No. 102. Washington, DC, 1989.
5. National Council on Radiation Protection and Measurements: Structural Shielding Design and Evaluation for Medical Use of X-rays and Gamma Rays of Energies up to 10 Mev. NCRP Publication No. 49. Washington, DC, 1976.
6. International Commission on Radiological Protection (ICRP): Radiation Protection. ICRP Publication No. 26. Oxford, Pergamon Press, 1977.
7. National Council on Radiation Protection and Measurements: Limitation of Exposure to Ionizing Radiation. NCRP Report No. 116. Washington, DC, 1993.
8. Code of Federal Regulations, Title 29, Part 16, Chapter 17, Section 1910.96. Washington, DC, U.S. Government Printing Office, 1971.
9. Code of Federal Regulations, Title 10, Part 20, Chapter 1, Section 20.1201. Washington, DC, U.S. Government Printing Office, 1991.
10. Bushong SC: Radiologic Science for Technologists: Physics, Biology, and Protection. St. Louis, CV Mosby, 1984.
11. Pizzarello DJ, Witcofski RC: Medical Radiation Biology. Philadelphia, Lea & Febiger, 1982.
12. Webster EW: Quality assurance in cine radiographic systems. In Waggener RG, Wilson CR (eds): Quality Assurance in Diagnostic Radiology: Medical Physics Monograph No. 4. New York, American Institute of Physics, 1980.
13. Gray JE, Winkler NT, Stears J, Frank ED: Quality Control in Diagnostic Imaging. Baltimore, University Park Press, 1983.
14. American Institute of Physics: Evaluation of Radiation Exposure Levels in Cine Cardiac Catheterization Laboratories. AAPM Report No. 12. New York, American Institute of Physics. 1984.
15. Houda W, Peters KR: Radiation-induced temporary epilation after a neuroradiologically guided embolization procedure. Radiology 193:642–644, 1994.
16. Wagner LK, Eifel PJ, Geise RA: Potential biological effects following high x-ray dose interventional procedures. J Vasc Interv Radiol 5:71–84, 1994.
17. Payne JT, Shope TB (eds): Proceedings of the ACR/FDA Workshop on Fluoroscopy: Strategies for Improvement in Performance, Radiation Safety, and Control. American College of Radiology, 1993.
18. Jeans SP, Faulkner K, Love HG, Bardsley RA: An investigation of the radiation dose to staff during cardiac radiological studies. Br J Radiol 58:419, 1985.

Pharmacology of Drugs Used with Radiographic Imaging

4

LOCAL ANESTHETICS

Local anesthetics prevent or relieve pain by interrupting nerve conduction. They bind to a specific receptor site within the pore of the Na^+ channels in nerves and block ion movement through this pore. In general, their action is restricted to the site of application and rapidly reverses on diffusion from the site of action in the nerve. The chemical and pharmacologic properties of each drug determine its clinical use. Local anesthetics can be administered by a variety of routes, including topical, infiltration, field or nerve block, intravenous regional, spinal, or epidural, as dictated by clinical circumstances.

EFFECTS ON SYSTEMS

In addition to blocking conduction in nerve axons in the peripheral nervous system, local anesthetics interfere with the function of all organs in which conduction or transmission of impulses occurs. Thus, they have important effects on the central nervous system (CNS), the autonomic ganglia, the neuromuscular junction, and all forms of muscle.[1-3] The danger of such adverse reactions is proportional to the concentration of local anesthetic achieved in the circulation.

Central Nervous System

Following absorption, local anesthetics may cause stimulation of the CNS, producing restlessness and tremor that may proceed to clonic convulsions. In general, the more potent the anesthetic, the more readily convulsions may be produced. Alterations of CNS activity are thus predictable from the local anesthetic agent in question and the blood concentration achieved. Central stimulation is followed by depression; death is usually caused by respiratory failure.

Although drowsiness is the most frequent complaint that results from the CNS actions of local anes-

thetics, lidocaine may produce dysphoria or euphoria and muscle twitching. Moreover, both lidocaine and procaine may produce a loss of consciousness that is preceded only by symptoms of sedation.[1] Whereas other local anesthetics also show the effect, cocaine has a particularly prominent effect on mood and behavior.

Cardiovascular System

Following systemic absorption, local anesthetics act on the cardiovascular system.[1] The primary site of action is the myocardium, where decreases in electrical excitability, conduction rate, and force of contraction occur. In addition, most local anesthetics cause arteriolar dilation. The cardiovascular effects usually are seen only after high systemic concentrations are attained and effects on the CNS are produced. However, on rare occasions lower doses cause cardiovascular collapse and death, probably due to either an action on the pacemaker or the sudden onset of ventricular fibrillation. However, ventricular tachycardia and fibrillation are relatively uncommon consequences of local anesthetics other than bupivacaine.

Neuromuscular Junction and Ganglionic Synapse

Local anesthetics also affect transmission at the neuromuscular junction. Procaine, for example, can block the response of skeletal muscle to maximal motor-nerve volleys and to acetylcholine at concentrations where the muscle responds normally to direct electrical stimulation. Similar effects occur at autonomic ganglia. These effects are due to blockade of the ion channel of the acetylcholine receptor.[4, 5]

Smooth Muscle

The local anesthetics depress contractions in the intact bowel and in strips of isolated intestine.[6] They also relax vascular and bronchial smooth muscle, although low concentrations may initially produce contraction.[1] Spinal and epidural anesthesia, as well as instillation of local anesthetics into the peritoneal cavity, cause sympathetic nervous system paralysis, which can result in increased tone of gastrointestinal musculature. Local anesthetics may increase the resting tone and decrease the contractions of isolated human uterine muscle; however, uterine contractions seldom are depressed directly during intrapartum regional anesthesia.

METABOLISM OF LOCAL ANESTHETICS

The metabolic fate of local anesthetics is of great practical importance, because their toxicity depends largely on the balance between their rates of absorption and elimination. As noted earlier, the rate of absorption of many anesthetics can be reduced considerably by the incorporation of a vasoconstrictor agent in the anesthetic solution. However, the rate of destruction of local anesthetics varies greatly, and this is a major factor in determining the safety of a particular agent. Since toxicity is related to the free concentration of drug, binding of the anesthetic to proteins in the serum and to tissues reduces the concentration of free drug in the systemic circulation and, consequently, reduces toxicity. For example, in intravenous regional anesthesia of an extremity, about half of the original anesthetic dose is still tissue bound 30 minutes after release of the tourniquet; the lungs also bind large quantities of local anesthetic.[7]

Ester Local Anesthetics

Ester-linked local anesthetics are hydrolyzed at the ester linkage in plasma by the plasma pseudocholinesterase. This plasma enzyme also hydrolyzes natural choline esters and the anesthetically administered drug succinylcholine. The rate of hydrolysis of ester-linked local anesthetics depends on the type and location of the substitution in the aromatic ring. For example, 2-chloroprocaine is hydrolyzed about four times faster than procaine, which in turn is hydrolyzed about four times faster than tetracaine. In the case of 2-chloroprocaine, the half-life in the normal adult is 45 seconds to 1 minute. In individuals with atypical plasma pseudocholinesterase, the rate of hydrolysis of all the ester-linked local anesthetics is markedly decreased, and a prolonged half-life of these drugs results. Therefore, whereas the potential for toxicity from plasma accumulation of the ester-linked local anesthetics (e.g., 2-chloroprocaine) is extremely remote with repeated dosing of the drug in normal individuals, this likelihood should be considered with the administration of large doses or repeated doses to individuals with the atypical pseudocholinesterase enzyme.[8]

The hydrolysis of all ester-linked local anesthetics leads to the formation of para-aminobenzoic acid (PABA) or a substituted PABA. PABA and its derivatives are associated with a low but real potential for allergic reactions.[9] A history of an allergic reaction to a local anesthetic agent should be considered primarily as resulting from the presence of PABA or derived from ester-linked local anesthetics. Allergic reactions may also develop from the use of multidose vials of amide-linked local anesthetics that contain PABA as a preservative. Allergic reactions to amide-linked local anesthetics without preservatives are rare.

Amide Local Anesthetics

In contrast to the ester-linked drugs, the amide-linked local anesthetics must be transported by the circulation to the liver before biotransformation can take place. The two major factors controlling the clearance of amide-linked local anesthetics by the liver are (1) hepatic blood flow (delivery of the drug to the liver) and (2) hepatic function (drug extraction by the liver). Factors that decrease hepatic blood flow or hepatic drug extraction result in an increased elimination half-life.

Renal clearance of unchanged local anesthetics is a minor route of elimination. For example, the amount of unchanged lidocaine excretion in the urine in the adult is small, roughly 3% to 5% of the total drug administered. For bupivacaine, the renal excretion of unchanged drug is also small but somewhat higher, in the 10% to 16% range of the administered dose.

Lidocaine metabolism occurs following uptake of the drug by the liver. The primary biotransformation step for lidocaine is a dealkylation reaction in which an ethyl group is cleaved from the tertiary amine (Fig. 4–1). Interestingly, this primary step in lidocaine's biotransformation appears to be only slightly slower in the newborn than in the adult, indicating functional maturity of this particular enzyme system in the newborn. However, an increase in the elimination half-life of lidocaine in the newborn of about twofold is seen, which is believed to result not from enzymatic immaturity but, instead, to reflect the larger volume of distribution for lidocaine in the newborn. A larger volume of distribution means that a given dose of drug achieves a lower plasma concentration; thus, less drug would be delivered to the liver for metabolism per unit time and to the kidney for excretion. Thus, it would take longer to clear a drug from the body when the drug has a larger volume of distribution.

As with the biotransformation of lidocaine, that of bupivacaine progresses with a dealkylation reaction as the primary step (Fig. 4–2). Again, in the newborn an increased volume of distribution is present for bupivacaine and a longer half-life is thus anticipated compared with that expected in the adult. Other reactions in the biotransformation of amide-linked local anesthetics include hydrolysis of the amide link and oxidation of the benzene ring portion of the drug. The metabolites thus formed can be cleared by the kidney as unchanged

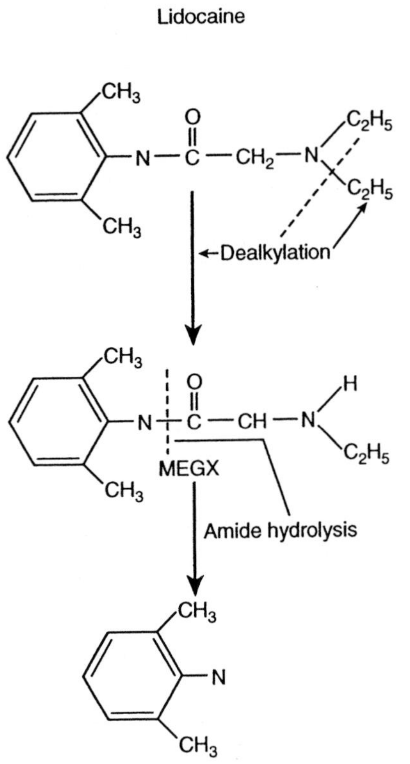

Lidocaine

FIGURE 4–1

Metabolism of lidocaine illustrating a deacylating reaction. (From Raj PP [ed]: Textbook of Regional Anesthesia, 3rd ed. Philadelphia, Churchill Livingstone, 2002.)

Bupivacaine

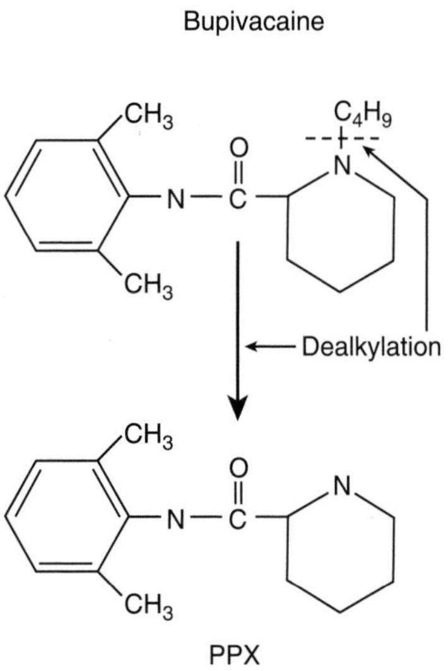

FIGURE 4–2

Metabolism of bupivacaine. (From Raj PP [ed]: Textbook of Regional Anesthesia, 3rd ed. Philadelphia, Churchill Livingstone, 2002.)

or conjugated compounds. For example, when hydroxy derivatives are formed from the oxidation of the benzene ring, they are conjugated and excreted as the glucuronide or sulfate conjugate.

With mepivacaine, the primary metabolic pathway is the oxidation of the benzene ring portion of the molecule, producing 3-hydroxy and 4-hydroxymepiva-

caine. Because this oxidation metabolic pathway is less well developed in the newborn, mepivacaine metabolism occurs much slower in the newborn than in the adult.

Ropivacaine metabolism in humans has been studied extensively (Fig. 4–3). At low plasma concentrations, the drug is primarily metabolized by ring oxidation to 3-hydroxyropivacaine, which is conjugated and excreted in the urine.[10] Significantly less drug is metabolized by dealkylation at low concentrations to PPX. At high concentrations in vitro, dealkylation to PPX becomes an important pathway.[11] The metabolites formed are much less active than the parent compound ropivacaine. Renal clearance of ropivacaine also is relatively small, with only about 1% of the administered dose excreted unchanged in the urine.

The metabolism of local anesthetics as well as that of many other drugs occurs in the liver by the cytochrome P-450 enzymes. This enzyme family has been subdivided into a number of isoenzymes, with those predominantly involved in local anesthetic biotransformation reactions being CYP-1A2 and CYP-3A4. The predominant cytochrome P-450 isoenzyme present in the human liver is CYP-3A4. This isoenzyme accounts for approximately 30% to 60% of the total cytochrome P-450 content in the liver. It is primarily responsible for the dealkylation reaction in drug metabolism, which, in the case of lidocaine, produces MEGX; with bupivacaine and ropivacaine, PPX is produced.

SPECIFIC LOCAL ANESTHETICS

Local anesthetics are classified as either ester or amide agents. Clinically useful ester agents are procaine, 2-chloroprocaine, and tetracaine.

Procaine

Procaine (Novocain), introduced in 1905 as the first synthetic local anesthetic, is an amino ester (Fig. 4–4). Although it formerly was used widely, it is now confined to infiltration anesthesia and occasionally to diagnostic nerve blocks. This is because of its low potency, slow onset, and short duration of action. While its toxicity is fairly low, it is hydrolyzed in vivo to produce PABA, which inhibits the action of sulfonamides. Thus, large doses should not be administered to patients taking sulfonamide drugs.

2-Chloroprocaine

2-Chloroprocaine (Nesacaine), an ester local anesthetic introduced in 1952, is a chlorinated derivative of procaine (see Fig. 4–4). Its major assets are its rapid onset and short duration of action and its reduced acute toxicity due to its rapid metabolism (plasma half-life of approximately 25 seconds). Enthusiasm for its use has been tempered by reports of prolonged sensory and

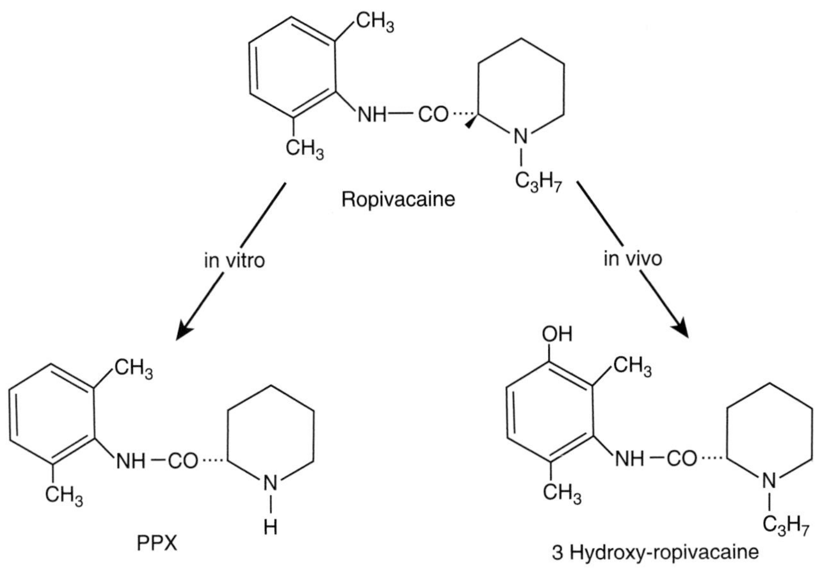

FIGURE 4-3

Schematic diagram showing the two major pathways of ropivacaine metabolism. (From Raj PP [ed]: Textbook of Regional Anesthesia, 3rd ed. Philadelphia, Churchill Livingstone, 2002.)

motor block after epidural or subarachnoid administration of large doses. This toxicity appears to have been a consequence of low pH and the use of sodium metabisulfite as a preservative in earlier formulations. There are no reports of neurotoxicity with newer preparations of chloroprocaine, which contain calcium EDTA as the preservative, although these preparations also are not recommended for intrathecal administration. A higher-than-expected incidence of muscular back pain following epidural anesthesia with 2-chloroprocaine also has been reported.[12] This back pain is thought to be due to tetany in the paraspinous muscles, which may be a consequence of Ca^{2+} binding by the EDTA included as a preservative; the incidence of back pain appears to be related to the volume of drug injected and its use for skin infiltration.

PHARMACOLOGY AND PHARMACODYNAMICS

2-Chloroprocaine is procaine with the addition of a chlorine group to the benzene ring. This drug has a very rapid onset of action and a short duration of activity (30 to 60 minutes). Once absorbed into the circulation, the drug is rapidly metabolized. The approximate half-life in plasma in adults is 45 seconds to 1 minute; hence, it is the most rapidly metabolized local anesthetic currently used. Because of this extremely rapid breakdown in plasma, it has very low potential for systemic toxicity and has been particularly attractive to obstetric anesthesiologists for use when elevated maternal blood levels of local anesthetic can cause major problems for the fetus and mother. This drug is also frequently used for epidural and peripheral blocks in an ambulatory care setting when short duration of anesthesia is needed and rapid recovery is highly desirable.

The epidural use of this drug, however, has been limited because of several reported problems. Prolonged and profound motor and sensory deficits occurred with the unintentional subarachnoid injection of the original 2-chloroprocaine commercial preparation marketed with the preservative bisulfite. The classic work by Gissen and coworkers[13] and Wang and colleagues[14] demonstrated that bisulfite in the presence of a highly acidic solution releases sulfur dioxide (SO_2), which equilibrates in solution into sulfurous acid, which is neurotoxic. Gissen postulated that the injection of the highly acidic commercial 2-chloroprocaine (pH 3) solution into the spinal sac resulted in the slow formation of and prolonged exposure to sulfurous acid, causing spinal cord damage. More recently, a 2-chloroprocaine preparation was released in which the bisulfite was removed

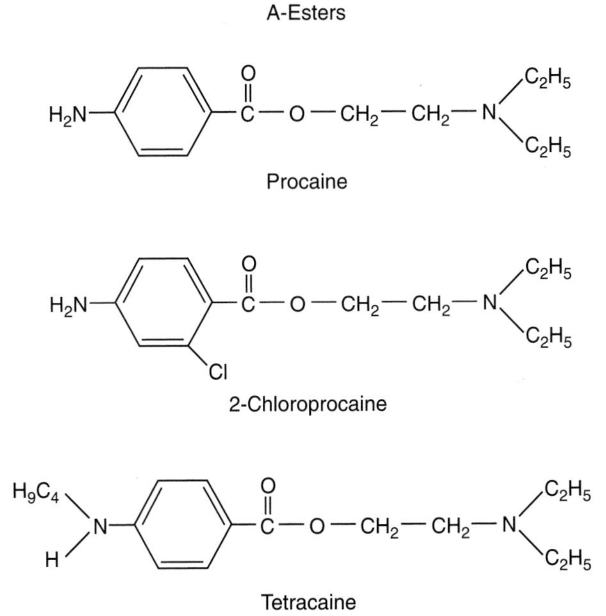

FIGURE 4-4

Local anesthetic chemical structures illustrating ester linkage. (From Raj PP [ed]: Textbook of Regional Anesthesia, 3rd ed. Philadelphia, Churchill Livingstone, 2002.)

and EDTA was substituted as the preservative. This change, however, has not been totally satisfactory because there appears to be a significant occurrence of back muscle spasm after epidural application of this formulation.[15] It has been postulated that the EDTA in this commercial preparation binds calcium and causes spasm in the paraspinal muscles.

A new 2-chloroprocaine commercial preparation has been released in which all preservatives have been removed. Initial studies with this formulation appear to be promising. No preparations of 2-chloroprocaine are recommended for either spinal or intravenous regional anesthesia.

Amide local anesthetics that are currently used are lidocaine, mepivacaine, bupivacaine, ropivacaine, and levobupivacaine.

Lidocaine

Lidocaine (Xylocaine), introduced in 1948, is now the most widely used local anesthetic. The chemical structure of lidocaine is shown in Figure 4–5.

PHARMACOLOGIC ACTIONS

The pharmacologic actions that lidocaine shares with other local anesthetic drugs has been described widely. Lidocaine produces faster, more intense, longer lasting, and more extensive anesthesia than does an equal concentration of procaine. Unlike procaine, it is an aminoethylamide and is the prototypical member of this class of local anesthetics. It is a good choice for patients sensitive to ester-type local anesthetics.

ABSORPTION, FATE, AND EXCRETION

Lidocaine is absorbed rapidly after parenteral administration and from the gastrointestinal and respiratory tracts. Although it is effective when used without any vasoconstrictor, in the presence of epinephrine the rate of absorption and the toxicity are decreased, and the duration of action usually is prolonged. Lidocaine is dealkylated in the liver by mixed-function oxidases to monoethylglycine xylidide and glycine xylidide, which can be metabolized further to monoethylglycine and xylidide. Both monoethylglycine xylidide and glycine xylidide retain local anesthetic activity. In humans, about 75% of xylidide is excreted in the urine as the further metabolite, 4-hydroxy-2,6-dimethylaniline.[7]

TOXICITY

The side effects of lidocaine seen with increasing dose include drowsiness, tinnitus, dysgeusia, dizziness, and twitching. As the dose increases, seizures, coma, and respiratory depression and arrest occur. Clinically significant cardiovascular depression usually occurs at serum lidocaine levels that produce marked CNS effects. The metabolite monoethylglycine cylidide and glycine xylidide may contribute to some of these side effects.

CLINICAL USES

Lidocaine has a wide range of clinical uses as a local anesthetic; it is useful in almost any application where a local anesthetic of intermediate duration is needed. Lidocaine also is used as an antiarrhythmic agent.

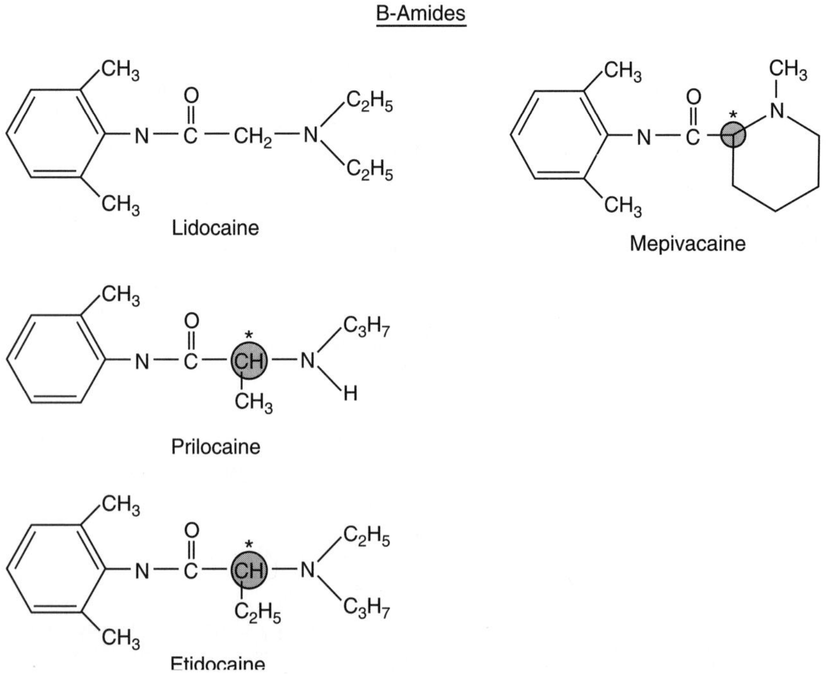

B-Amides

Lidocaine

Mepivacaine

Prilocaine

Etidocaine

FIGURE 4–5

Local anesthetic chemical structures illustrating amide linkage and indicating an asymmetric carbon atom (asterisk) when present. (From Raj PP [ed]: Textbook of Regional Anesthesia, 3rd ed. Philadelphia, Churchill Livingstone, 2002.)

Mepivacaine

Mepivacaine (Carbocaine, others), introduced in 1957, is an intermediate-acting amino amide (see Fig. 4–5). Its pharmacologic properties are similar to those of lidocaine. Mepivacaine, however, is more toxic to the neonate and thus is not used in obstetric anesthesia. The increased toxicity of mepivacaine in the neonate is related not to its slower metabolism in the neonate but to ion trapping of this agent because of the lower pH of neonatal blood and the pKa of mepivacaine. Despite its slow metabolism in the neonate, it appears to have a slightly higher therapeutic index in adults than lidocaine. Its onset of action is similar to that of lidocaine and its duration slightly longer (about 20%) than that of lidocaine in the absence of a coadministered vasoconstrictor. Mepivacaine is not effective as a topical anesthetic.

Bupivacaine

Bupivacaine (Marcaine, Sensorcaine), introduced in 1963, is a widely used amide local anesthetic; its structure is similar to that of lidocaine, except the amine-containing group is a butyl piperidine (see Fig. 4–5). It is a potent agent capable of producing prolonged anesthesia. Its long duration of action plus its tendency to provide more sensory than motor block has made it a popular drug for providing prolonged analgesia during labor or the postoperative period. By taking advantage of indwelling catheters and continuous infusions, bupivacaine can be used to provide several days of effective analgesia.

Bupivacaine was developed as a modification of mepivacaine. Its structural similarities with mepivacaine are readily apparent. Bupivacaine has a butyl (four-carbon substitution) group on the hydrophilic nitrogen.

Bupivacaine has made a contribution to regional anesthesia second in importance only to lidocaine. It is one of the first of the clinical used local anesthetic drugs that provides good separation of motor and sensory blockade after its administration. The onset of anesthesia and the duration of action are long and can be further prolonged by the addition of epinephrine in areas with a low fat content. Only small increases in duration are seen when bupivacaine is injected into areas with a high fat content. For example, a 50% increase in duration of brachial plexus blockade (an area of low fat content) follows the addition of epinephrine to bupivacaine solutions; in contrast, only a 10% to 15% increase in duration of epidural anesthesia results from the addition of epinephrine to bupivacaine solutions, since the epidural space has a high fat content.

TOXICITY

Bupivacaine is more cardiotoxic than equieffective doses of lidocaine. Clinically, this is manifested by severe ventricular arrhythmias and myocardial depression after inadvertent intravascular administration of large doses of bupivacaine. The enhanced cardiotoxicity of bupivacaine probably is due to multiple factors. Lidocaine and bupivacaine both block cardiac Na^+ channels rapidly during systole. However, bupivacaine dissociates much more slowly than does lidocaine during diastole, so a significant fraction of Na^+ channels remains blocked at the end of diastole (at physiologic heart rates) with bupivacaine.[16] Thus the block by bupivacaine is cumulative and substantially more than would be predicted by its local anesthetic potency. At least a portion of the cardiac toxicity of bupivacaine may be mediated centrally, as direct injection of small quantities of bupivacaine into the medulla can produce malignant ventricular arrhythmias.[17] Bupivacaine-induced cardiac toxicity can be difficult to treat, and its severity is enhanced in the presence of acidosis, hypercarbia, and hypoxemia.

NEWER LOCAL ANESTHETICS

Chiral Forms of Lidocaine

An area of newfound importance for anesthesiologists is in the use of *stereoisomers* of drugs to take advantage of differences in activity or toxicity of the isomers. For stereoisomerism to be present, an *asymmetric carbon* (a carbon atom in the molecule that has four distinctly different substitution groups) must be present in the molecule. Stereoisomers are possible for the local anesthetics etidocaine, mepivacaine, bupivacaine, prilocaine, and ropivacaine, and some of these drugs have differences in potency or toxicity for the isomers. For these local anesthetics, the asymmetric carbons are indicated in Figure 4–6 with an asterisk.

In the older literature, isomers were described as *L* and *D* on the basis of chemical configuration and as (+) or (–) on the basis of topical rotation, i.e., *L* (+) or *D* (-). More recent literature describes isomers as *R* or *S*, and the optical rotation is still included in the parentheses as (+) and (–). *R* and *S* basically correspond to the *D* and *L* in the older nomenclature.

As a rule, when differences between the activity of isomers are present for local anesthetics, the *S* form is less toxic and has a longer duration of anesthesia.[18, 19] For instance, anesthesia produced by bupivacaine infiltration was of longer duration when the *S* isomer was used compared with the *R* isomer. Also the *S* isomer had lower systemic toxicity. The mean convulsant dose of *R* bupivacaine was 57% of the *S* bupivacaine convulsant dose.[20] When the isomers of ropivacaine were evaluated, the *S* isomer of the drug had a longer duration of blockade and a lower toxicity than its *R* isomer.[21] Additionally, when cardiac electrophysiologic toxicity was evaluated in animal studies, ropivacaine (the commercial preparation is the *S* form of drug) at equipotent nerve blocking doses appears to have a safety margin

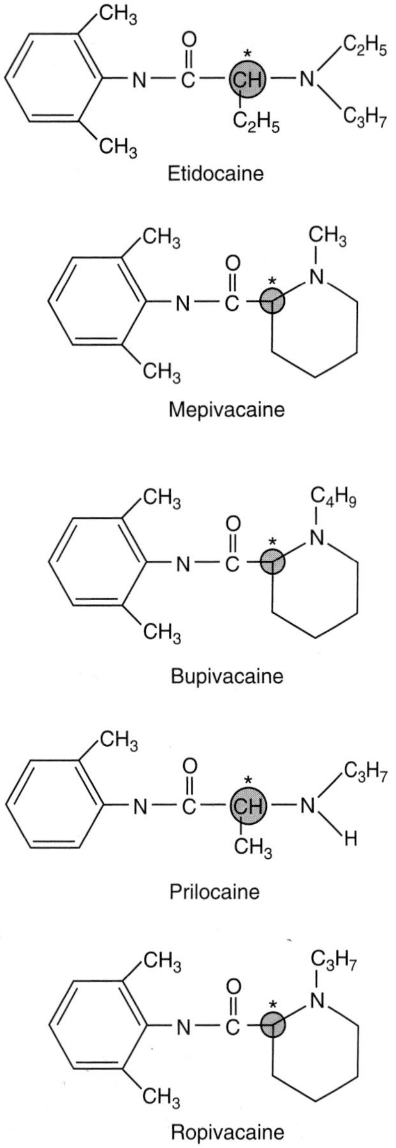

Etidocaine

Mepivacaine

Bupivacaine

Prilocaine

Ropivacaine

FIGURE 4–6

Stereoisomers are possible for local anesthetics: etidocaine, mepivacaine, bupivacaine, prilocaine, and ropivacaine. The asymmetric carbons are indicated with an asterisk. (From Raj PP [ed]: Textbook of Regional Anesthesia, 3rd ed. Philadelphia, Churchill Livingstone, 2002.)

Ropivacaine

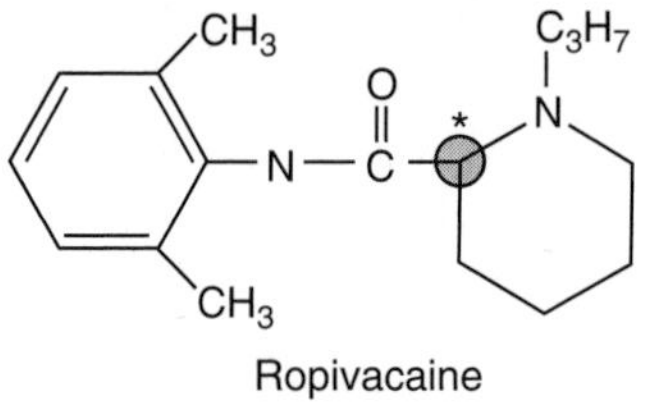

FIGURE 4–7

This chemical structure is the *S*-enantiomer of 1-propyl-2',6'-pipecolo-cyclidide. (From Raj PP [ed]: Textbook of Regional Anesthesia, 3rd ed. Philadelphia, Churchill Livingstone, 2002.)

tiomer, like most local anesthetics with a chiral center, was chosen because it has a lower toxicity than the *R* isomer. This is presumably due to slower uptake, resulting in lower blood levels for a given dose. Ropivacaine is slightly less potent than bupivacaine in producing anesthesia. In several animal models, it appears to be less cardiotoxic than equieffective doses of bupivacaine. In clinical studies, ropivacaine appears to be suitable for both epidural and regional anesthesia, with duration of action similar to that of bupivacaine. Interestingly, it seems to be even more motor sparing than bupivacaine.

Ropivacaine is a long-acting, enantiomerically pure (*S*-enantiomer) amide local anesthetic with a high pKa and low lipid solubility that blocks nerve fibers involved in pain transmission (Aδ and C fibers) to a greater degree than those controlling motor function (Aß fibers). The drug was less cardiotoxic than equal concentrations of racemic bupivacaine but more so than lidocaine (lignocaine) in vitro and had a significantly higher threshold for CNS toxicity than racemic bupivacaine in healthy volunteers (mean maximum tolerated unbound arterial plasma concentrations were 0.56 and 0.3 mg/L, respectively).

Extensive clinical data have shown that epidural ropivacaine 0.2% is effective for the initiation and maintenance of labor analgesia and provides pain relief after abdominal or orthopedic surgery, especially when given in conjunction with opioids (coadministration with opioids may also allow for lower concentrations of ropivacaine to be used). The drug had an efficacy generally similar to that of the same dose of bupivacaine with regard to pain relief but caused less motor blockade at low concentrations.

Levobupivacaine (Chirocaine)

Levobupivacaine (Chirocaine) injection contains a single enantiomer of bupivacaine hydrochloride that is chemically described as *S*-1-butyl-2-piperidylformo-2',6'-xylidide hydrochloride and it is related chemically and pharmacologically to the amino amide class of local anesthetics (Fig. 4–8).

Levobupivacaine hydrochloride, the *S*-enantiomer of bupivacaine, is a white crystalline powder with a

that is almost twice that of commercial bupivacaine, which is a mixture of the *R* and *S* isomers.[21] Recent studies with the *R* and *S* bupivacaine isomers indicate that the *R* form is apparently more arrhythmogenic and more cardiotoxic.[22, 23] Further evaluation of the isomers of bupivacaine is necessary before commercial use can be achieved.

Ropivacaine

The cardiac toxicity of bupivacaine stimulated interest in developing a less toxic, long-lasting local anesthetic. The result of that search was the development of a new amino ethylamine, ropivacaine (Fig. 4–7), the *S*-enantiomer of 1-propyl-2',6'-pipecolocylidide. The *S*-enan-

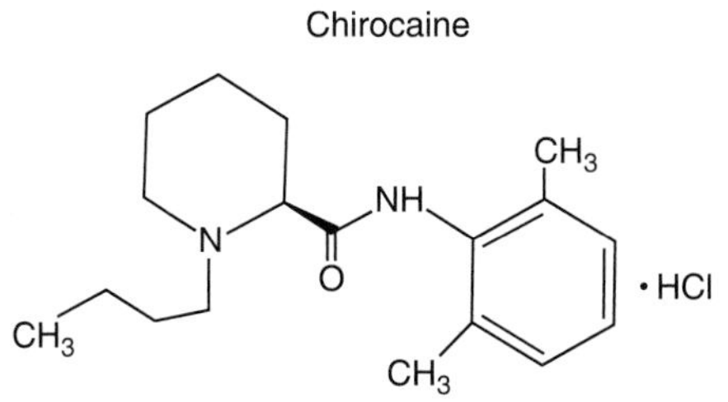

Chirocaine

FIGURE 4–8

A single enantiomer of levobupivacaine hydrochloride (Chirocaine) chemically described as *S*-1-butyl-2-piperidylformo-2',6'-xylidide hydrochloride. (From Raj PP [ed]: Textbook of Regional Anesthesia, 3rd ed. Philadelphia, Churchill Livingstone, 2002.)

molecular formula of $C_{18}H_{28}N_2O \bullet HCl$, a molecular weight of 324.9.

The solubility of levobupivacaine hydrochloride in water is about 100 mg/mL at 20°C and the partition coefficient (oleyl alcohol/water) is 1624; the pKa of levobupivacaine hydrochloride is the same as that of bupivacaine hydrochloride, and the partition coefficient is very similar to that of bupivacaine hydrochloride (1565).

Chirocaine is a sterile, nonpyrogenic, colorless solution (pH 4.0 to 6.5) containing levobupivacaine hydrochloride equivalent to 2.5 mg/mL, 5.0 mg/mL, and 7.5 mg/mL of levobupivacaine, sodium chloride for isotonicity, and water for injection. Sodium hydroxide and/or hydrochloric acid may be added to adjust the pH. Chirocaine is preservative free and is available in 10- and 30-mL single-dose vials.

CLINICAL PHARMACOLOGY

Mechanism of Action. Chirocaine is a member of the amino amide class of local anesthetics. Local anesthetics block the generation and the conduction of nerve impulses by increasing the threshold for electrical excitation in the nerve, by slowing propagation of the nerve impulse, and by reducing the rate of rise of the action potential. In general, the progression of anesthesia is related to the diameter, myelination, and conduction velocity of affected nerve fibers. Clinically, the order of loss of nerve function is as follows: (1) pain, (2) temperature, (3) touch, (4) proprioception, and (5) skeletal muscle tone.

Pharmacokinetics. After intravenous infusion of equivalent doses of levobupivacaine and bupivacaine, the mean clearance, volume of distribution, and terminal half-life values of levobupivacaine and bupivacaine were similar. No detectable levels of *R*(+)-bupivacaine were found after the administration of levobupivacaine.

Distribution. Plasma protein binding of levobupivacaine evaluated in vitro was found to be greater than 97% at concentrations between 0.1 and 1 µg/mL. The association of levobupivacaine with human blood cells

was very low (0 to 2%) over the concentration range 0.01 to 1 µg/mL and increased to 32% at 10 µg/mL. The volume of distribution of levobupivacaine after intravenous administration was 67 L.

Metabolism. Levobupivacaine is extensively metabolized with no unchanged levobupivacaine detected in urine or feces. In vitro studies using [^{14}C]levobupivacaine showed that CYP3A4 isoform and CYP1A2 isoform mediate the metabolism of levobupivacaine to desbutyl levobupivacaine and 3-hydroxy levobupivacaine, respectively. In vivo, the 3-hydroxylevobupivacaine appears to undergo further transformation to glucuronide and sulfate conjugates. Metabolic inversion of levobupivacaine to *R*(+)-bupivacaine was not evident both in vitro and in vivo.

Elimination. Following intravenous administration, recovery of the radiolabeled dose of levobupivacaine was essentially quantitative, with a mean total of about 95% being recovered in urine and feces in 48 hours. Of this 95%, about 71% was in urine whereas 24% was in feces. The mean elimination half-life of total radioactivity in plasma was 3.3 hours. The mean clearance and terminal half-life of levobupivacaine after intravenous infusion were 39 L/hr and 1.3 hours, respectively.

Pharmacodynamics. Chirocaine can be expected to share the pharmacodynamic properties of other local anesthetics. Systemic absorption of local anesthetics can produce effects on the central nervous and cardiovascular systems. At blood concentrations achieved with therapeutic doses, changes in cardiac conduction such as excitability, refractoriness, contractility, and peripheral vascular resistance have been reported. Toxic blood concentrations depress cardiac conduction and excitability, which may lead to atrioventricular block, ventricular arrhythmias, and cardiac arrest, sometimes resulting in death. In addition, myocardial contractility is depressed and peripheral vasodilation occurs, leading to decreased cardiac output and arterial blood pressure.

POTENCY OF BUPIVACAINE STEREOISOMERS

Chiral local anesthetics, such as ropivacaine and levobupivacaine, have the potential advantage over racemic mixtures in showing reduced toxic side effects. However, these isomers also have reportedly lower potency than their optical antipode, possibly resulting in no advantage in therapeutic index. Potency for local anesthetics inhibiting Na^+ channels or action potentials depends on the pattern of membrane potential, and so also does the stereopotency ratio. Here the authors have quantitated the stereopotencies of *R*-, *S*-, and racemic bupivacaine, comparing several in vitro assays of neuronal Na^+ channels with those from in vivo functional nerve block, to establish relative potencies and to understand better the role of different modes of channel inhibition in overall functional anesthesia.

CHEMICAL NEUROLYTIC AGENTS

Prolonged interruption of painful pathways may be accomplished by the injection of neurolytic agents. This form of chemical neurolysis has been performed for many years. The first reported injection of a neurolytic solution in the treatment of pain was probably by Luton,[24] who in 1863 administered subcutaneous injections of irritant substances into painful areas. Levy and Baudouin (1906) were the first to administer the injection of neurolytic agents percutaneously.[25] Doppler, in 1925, was the first to report the use of phenol for neurolysis.[1] The first use of phenol for subarachnoid neurolysis was reported by Maher in 1955.[25, 26] Today, phenol and ethyl alcohol (ethanol) are the most commonly used agents. It is indicated for patients with limited life expectancy and patients who have recurrent or intractable pain after a series of analgesic blocks.[27]

CONSIDERATIONS PRIOR TO USE OF NEUROLYTIC AGENTS

Diagnostic blocks are considered of prime importance due to the undesirable side effects of the neurolytic agents combined with a limited duration of analgesia. Potential side effects of neurolytic agents include neuritis and deafferentation pain, motor deficit when mixed nerves are ablated, and unintentional damage to non-targeted tissue.[27] Therefore, careful selection of patients combined with clinical expertise is of the essence. The following criteria should be considered before peripheral neurolysis is performed[27]:

- Determine and document that the pain is severe.
- Document that the pain will not be relieved by less invasive therapies.
- Document that the pain is well localized and in the distribution of an identifiable nerve.[28]
- Confirm that the pain is relieved with a diagnostic block performed with local anesthetic.
- Document the absence of undesirable deficits after the local anesthetic blocks.[27]

ETHYL ALCOHOL

Ethyl alcohol is commercially available in 1- or 50-mL ampules as a colorless solution that can be injected readily through small-bore needles.[27] It is hypobaric with respect to cerebrospinal fluid (CSF). However, specific gravity is not of concern when injecting on the peripheral nerve because injection takes place in a nonfluid medium.[27] It is usually used undiluted (absolute or >95% concentration). The perineural injection of alcohol is followed immediately by severe burning pain along the nerve's distribution, which lasts about a minute before giving way to a warm, numb sensation. Pain on injection may be diminished by the prior injection of a local anesthetic.[27] To precede the injection of any neurolytic drug with an injection of local anesthetic optimizes comfort and serves as a "test dose."[27] The alcohol spreads rapidly from the injection site. When injected in the CSF, only 10% of the initial dose remains at the site of the injection after 10 minutes, and about 4% remains after 30 minutes.[29] Between 90% and 98% of the ethanol that enters the body is completely oxidized.[30] This occurs chiefly in the liver and is initiated principally by alcohol dehydrogenase.[31] Denervation and pain relief accrue over a few days after injection, usually after 1 week. If no pain relief is present in weeks, then the neurolysis is incomplete and needs repetition.[27]

Various concentrations and mixtures of alcohol have been studied in an attempt to determine selectivity for sensory nerves.[32, 33] Schlosser[32] studied the effect of alcohol on somatic nerves. He reported that alcoholization was followed by degeneration and absorption of all the components of the nerve except the neurilemma. There is general agreement that with 95% absolute alcohol, the destruction involves the sympathetic, sensory, and motor components of a mixed somatic nerve, and therefore it is undesirable to block a mixed nerve with such concentrations of alcohol. However, there is a great discrepancy in determining the effects when the alcohol is placed on motor fibers at less than 80% concentration.

Despite the inconsistency in results for varying concentrations of alcohol, there is consensus regarding maximum and minimum concentrations. For complete paralysis, the concentration must be stronger than 95%. From Labat and Greene,[34] it may be concluded that a minimum concentration of 33% alcohol is necessary to obtain satisfactory analgesia without any motor paralysis.

Mechanism of Action of Alcohol

Histopathologic studies have shown that alcohol extracts cholesterol, phospholipids, and cerebrosides from the nerve tissue and causes precipitation of lipoproteins and mucoproteins.[35, 36] This results in sclerosis of the nerve fibers and myelin sheath.[37, 38] Alcohol produces nonselective destruction of nervous tissue by precipitating cell membrane proteins and extracting lipid compounds, resulting in demyelination and subsequent wallerian degeneration. Because the basal lamina of the Schwann cell tube is often spared, however, the axon often regenerates along its former course.[38] If injection is into a ganglion, it may produce cell body destruction without subsequent regeneration.[38] Topical application of alcohol to peripheral nerves produces changes typical of wallerian degeneration. A subarachnoid injection of absolute alcohol causes similar changes in the rootlets.[36, 39] Mild focal inflammation of meninges and patchy areas of demyelination are seen in posterior columns, Lissauer's tract, and dorsal roots and rootlets. Later, wallerian degeneration is seen to extend into the dorsal horns. Injection of a larger volume can result in degeneration of the spinal cord.[36] When alcohol is injected near the sympathetic chain, it destroys the ganglion cells and thus blocks all postganglionic fibers to all effector organs.[40] A temporary and incomplete block results if the injection affects only the rami communicantes of preganglionic and postganglionic fibers. Histopathologically, wallerian degeneration is evident in the sympathetic chain fibers.[36]

For subarachnoid block, concentrations between 50% and 100% are generally selected (Fig. 4–9). Alcohol is hypobaric in nature relative to CSF. Therefore, the position of the patient must be in the lateral decubitus position with the painful site uppermost. Then, the patient must be rolled anteriorly approximately 45 degrees to place the dorsal (sensory) root uppermost.[41] The reported volumes required for neurolysis have ranged from 0.3 mL to a maximum of 0.7 mL of absolute alcohol per segment[29] to 0.5 to 1 mL to a maximum of 1.5 mL per segment.[33, 37] For celiac plexus block, volumes of 10 to 20 mL of absolute alcohol bilaterally may be used.[27] Similar volumes have been reported for lumbar sympathetic block. Often, 100% alcohol is diluted 1:1 with a local anesthetic prior to injection.[33]

The most ominous complication associated with the use of alcohol is the possible occurrence of alcoholic neuritis. It has been postulated that alcoholic neuritis is due to incomplete destruction of somatic nerves. This seems plausible, in that neuritis has not been observed following the intraneural injection of a cranial or somatic nerve that produces a complete block.[33] Alcoholic neuritis occurs frequently following paravertebral block of the thoracic sympathetics. This may be due to the close proximity of the sympathetic ganglia to the intercostal nerves. The alcohol, which is intended for the ganglion, inadvertently bathes and partially destroys the somatic nerve.[33] During the period of regeneration, hyperesthesia and intense burning pain with occasional sharp, shooting pain occurs. These pains may be more intense than the original pain complaint. Fortunately, in most instances, these symptoms subside within a few weeks or a month. Occasionally, however, this complication persists for many months, requiring sedation, and in some instances, the performance of a subsequent rhizotomy or sympathectomy.[33] As a prophylactic measure, Mandl recommends the injection of a local anesthetic during the insertion of the needle, at the site of injection before the alcohol is injected, and on withdrawing the needle.[42] With this technique he has observed only two instances of alcoholic neuritis.

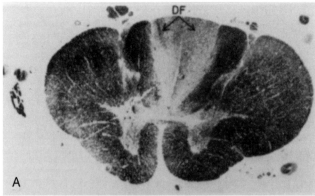
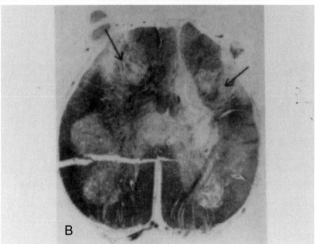

FIGURE 4–9

A, Effect of alcohol on the spinal cord 4 days after neurolytic block. A cross section through the spinal cord at T4 shows degeneration of the dorsal fascicularis (DF) after injection of 100% alcohol several interspaces lower. *B,* Effect of alcohol on the spinal cord 50 days after direct cord injection. Note the necrosis and degeneration *(arrows)* following accidental injection of 100% alcohol into the spinal cord. (From Gallagher HS, Yonexawa T, Hay RC, et al: Subarachnoid alcohol block: II. Histologic changes in the central nervous system. Am J Pathol 35:679, 1961.© American Society for Investigative Pathology.)

Mild cases of alcoholic neuritis are treated conservatively with mild analgesics such as aspirin or with small doses of codeine.[33] Moderate cases of alcoholic neuritis may require more active therapy. In some cases, the administration of intravenous local anesthetics has been helpful. Bonica determined that 250 mg of Pontocaine dissolved in 500 mL of fluid was superior to procaine.[43] In one case in which intravenous procaine had been administered several times with only transient relief of pain, one infusion of tetracaine effected prolonged pain relief. In some cases, daily sympathetic blocks have been employed, with excellent results.[33] In the case of lumbar nerve neuritis following lumbar sympathetic blocks, serial caudal blocks done at regular intervals can effect complete relief of pain.[33] Severe cases of alcoholic neuritis that do not respond to these conservative methods may require sympathectomy or rhizotomy. De Takats[44] reported three such cases in which sympathectomy was required.

Another complication associated with alcohol nerve block includes hypesthesia or anesthesia of the dermatomal distribution of the nerve roots treated with neurolysis. The lack of sensation can overshadow the pain relief obtained by the procedure. Fortunately, this complication is rare and recovery is relatively quick.[36] Loss of bowel or bladder sphincter tone, leading to bowel or urinary incontinence, has also been reported with intrathecal alcohol neurolysis in the lower lumbar and sacral areas.[36] To decrease the risk of this complication, it is recommended that during sacral neurolysis, only one side should be blocked at a time.[36] A complication of lumbar sympathetic neurolysis with alcohol is the development of genitofemoral neuralgia, which can cause severe groin pain. This is referred pain caused by the degeneration of the rami communicantes from the L2 nerve root to the genitofemoral nerve.[36–47] Paraplegia can result if injection of alcohol causes spasm of the artery of Adamkiewicz.[36]

PHENOL

Phenol is a combination of carbolic acid, phenic acid, phenylic acid, phenyl hydroxide, hydroxybenzene, and oxybenzene. It is not available commercially in the injectable form but can be prepared by the hospital pharmacy. One gram of phenol dissolves in about 15 mL of water (6.67%). It is very soluble in alcohol, glycerol, and a number of other organic substances. It is usually mixed with saline or glycerin. It may be mixed with sterile water or material used for contrast radiography.[30] Because it is highly soluble in glycerin, it diffuses from it slowly. This is an advantage when injecting intrathecally because it allows for limited spread and highly localized tissue fixation. This also makes it hyperbaric relative to CSF. When mixed with glycerin, it is so viscid that even when warmed, injection must be through at least a 20-gauge needle. This mixture must be free of water or the necrotizing effect will be much greater than anticipated.[30] When phenol is mixed in an aqueous mixture, it is a far more potent neurolytic.[36] Phenol oxidizes and turns red when exposed to air and light.[30] It has a shelf life that is said to exceed 1 year when preparations are refrigerated and not exposed to light. Phenol acts as a local anesthetic at lower concentrations and as a neurolytic agent in higher concentrations. It has an advantage over alcohol in that it causes minimal discomfort on injection.

Doppler was the first to use phenol to deliberately destroy nervous tissue in 1925.[48] After painting it on human ovarian vessels, he noted downstream vasodilation and flush. Later, he reported treating peripheral vascular disease in the lower extremity by exposing and painting the femoral arteries with a 7% aqueous solution. In 1933, Binet[48] in France reported painting ovarian vessels with 7% phenol. Both researchers attributed their good results to destruction of perivascular sympathetic fibers.[33] In 1933, Nechaev[49] reported the use of phenol as a local anesthetic. This was followed in 1936 by Putnam and Hampton,[50] who used an injection of phenol to perform a neurolysis of the gasserian ganglion.

In 1947, Mandl suggested the injection of phenol to obtain permanent sympathectomy.[51] In 1950, he reported its use in 15 patients without complications, suggesting that it was preferable to alcohol.[33, 42] The paravertebral injection of phenol for peripheral vascular disease was also reported by Haxton[52] and Boyd and coworkers[53] in 1949. In 1955, Maher[54] introduced it as a hyperbaric solution for intrathecal use in intractable cancer pain, with the famous remark that "it is easier to lay a carpet than to paper a ceiling." Thereafter he reported its epidural use as well.

By 1959, phenol was established as a neurolytic agent for the relief of chronic pain.[33] Then Kelly and Gautier-Smith[55] and Nathan[56] simultaneously reported the use of phenol for the relief of spasticity caused by upper motor neuron lesions. Phenol, in hyperbaric solution, was injected intrathecally with proper patient positioning to "fix" it on the anterior nerve roots, thus relieving the spasticity (Fig. 4–10).

Maher studied varying concentrations (10% to 3.3%) of phenol in glycerin in the subarachnoid space in an effort to determine the ideal neurolytic strength solution.[54] There was a graduation of block according to the concentration. The stronger concentration produced motor damage. Pain sensation was blocked at lower concentrations (5%) than were touch and proprioception. The 3.3% concentration was ineffective. Iggo and Walsh[57] determined that 5% phenol in either Ringer's solution or oil contrast medium produced selective block of the smaller nerve fibers in cat spinal rootlets. The same conclusions were drawn from the investigations by Nathan and Sears.[58] For a long time thereafter, the idea prevailed that phenol caused selective destruction of smaller nerve fibers with slower conduction rates, the C afferents carrying slow pain, the Aδ afferents carrying fast pain, and the Aγ controlling muscle tone.[33]

Mechanism of Action of Phenol

Histopathologic studies by Stewart and Lourie[59] demonstrated nonselective degeneration in cat rootlets, the severity being parallel to the concentration.[33] Nathan and associates[60] found evidence of Aδ and Aβ damage in the electrophysiologic experiments and confirmed the nonselectivity of damage by histologic examination.

At concentrations less than 5%, phenol produces protein denaturation. Concentrations greater than 5% cause protein coagulation and nonspecific segmental demyelination and orthograde degeneration (i.e., wallerian degeneration).[38] Concentrations of 5% to 6% produce destruction of nociceptive fibers with minimum side effects. Higher concentrations result in axonal abnormalities, nerve root damage, spinal cord infarcts, and arachnoiditis or meningitis.[38, 61] These char-

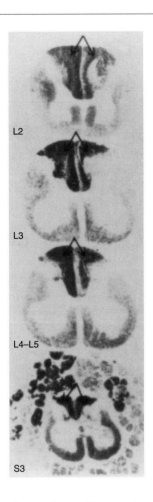

FIGURE 4–10

Effect of phenol on the spinal cord. Micrographs of transverse section at levels L2, L3, L4–5, and S3 show degeneration of the posterior column following subarachnoid injection of phenol at L3–L4. (From Smith MC: Histological findings following intrathecal injections of phenol solutions for relief of pain. Br J Anaesth 36:387, 1964. Copyright © The Board of Management and Trustees of the British Journal of Anesthesia. Reproduced by permission of Oxford University Press, British Journal of Anesthesia.)

acteristics may explain the long-lasting results of neurolytic blocks performed with 10% phenol in the sympathetic axis.[38]

The block produced by phenol tends to be less intense and of shorter duration than that produced by alcohol. Moller and associates[62] compared various concentrations of alcohol with phenol and concluded that 5% phenol equaled 40% alcohol in neurolytic potency. Axons of all sizes are affected by therapeutic concentrations and, as described by ethyl alcohol, appear edematous. The posterior root ganglia are unaffected by phenol.[63] Similar pathologic changes occur in peripheral nerves when exposed to phenol.[33] The process of degeneration takes about 14 days, and regeneration is completed in about 14 weeks. After an intrathecal injection of phenol, its concentration decreases rapidly—to 30% of the original concentration in 60 seconds and to 0.1% within 15 minutes.[36, 64]

Phenol is efficiently metabolized by liver enzymes. The principal pathways are conjugation to the glucuronides and oxidation to equinal compounds or to carbon dioxide and water. It is then excreted as a variety of conjugates via the kidney.[33]

A higher affinity for vascular tissue than for neuronal tissue has been suggested by Wood.[61] The interference with blood flow is believed to be the etiology for the observed neuropathy.[65, 66] However, Racz and associates[67] studied the morphologic changes that occurred following epidural and subarachnoid injection. They found that massive tissue destruction was present after subarachnoid injection as compared with epidural injection despite intact vasculature in areas of spinal cord destruction.[67] These findings support a direct neurotoxic effect of phenol rather than an effect secondary to vascular destruction.[38, 68]

Large systemic doses of phenol (≥8.5 g) cause convulsions and then CNS depression and cardiovascular collapse. Chronic poisoning results in skin eruptions, gastrointestinal symptoms, and renal toxicity.[38] Clinical doses between 1 and 10 mL of 1% to 10% solutions (up to 1000 mg) are unlikely to cause serious toxicity.[38, 69]

GLYCEROL

Glycerol is used mostly for neurolysis of the gasserian ganglion to treat idiopathic trigeminal neuralgia.[70] Considered a mild neurolytic, like other alcohols, it produces localized perineurial damage, whereas intraneural injection results in Schwann cell edema, axolysis, and wallerian degeneration.[38] In one histologic study, intraneural injection of glycerol was more damaging than topical application, although significant, localized, subperineurial damage occurred after local application of a 50% glycerol solution.[38, 71] Histologic changes included the presence of many inflammatory cells, extensive myelin swelling, and axolysis. Myelin disintegration occurs weeks after the injury along with ongoing axolysis during periods of myelin restitution, indicating an ongoing nerve fiber injury possibly caused by secondary events such as compression of transperineal vessels and ischemia.[38, 71, 72] Electron microscopy shows evidence of wallerian degeneration; with intraneural injection, all nerve fibers are destroyed.[37]

Mechanism of Action

The mechanism of action is not clear. Sweet and colleagues[73] suggested that glycerol affected primarily small myelinated and unmyelinated fibers.[38] Bennett and Lunsford, using trigeminal evoked-potential studies, concluded that glycerol more specifically affects the damaged myelinated axons implicated in the pathogenesis of trigeminal neuralgia.[74, 75] Because there is no permanent injury to surrounding structures and facial sensation is preserved in most patients, Feldstein[76] thought that glycerol was superior to radiofrequency rhizotomy for the treatment of tic douloureux. However, potential spread to the subarachnoid space, the risk of neuropathy, and poor control of the spread of a fluid agent have made radiofrequency a continued attractive alternative. With the recent use of pulsed radiofrequency, the advantage of a discrete, controlled lesion remains without the concern for neuritis or loss of facial sensation. However, long-term follow-up on its effectiveness has not been reported.

HYPERTONIC AND HYPOTONIC SOLUTIONS

Hypertonic or hypotonic subarachnoid injections have been used for achieving neurolysis.[77] The intrathecal injection of cold (2° to 4ºC) 0.9% NaCl is supposed to have a specific action on the pain-carrying C fibers, sparing the larger fibers that subserve sensory, motor, and autonomic functions.[78] The technique requires the spinal fluid to be withdrawn and replaced with cold saline as rapidly as possible.[33] Up to 40 to 60 mL of saline has been injected. Local anesthetic should be used concomitantly or the procedure can be quite painful. The pain relief is usually brief.[33]

Injections of hypertonic saline can be quite painful; therefore, local anesthetics are generally injected before the saline.[30] The intrathecal injection of hypertonic saline can produce a variety of complications.[79] Some degree of complications occurred in 11% and significant morbidity in 1% of patients. Two deaths have been reported secondary to myocardial infarction. During saline injection, sinus tachycardia or premature ventricular contraction have been seen,[80] and localized paresis lasting for many hours and paresthesia extending for weeks have been observed.[81] Other complications reported include hemiplegia, pulmonary edema, pain in the ear, vestibular disturbances, and loss of sphincter control with sacral anesthesia.[33, 82]

Mechanism of Action

Pathologic changes due to hypertonic and hypotonic solutions have been extensively studied.[33, 83, 84] Microscopic changes seen on the peripheral nerves do not correlate with clinical effects of differential C fiber block.[83, 84] However, application of distilled water on the dorsal root ganglia for 5 minutes produced a differential C fiber block similar to that seen with in vitro hypertonic saline. The mechanism of action seems to be the intracellular shifts of water with extracellular change in osmolarity.[33]

AMMONIUM SALTS

In 1935, Judovich used pitcher plant distillate for prolonged analgesia. The active component of the distillate was determined to be ammonium sulfate, ammonium chloride, or ammonium hydroxide, depending on the acid used to neutralize the distillate and on the pH.[33, 86] Limited pathologic studies suggested that ammonium

salts in concentrations of greater than 10% caused acute degenerative neuropathy. This degeneration is nonselective, affecting all types of nerve fibers.[33] More recent in vitro studies with pitcher plant distillate attributed the effects to benzyl alcohol contained in the vehicle.[33, 87] Associated complications such as nausea and vomiting, headache, paresthesia, and spinal cord injury have led to the clinical abandonment of ammonium salt solutions, including pitcher plant distillate.[33]

The action of ammonium salts on nerve impulses produces obliteration of C fiber potentials with only a small effect on A fibers.[88, 89] Limited pathologic studies suggest that injection of ammonium salts around a peripheral nerve causes an acute degenerative neuropathy affecting all fibers.[32]

Hand[90] reported the use of subarachnoid ammonium salts in 50 patients. Transient complications were nausea and headache, whereas paresthesias or burning sensation occurred in 30% of patients at doses of 500 mg of ammonium salt and lasted 2 to 14 days.[33]

SUMMARY

The use of chemical neurolytic agents for the interruption of painful pathways is one option for the treatment of intractable chronic pain. Owing to the undesirable side effects, it is imperative this method be used by an experienced clinician. The use of fluoroscopic or radiographic guidance is strongly encouraged for accurate placement of the needle and the injection of the solution because the lesion created is not discrete. The patients must be carefully selected and give fully informed consent.

WATER-SOLUBLE MYELOGRAPHIC AGENTS (Tables 4–1 and 4–2)

The first report in 1931 describing a water-soluble contrast agent for myelography was published.[91] Its lower viscosity and density and improved miscibility with CSF allowed finer detail to be detected. Methiodal was spontaneously absorbed, which eliminated the need for removal following each investigation. Sodium methiodal was highly irritating.

Meglumine iothalamate was too toxic for use above the lumbar region.[92] A major improvement in contrast agent design occurred in 1972 with the introduction of the first nonionic, water-soluble contrast medium, metrizamide (Amipaque). Metrizamide also proved to be far less neurotoxic than the ionic agents and was less likely to induce arachnoiditis.[93] It was the first water-soluble contrast agent used for investigation of the entire subarachnoid space.

The adverse reactions associated with metrizamide are minor, such as headache (reported in 21% to 68% of

▽ TABLE 4–1 Recommended Concentration and Doses of Iohexol

Procedure	Formulations*	Concentration (mg/mL)	Volume (mL)	Dose (g)
Lumbar				
myelography (via lumbar injection)	Omnipaque 180	180	10–17	1.8–3.06
	Omnipaque 240	240	7–12.5	1.7–3
Thoracic				
myelography (via lumbar or cervical	Omnipaque 240	240	6.12.5	1.7–3
injection)	Omnipaque 300	300	6–10	1.8–3
Cervical				
myelography (via lumbar injection)	Omnipaque 240	240	6–12.5	1.4–3
	Omnipaque 300	300	6–10	1.8–3
Cervical	Omnipaque 180	180	7–10	1.3–1.8
myelography (via C1–2 injection)	Omnipaque 240	240	6–12.5	1.4–3
	Omnipaque 300	300	4–10	1.2–3
Total columnar				
myelography (via lumbar injection)	Omnipaque 240	240	6–12.5	1.4–3
	Omnipaque 300	300	6–10	1.8–3

* Iohexol is the generic name for Omnipaque.

▽ TABLE 4–2 Pharmacologic Properties of Iohexol

Concentration (mg Iodine/mL)	Osmolality* (mOsm/kg water)	Osmolarity (mOsm/L)	Absolute Viscosity (cp) 20°C	Absolute Viscosity (cp) 37°C	Specific Gravity at 37°C
140	322	273	2.3	1.5	1.164
180	408	661	3.1	2.0	1.209
210	460	362	4.2	2.5	1.244
300	672	465	11.8	6.3	1.349
350	844	541	20.4	10.4	1.406

* By vapor-pressure osmometry

patients)[94] and nausea (reported in 25% to 40% of patients),[95, 96] but there have also been a significant number of more serious reactions, such as mental disturbances, cortical blindness, aphasia, encephalopathy, and seizures.[97–103]

REFERENCES

1. Butterworth JF, Strichartz CR: The molecular mechanisms by which local anesthetics produce impulse blockade: A review. Anesthesiology 72:711–734, 1990.
2. Catterall WA: Cellular and molecular biology of voltage-gated sodium channels. Physiol Rev 72:S15–848, 1992.
3. Ragsdale DR, McPhee JO, Scheuer T, et al: Molecular determinants of state-dependent block of Na+ channels by local anesthetics. Science 265:1724–1728, 1994.
4. Gasser HS, Erlanger J: The role of fiber size in the establishment of a nerve block by pressure or cocaine. Am J Physiol 88:581–591, 1929.
5. Raymond SA, Gissen AJ: Mechanism of differential nerve block: Local anesthetics. In Strichartz CR (ed): Handbook of Experimental Pharmacology, Vol 81. Berlin, Springer-Verlag, 1987, pp 95–164.
6. Carpenter RI, Mackey DC: Local anesthetics. In Barash PC, Cullen BF, Stoelting RK (eds): Clinical Anesthesia, 2nd ed. Philadelphia, JB Lippincott, 1992, pp 509–541.
7. Ritchie JM, Greengard P: On the mode of action of local anesthetics. Annu Rev Pharmacol 6:405–430, 1966.
8. Lynch C III: Depression of myocardial contractility in vitro by bupivacaine, etidocaine, and lidocaine. Anesth Analg 65:551, 1986.
9. Feldman HS, Covino BC, Sage DJ: Direct chronotropic and inotropic effects of local anesthetic agents in isolated guinea pig atria. Reg Anesth 7:149, 1982.
10. Stevens MF, Klement W, Lipfert P: Conduction block in man is stimulation frequency dependent. Anesthetists 45:533–537, 1996.
11. Huang YF, Pryor ME, Mather LE, et al: Cardiovascular and central nervous system effects of intravenous levobupivacaine and bupivacaine in sheep. Anesth Analg 86:797–804, 1998.
12. Bromage PR: A comparison of the hydrochloride and carbon dioxide salts of lidocaine and prilocaine in epidural analgesia. Acta Anaesth Scand Suppl 16:55–69, 1965.
13. Gissen AJ, Datta S, Lambert D: The chloroprocaine controversy: II. Is chloroprocaine neurotoxic? Reg Anesth 9:135–145, 1984.
14. Wang BC, Hillman DE, Spielholz NI, et al: Chronic neurological deficits and nesacaine-CE: An effect to the anesthetic, 2-chloroprocaine, or the antioxidant, sodium bisulfite? Anesth Analg 63:445–447, 1984.
15. Tarkkila P, Huhtala J, Tuominen M: Transient radicular irritation after spinal anesthesia with hyperbaric 5% lidocaine. Br J Anaesth 74:328–329, 1995.
16. DiFazio CA, Carron H, Grosslight KR, et al: Comparison of pH-adjusted lidocaine solutions for epidural anesthesia. Anesth Analg 65:760–764, 1986.
17. Hilgier M: Alkalinization of bupivacaine for brachial plexus block. Reg Anesth 10:59–61, 1985.
18. Selander D: Neurotoxicity of local anesthetics: Animal data. Reg Anesth 18:461–468, 1993.
19. Rigler ML, Drasner K, Krejcie TC, et al: Cauda equina syndrome after continuous spinal anesthesia. Anesth Analg 72:275–281, 1991.
20. Schneider M, Ettlin T, Kaufmann M, et al: Transient neurologic toxicity after hyperbaric subarachnoid anesthesia with 5% lidocaine. Anesth Analg 76:1154–1157, 1993.
21. Hampl KF, Schneider MC, Ummenhofer W, et al: Transient neurologic symptoms after spinal anesthesia. Anesth Analg 81:1148–1153, 1995.
22. Carpenter RL: Hypobaric lidocaine spinal anesthesia: Do we need an alternative? Anesth Analg 81:1125–1128, 1995.

23. Pollock J, Neal J, Stephenson C, et al: Prospective study of the incidence of transient radicular irritation in patients undergoing spinal anesthesia. Anesthesiology 84:1361–1367, 1996.

24. Luton A: Etudes sur la medication substitutive. Premiere partie, de la substitution parenchymapeuse. Deuxieme partie de la medication substitutive: son Entendue, ses divisions. Arch Gen Med 2:57, 1863.

25. Jain S: The role of neurolytic procedures. In Parris WCV (ed): Cancer Pain Management: Principles and Practice. Boston, Butterworth-Heinemann, 1997, pp 231–244.

26. Arter OE, Racz GB: Pain management of the oncologic patient. Semin Surg Oncol 6:162, 1990.

27. Raj PP, Patt RB: Peripheral neurolysis. In Raj PP (ed): Pain Medicine: A Comprehensive Review. St. Louis, Mosby–Year Book, 1996, pp 288–296.

28. Ferrer-Brecher T. Anesthetic techniques for the management of cancer pain. Cancer 63:2343, 1989.

29. Matsuki M, Kato Y, Ichiyangi L: Progressive changes in the concentration of ethyl alcohol in the human and canine subarachnoid space. Anesthesiology 36:617, 1972.

30. Heavner JE: Neurolytic agents. In Raj PP (ed): Pain Medicine: A Comprehensive Review. St. Louis, Mosby–Year Book, 1996, pp 285–286.

31. Rall TW: Hypnotics and sedatives: Ethanol. In Gilman AG, et al (eds): The Pharmacological Basis of Therapeutics, 8th ed. New York, Pergamon Press, 1990.

32. Schlosser H: Erfahrungen in der Neuralgiebehandlung mit Alkoholeinspritzungen. Verh Dtsch Ges Inn Med 24:49, 1907.

33. Raj PP, Denson DD: Neurolytic agents. In Raj (ed): Clinical Practice of Regional Anesthesia. New York, Churchill Livingstone, 1991, pp 135–152.

34. Labat G, Greene MB: Contributions to the modern method of diagnosis and treatment of so-called sciatic neuralgias. Am J Surg 11:435, 1931.

35. Rumbsy MG, Finean JB: The action of organic solvents on the myelin sheath of peripheral nerve tissue: II. Short-chain aliphatic alcohols. J Neurochem 13:1509, 1966.

36. Jain S, Gupta R: Neurolytic agents in clinical practice. In Waldman SD (ed): Interventional Pain Management, 2nd ed. Philadelphia, WB Saunders, 2001, pp 220–225.

37. Dwyer B, Gibb D: Chronic pain and neurolytic blockade. In Cousins MJ, Bridenbaugh PO (eds): Neural Blockade in Clinical Anesthesia and Management of Pain. Philadelphia, JB Lippincott, 1980.

38. de Leon-Casasola OA, Ditonto E: Drugs commonly used for nerve blocking: Neurolytic agents. In Raj PP (ed): Practical Management of Pain, 3rd ed. St. Louis, Mosby, 2000, pp 575–578.

39. Gallagher HS, Yonezawa T, Hoy RC, Derrick WS: Subarachnoid alcohol block: I. Histological changes in the central nervous system. Am J Pathol 35:679, 1961.

40. Merrick RL: Degeneration and recovery of autonomic neurons following alcoholic block. Ann Surg 113:298, 1941.

41. Swerdlow M: Neurolytic blocks. In Patt RB (ed): Cancer Pain. Philadelphia, JB Lippincott, 1993, p 435.

42. Mandl F: Aqueous solution of phenol as a substitute for alcohol in sympathetic block. J Int Coll Surg 13:566, 1950.

43. Bonica JJ: Regional anesthesia with tetracaine. Anesthesiology 11:606, 716, 1950.

44. De Takats G: Discussion of paper by HS Ruth: Diagnostic, prognostic, and therapeutic nerve blocks. JAMA 102:419, 1934.

45. Rocco A: Radiofrequency lumbar sympatholysis: The evolution of a technique for managing sympathetically mediated pain. Reg Anesth 20:3–12, 1995.

46. Bogduk N, Tynan W, Wilson SS: The nerve supply to the human intervertebral discs. J Anat 132:39–56, 1981.

47. Edwards EA: Operative anatomy of the lumbar sympathetic chain. Angiology 12:184–198, 1951.

48. Binet A: Valeur de la sympathectomie chimique en gynecologie. Gynecol Obstet 27:393, 1933.

49. Nechaev VA: Solutions of phenol in local anesthesia. Soviet Khir 5:203, 1933.

50. Putnam TJ, Hampton AO: A technique of injection into the gasserian ganglion under roentgenographic control. Arch Neurol Psychiatry 35:92, 1936.

51. Mandl F: Paravertebral Block. Orlando, Grune & Stratton, 1947.

52. Haxton HA: Chemical sympathectomy. Br Med J 1:1026, 1949.

53. Boyd AM, Ratcliff AH, Jepson RP, et al: Intermittent claudication. J Bone Joint Surg Br 3:325, 1949.

54. Maher RM: Phenol for pain and spasticity. In Pain: Henry Ford Hospital International Symposium. Boston, Little, Brown, 1966, p 109.

55. Kelly RE, Gautier-Smith PC: Intrathecal phenol in the treatment of reflex spasms and spasticity. Lancet 2:1102, 1959.

56. Nathan PW: Intrathecal phenol to relieve spasticity in paraplegia. Lancet 2:1099, 1959.

57. Iggo A, Walsh EG: Selective block of small fibres in the spinal roots by phenol. Brain 83:701, 1960.

58. Nathan PW, Sears TA: Effects of phenol on nervous conduction. J Physiol (Lond) 150:565, 1960.

59. Stewart WA, Lourie H: An experimental evaluation of the effects of subarachnoid injection of phenol-pantopaque in cats. J Neurosurg 20:64, 1963.

60. Nathan PW, Sears TA, Smith MC: Effects of phenol solutions on the nerve roots of the cat: An electrophysiologic and histologic study. J Neurol Sci 2:7, 1965.

61. Wood KM: The use of phenol as a neurolytic agent: A review. Pain 5:205, 1978.

62. Moller JE, Helweg-Larson J, Jacobson E: Histopathological lesions in the sciatic nerve of the rat following perineural application of phenol and alcohol solutions. Dan Med Bull 16:116–119, 1969.

63. Smith MC: Histological findings following intrathecal injection of phenol solutions for the relief of pain. Anaesthesia 36:387, 1964.

64. Bates W, Judovich BD: Intractable pain. Anesthesiology 3:363, 1942.

65. Nour-Eldin F: Uptake of phenol by vascular and brain tissue. Microvasc Res 2:224, 1970.

66. Totoki T, Kato T, Nomoto Y, et al: Anterior spinal artery syndrome—a complication of cervical intrathecal phenol injection. Pain 6:99, 1979.

67. Racz GB, Heavner J, Haynsworth R: Repeat epidural phenol injections in chronic pain and spasticity. In Lipton S, Miles J (eds): Persistent Pain, 2nd ed. New York, Grune & Stratton, 1985, p 157.

68. Heavner JE, Racz GB: Gross and microscopic lesions produced by phenol neurolytic procedures. In Racz GB (ed): Techniques of Neurolysis. Boston, Kluwer, 1989, p 27.

69. Cousins MJ: Chronic pain and neurolytic neural blockade. In Cousins MJ, Bridenbaugh PO (eds): Neural Blockade in Clinical Anesthesia and Management of Pain, 2nd ed. Philadelphia, JB Lippincott, 1988, p 1053.

70. Hakanson S: Trigeminal neuralgia treated by the injection of glycerol into the trigeminal cistern. Neurosurgery 9:638, 1981.

71. Rengachary SS, Watanabe IS, Singer P, Bopp WJ: Effect of glycerol on peripheral nerve: An experimental study. Neurosurgery 13:681, 1983.

72. Myers RR, Katz J: Neuropathy of neurolytic and semidestructive agents. In Cousins MJ, Bridenbaugh PO (eds): Neural Blockade in Clinical Anesthesia and Management of Pain, 2nd ed. Philadelphia, JB Lippincott, 1988, p 76.

73. Sweet WH, Poletti CE, Macon JB: Treatment of trigeminal neuralgia and other facial pains by retrogasserian injection of glycerol. Neurosurgery 9:3647, 1981.

74. Bennett MH, Lunsford LD: Percutaneous retrogasserian glycerol rhizotomy for tic douloureux: II. Results and implications of trigeminal evoked potentials. Neurosurgery 14:431, 1984.

75. Lunsford LD, Bennett MH: Percutaneous retrogasserian glycerol rhizotomy for tic douloureux: I. Technique and results in 112 patients. Neurosurgery 14:424, 1984.

76. Feldstein GS: Percutaneous retrogasserian glycerol rhizotomy in the treatment of trigeminal neuralgia. In Racz GB (ed): Techniques of Neurolysis. Boston, Kluwer, 1988, p 125.

77. Hitchcock E: Osmolytic neurolysis for intractable facial pain. Lancet 1:434, 1969.

78. Lund PC: Principles and Practice of Spinal Anesthesia. Springfield, IL, Charles C Thomas, 1971.

79. Lucas JT, Ducker TB, Perok PL: Adverse reactions to intrathecal saline injection for control of pain. J Neurosurg 42:557, 1975.

80. McKean MC, Hitchcock E: Electrocardiographic changes after intrathecal hypertonic saline solution. Lancet 2:1083, 1968.

81. Ventafridda V, Spreafico R: Subarachnoid saline perfusion. Adv Neurol 4:477, 1974.

82. O'Higgins JW, Padfield A, Clapp H: Possible complications of hypothermic saline subarachnoid injection. Lancet 1:567, 1970.

83. Hewett DL, King JS: Conduction block of monkey dorsal rootlets by water and hypertonic solutions. Exp Neurol 33:225, 1971.

84. Nicholson MF, Roberts FW: Relief of pain by intrathecal injection of hypothermic saline. Med J Aust 1:61, 1968.

85. Thompson GE: Pulmonary edema complicating intrathecal hypertonic saline injection for intractable pain. Anesthesiology 35:425, 1971.

86. Walti A: Determination of the nature of the volatile base from the rhizome of the pitcher plant, *Sarracenia purpurea*. J Am Chem Soc 67:22, 1945.

87. Ford DJ, Phero JC, Denson D: Effect of pitcher plant distillate on frog sciatic nerve. Reg Anesth 5:16, 1980.

88. Davies JI, Steward PB, Fink P: Prolonged sensory block using ammonium salts. Anesthesiology 28:244, 1967.

89. Judovich BD, Bates W, Bishop K: Intraspinal ammonium salts for the intractable pain of malignancy. Anesthesiology 5:341, 1944.

90. Hand LV: Subarachnoid ammonium sulfate therapy for intractable pain. Anesthesiology 5:354, 1944.

91. Arndll S, Lidstrom F: Myelography with skiodan (Abrodil). Acta Radiol 12:287–288, 1931.

92. Campbell RI, Campbell IA, Heimburger RE, et al: Ventriculography and myelography with absorbable radiopaque medium. Radiology 82:286–289, 1964.

93. Haughton VM, Eldevik OP: Complications from aqueous myelographic media: Experimental studies. In Sackett IF, Strother CM (eds): New Techniques in Myelography. New York, Harper & Row, 1979, pp 184–194.

94. Skalpe LO: Adverse effects of water-soluble contrast media in myelography, cisternography, and ventriculography: A review with special reference to metrizamide. Acta Radiol 355(Suppl):359–370, 1977.

95. Sackett JF, Strother CM, Quaglieri CE, et al: Metrizanide: Cerebrospinal fluid contrast medium. Radiology 123:779–782, 1977.

96. Bergstrom K, Mostrum U: Technique for cervical myelography with metrizamide. Acta Radiol 355(Suppl):105–109, 1977.

97. Junck L, Marshall WH: Neurotoxicity of radiological contrast agents. Ann Neurol 13:469–484, 1983.

98. Ekholm SE: Adverse reactions to intravascular and intrathecal contrast medium. In Preger L (ed): Iatrogenic Diseases, Vol 1. Boca Raton, FL, CRC Press, 1986, pp 111–136.

99. Gonsette RE: Cervical myelography with a new resorbable contrast medium: Amipaque. Acta Neurol Belg 76:283–285, 1976.

100. Amundsen P: Metrizamide in cervical myelography: Survey and present state. Acta Radiol 355(Suppl):85–97, 1977.

101. Dugstad G, Eldevik P: Lumbar myelography. Acta Radiol 355(Suppl):17–30, 1977.

102. Nickel AR, Salem JJ: Clinical experience in North America with metrizamide. Acta Radiol 355(Suppl):409–416, 1977.

103. Budny IL, Hopkins LN: Ventriculitis after metrizamide lumbar myelography. Neurosurgery 17:467–468, l985.

Physics and Principles of Cryoneurolysis and Radiofrequency Lesioning

This chapter provides an overview of both cryoneurolysis and radiofrequency lesioning. Both procedures are best used when a single nerve or site is involved; they are not suitable for diffuse processes in multiple sites. In certain conditions, one technique may be superior to the other. For example, for trigeminal neuralgia, the cryoneurolysis results are poorer than those obtained by radiofrequency lesioning.[1, 2]

After failure of more conservative measures, diagnostic microinjections of local anesthetic are performed at the peripheral nerve or nerves. A favorable response to diagnostic injections does not always predict a successful result with radiofrequency or cryoneurolysis. Failure of palliation of symptoms by neurodestruction after successful diagnostic block may occur in up to 30% of cases.[3] Reasons for this include the following:

- Placebo response
- Poor needle placement
- Excessive volumes of local anesthetic, which cause a diffuse neural blockade without specificity
- Systemic effects of absorbed local anesthetics
- Technical problems that prevent generation of the lesion

Contraindications to the procedures include the following:

- Undiagnosed condition
- Coagulopathy
- Infection
- Unwillingness or inability to cooperate
- Psychopathology, including anxiety that makes toleration of the procedure unlikely

CRYONEUROLYSIS

Cryoneurolysis is a technique in which the application of low temperatures produced by cryosurgical equipment achieves anesthesia or analgesia by blocking peripheral nerves or destroying nerve endings.

HISTORY

The analgesic effect of low temperatures has been recorded since Hippocrates (460–377 BC).[4-7] Avicenna of Persia (980–1070) and Severino of Naples (1580–1656) recorded their use of cold for preoperative analgesia.[8, 9] James Arnott (1797–1883) advocated local cooling during surgery and in the treatment of headache and cancer pains.[10] In 1777, John Hunter studied the reversible destructive effects of freezing on animal tissues. More practical and portable methods of cooling used ether spray and ethyl chloride to reduce temperatures locally as low as −12ºC.[8, 9] In 1917, Trendelenburg[10] demonstrated that freezing caused severe but reversible damage to nerves without scar or neuroma formation.

Interest in cryotherapy was revived in 1939, when Smith and Fay[11] reported evidence of tumor regression after localized freezing.[12] Cooper developed the first cryoprobe in 1961.[13] He was able to produce a temperature of −196ºC by using liquid nitrogen. Amoils[14] introduced the enclosed gas expansion cryoprobe in which carbon dioxide was used. Since then, nitrous oxide has also been used as the refrigerant. Lloyd and colleagues[15] introduced the technique termed *cryoanalgesia*, with which prolonged analgesia could be obtained after a single freezing of a peripheral nerve. They reported that this was a safe procedure, nerve function always returned, and neuroma formation did not occur. The present generation of thin, long probes incorporates thermocouples and stimulators.

PHYSICS OF CRYOANALGESIA

Expansion of gas enclosed in the cryoprobe results in the Joule-Thompson or Kelvin effects; that is, gas under

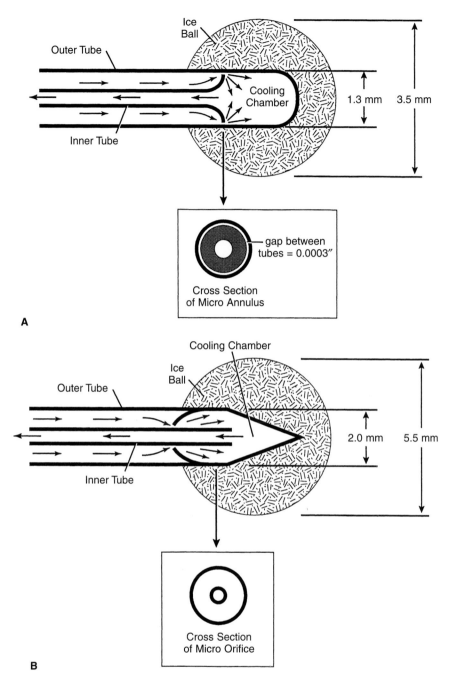

FIGURE 5–1

A and *B*, Two typical cryoprobe designs. High-pressure gas flows through the outer tube and expands after passing through the orifice. The gas is vented through the center tube. (From Saberski LR: Cryoneurolysis in clinical practice. In Waldman SD, Winnie AP [eds]: Interventional Pain Management. Philadelphia, WB Saunders, 1996, pp 172–184.)

pressure escaping through a small orifice expands and cools (Fig. 5–1). The probes are made of stainless steel insulated with a coating of polytetrafluoroethylene (Teflon) and are of coaxial design. A thin outer tube carries the gas under pressures between 4000 and 6000 kPa to the tip, where it passes through a narrow orifice, leading to a pressure drop to 50 to 75 kPa. The gas subsequently expands and cools, achieving temperatures between -50° and -70°C at the tip, and returns through an inner tube. The inner tube acts as an exhaust conduit to vent the gas. Modern probes use either nitrous oxide or carbon dioxide. The shaft diameter has now been reduced to 1.3 mm and the length increased to 120 mm.

The tip can be trocar shaped or hemispherical. Thermocouples and stimulators with variable voltages and frequencies are built into the exposed tip surface, and by using a console with a variable flow control it is possible to achieve a wide range of subzero temperatures (Fig. 5–2).

The ice ball encompasses the end of the probe and is about 3.5 mm in diameter for a 1.3-mm tipped probe. The variables involved in ice ball size include probe size, freeze time, tip temperature, tissue thermal conductivity, tissue permeability to water, and presence or absence of vascular structure (i.e., a heat sink). When thermal equilibrium between the probe and tissues is

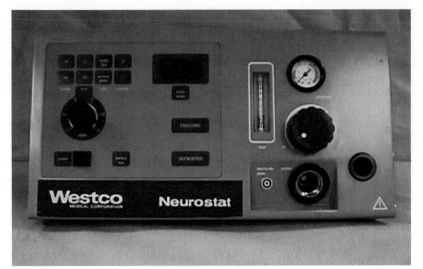

FIGURE 5–2

Typical cryodenervation incorporating a variable flow control, a thermocouple, and a nerve stimulator. (From Raj PP [ed]: Practical Management of Pain, 3rd ed. St. Louis, Mosby, 2000.)

achieved, there is no further increase in the size of the ice ball; however, repetition of the freeze-thaw cycle increases the size of the cryolesion.[16]

When the probe is used percutaneously, it is difficult to ensure close proximity to the nerve, and large ice balls have a greater chance of producing the desired lesion. For myelinated fibers a direct lesion 3 mm in diameter with a freeze time of 1 minute produces a conduction block.[17] Where the nerve is frozen amid other tissues, the duration of exposure should be approximately 90 to 120 seconds. Rapid defrosting aids removal of the probe from tissues.

PATHOLOGY OF THE LESION

Freezing involves removal of pure water from solution and its isolation into biologically inert ice crystals. The extent of the lesion depends primarily on the rates of freezing and thawing.[18] When cooling is slow, ice crystal nucleation occurs in the extracellular fluid. When freezing is rapid, crystal nuclei develop uniformly throughout the tissue. The central zone close to the probe tip cools rapidly compared with the peripheral zone, which is influenced by heat generated by the surrounding tissues. Intracellular ice is formed at the center of the lesion and extracellular crystals are formed at the periphery.[19, 20] Tissue destruction is more complete at the center of a cryolesion. It is also likely that the areas at the edge of the cryolesion undergo ischemic necrosis.

Application of cold to peripheral nerves induces a reversible block of conduction similar to that produced by local anesthesia. The extent and duration of the effect depend on the temperature attained in the tissue and the duration of exposure. Large myelinated fibers are initially affected with relative sparing of smaller sensory nerves.

A prolonged conduction block occurs when the nerve is frozen at temperatures between $-5°$ and $-20°C$.[21, 22] This causes axonal disintegration and breakdown of myelin sheaths. Wallerian degeneration occurs with the perineurium and epineurium remaining intact. The absence of external damage to the nerve and the minimal inflammatory reaction following freezing ensure that regeneration is accurate and complete. Recovery depends on the rate of axonal regeneration and the distance of the cryolesion from the end organ. All elements of the nerve are involved. The rate of axonal regrowth is 1 to 3 mm per day. Histologic sectioning of nerve suggests that regeneration is still occurring in functionally intact nerves.

TECHNIQUE

The cryolesion is attempted only after successful temporary reduction of symptoms by a diagnostic block. After a small skin wheal is raised with local anesthetic, a 1.3- or 2-mm probe is passed via a 16- or 12-gauge catheter, respectively, depending on the nerve size (Fig. 5–3). Larger probes counteract arterial warmth where heat sinks are expected. Localization is facilitated with stimulation between 50 and 100 Hz at less than 0.5 V for sensory nerves or at 2 to 5 Hz for motor nerves. Two or three 2-minute cycles are usually sufficient. During the freezing, care is taken to prevent frostbite if the probe comes in direct contact with the skin. Continuous irrigation with 0.9% saline solution at room temperature reduces the possibility of skin injury.

COMMON PROCEDURES

Detailed descriptions of all recognized cryoneurolysis procedures are beyond the scope of this chapter. Indication for cryoneurolysis is mentioned in the chapters as applicable.

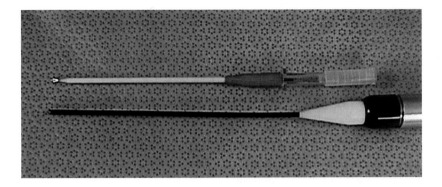

FIGURE 5–3

Lloyd probe. (From Raj PP [ed]: Practical Management of Pain, 3rd ed. St. Louis, Mosby, 2000.)

RADIOFREQUENCY

The first attempts to use direct current (DC) electricity experimentally were made in the 1870s, and it was introduced into clinical practice in the 1940s. The DC generators produced irregular unpredictable lesions. Tissue temperature and thus lesion characteristics were difficult to control. Excess temperature often led to tissue burning, gas formation, and excessive tissue destruction. Cushing and Bovie developed surgical thermocoagulation for hemostasis in the 1920s. This radiofrequency technique was adapted for generating neural lesions in the 1950s by Aranow and Cosman. These generators were a great improvement over older DC lesion generators. In contrast to DC generators, radiofrequency generators use continuous high-frequency waves of about 1 MHz.

The current generators represent several important advances over earlier DC generators.

1. The mechanism of lesion generation is different. With DC generators, the lesions were generated by dielectric mechanisms. With radiofrequency the lesions are generated by ionic means. These lesions are more predictable.
2. The tissue temperature and thus the extent of the lesion are more controllable. Modern generators have automatic temperature controls that prevent overheating and boiling of tissue. Active electrode design has improved. Most electrodes have low thermal coefficients, which lead to faster warming of the electrode and thus more accurate depiction of the tissue temperature.
3. Electrical stimulation can be used to locate the nerve and also to prevent unwanted nerve damage.
4. Tissue resistance (impedance) can be measured. Low tissue impedance may affect the size and characteristics of the lesion generated.

PHYSICS OF RADIOFREQUENCY

The circuit consists of an active electrode, which delivers the current; a method for measuring tissue temperature (thermistor or thermocouple); a radiofrequency generator; and a passive electrode with a large surface area. Current in the region of the active electrode generates heat. The heat generated is a function of the amount of current per unit area (current density) that flows in the region of the electrode. The active electrode itself does not generate heat but is heated as a result of local tissue warming. The current flows from the active to the passive electrode. Because of the much greater surface area of the passive electrode, the current density is much less. Therefore, heating and tissue damage do not usually occur at the passive electrode.

Heating of the active electrode is an important safety feature of this system, because tissue damage is related to the temperature generated. The newer electrodes have a low thermal coefficient, meaning that the electrode absorbs heat well and heats rapidly, leading to a faster response and improved safety of the system. Excessive heating causes more diffuse and permanent tissue damage. It is possible to boil tissues, and these tissues may then adhere to the electrode and be avulsed when the electrode is removed. The thermocouple lends itself better to miniaturization than the thermistor and is therefore more widely used.

Most electrodes are available in a number of sizes and lengths. Both reusable and disposable needles are used. Most have varying lengths of the exposed tip, and the electrode must be selected for the desired purpose. For example, an 18-gauge reusable electrode with a 2-mm exposed tip is suitable for radiofrequency denervation of the trigeminal nerve, whereas a 22-gauge electrode with a 4-mm exposed tip is appropriate for lumbar facet denervation. In some neurosurgical procedures, curved needles are used to generate eccentric lesions.

LESION CHARACTERISTICS

It is critical to control lesion size. The size and consistency of the lesion are governed by four major factors:

1. *Temperature generated:* At higher temperatures, the local tissue reaction is greater.
2. *Rate of thermal equilibrium:* If there is more rapid equilibrium between tissues, the lesion is more uniform. Conversely, if there is slow and incomplete equilibrium, the lesion is erratic. Usually thermal equilibrium is complete by 60 seconds. The lesion size initially rises exponentially with time but becomes independent of time after approximately 30 seconds (Fig. 5–4).
3. *Electrode size and configuration:* Larger electrodes generate larger lesions. For example, an 18-gauge electrode generates a lesion with a radius of 2.2 mm, whereas a 22-gauge electrode generates a radius of only 1.9 mm. Larger electrodes generate bigger lesions but at the expense of more tissue trauma on insertion, unwanted neural destruction, and larger reversible zones (Fig. 5–5).
4. *Local tissue characteristics:* Lesions in tissues in contact with tissues of low electrical resistance such as blood and cerebrospinal fluid may be reduced or irregular in size and shape. Blood may also act as a heat sink, removing heat from the area and thereby limiting local tissue temperature rise and lesion size.

The size of the lesion does not correlate well with either the time or the power used, because the temperature generated depends on tissue characteristics. The lesion generated is usually an inverted cone. In vitro evidence suggests that the lesion radius is maximal at the part of the exposed electrode farthest from the tip.[23] The actual tip may not even be incorporated in the lesion, and this has important clinical implications. Nerves in contact with the tip may be only partially blocked, and an electrode placed tangential to the nerve generates a more effective lesion. The effect on tissues depends on the temperature generated. Above 45ºC, irreversible tissue injury occurs. Between 42° and 45ºC, temporary neural blockade occurs. In general, the larger the lesion, the larger the zone of reversibility (see Fig. 5–5).

The histologic appearance of lesions generated by radiofrequency is one of local tissue burn. Nerve architecture is destroyed. After the lesion is created, wallerian degeneration becomes apparent. The perineurium may also be destroyed. In radiofrequency lesioning, unlike cryoneurolysis, neuroma formation is possible. Clinically, it appears that there is relative selectivity for small, unmyelinated fibers at lower temperatures. Therefore, by limiting the temperature, it may be possible to damage pain fibers selectively. This selectivity has

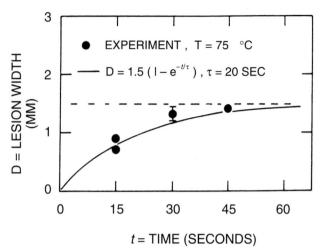

DREZ LESION WIDTH VS. TIME

FIGURE 5–4

The radiofrequency lesion size rises exponentially initially but plateaus after approximately 30 seconds. (From Cosman ER, Nashold BS, Ovelman-Levitt J: Theoretical aspects of radiofrequency lesions in the dorsal root entry zone. Neurosurgery 15:945–950, 1984.)

not been borne out during in vitro experiments. There is no evidence of selectivity for white or gray matter.[24, 25]

TECHNIQUE

Minimal sedation is used so that the patient can participate fully and accurately report the stimuli. All of the equipment, particularly the cables and thermocouple or thermistor, is checked before beginning the procedure. The lesion parameters, especially the maximal temperature, are preset. The radiofrequency probe must be of the appropriate size and length for the needle. In particular, the correct exposed tip length, needle diameter, and length are critical in improving the efficacy of the procedure and reducing the risk of inadvertent tissue injury. Fluoroscopy is mandatory.

The most common reason for failure to generate a lesion is a poor electrical connection, usually related to cable damage. Occasionally, the insulation on the active electrode is disrupted, with a subsequent reduction of current density and poor lesion generation. This may also lead to lesions farther up along the shaft in other tissues traversed by the needle. Poor connection may also occur at the passive electrode, leading to poor conduction or even local tissue burning. The newer machines all measure impedance and can help isolate the source of the problem. Very high impedance (>2000 Ω) suggests electrical disconnection, whereas very low impedance (<200 Ω) implies a short circuit.

Inadequate temperature generation may occur if the temperature selected is too low. Lesions tend to be smaller when lower temperatures are used (see Fig. 5–5). Poor needle placement accounts for many

TISSUE TEMPERATURE VS. DISTANCE FROM ELECTRODE

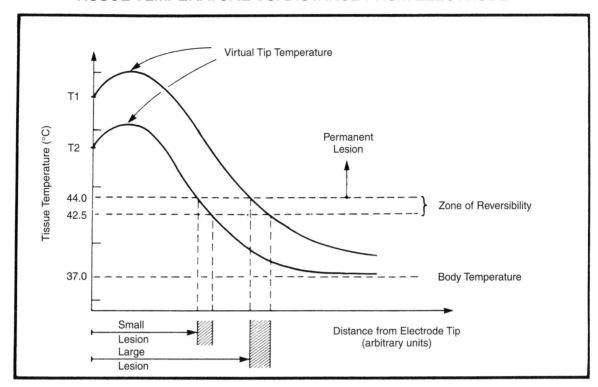

FIGURE 5–5

Tissue injury after radiofrequency lesioning. Note the shape of the lesion and the large area of reversibility. (From Cosman ER, Nashold BS, Ovelman-Levitt J: Theoretical aspects of radiofrequency lesions in the dorsal root entry zone. Neurosurgery 15:945–950, 1984.)

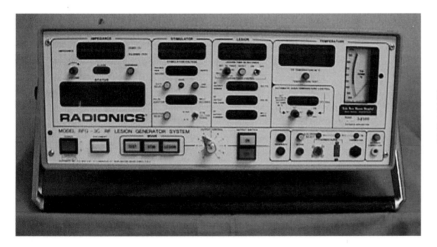

FIGURE 5–6

Typical radiofrequency generator incorporating a nerve stimulator. (From Raj PP [ed]: Practical Management of Pain, 3rd ed. St. Louis, Mosby, 2000.)

technical failures. Newer lesion generators incorporate an electrical nerve stimulator to help locate the nerve (Fig. 5–6).

COMMON PROCEDURES

Detailed descriptions of all the recognized radiofrequency procedures are beyond the scope of this chapter. Its indications are described in each chapter.

REFERENCES

1. Zakrzewska JM: Cryotherapy for trigeminal neuralgia: A 10-year audit. Br J Oral Maxillofac Surg 29:1–4, 1991.
2. Zakrzewska JM, Thomas DG: Patient's assessment of outcome after three surgical procedures for the management of trigeminal neuralgia. Acta Neurochir 122:225–230, 1993.
3. North RB, Kidd DH, Zahurak M, Piantadosi S: Specificity of diagnostic nerve blocks: A prospective, randomized study of sciatica due to lumbosacral spine disease. Pain 65:77–85, 1996.
4. Hippocrates: Aphorism: Heracleitus on the Universe. London, Heinemann, 1931.

5. Gruner OC: A Treatise on the Canon of Medicine of Avicenna. London, Luzac, 1930.

6. Bartholini T: De Nivis Usu Medico Observationes Variae. Copenhagen, Hafniae, 1661.

7. Bird HM: James Arnott, MD, 1797–1883: A pioneer in refrigeration analgesia. Anaesthesia 4:10–17, 1949.

8. Richardson B: On a new and ready method of producing local anaesthesia. Med Times Gaz 1:115–117, 1866.

9. Redar C: Nouvelle methode d' anesthesie locale par le chlorure d'ethyle: Congres francais de chirurgie, Se session. Germer Bailhere, 1891.

10. Trendelenburg W: Über langdauernde Nervenausschaltung mit sicherer Regenerationsfahigkeit. Z Gesamte Exp Med 5:371–374, 1917.

11. Smith LW, Fay T: Temperature factors in cancer and embryonal cell growth. JAMA 113:653–660, 1939.

12. Fay T: Observations on prolonged human refrigeration. N Y State J Med 40:1351–1354, 1940.

13. Garamy G: Engineering Aspects of Cryosurgery. Springfield, IL, Charles C Thomas, 1968.

14. Amoils SP: The Joule-Thomson cryoprobe. Arch Ophthalmol 78:201–207, 1967.

15. Lloyd JW, Barnard JD, Glynn CI: Cryoanalgesia: A new approach to pain relief. Lancet 2:932–934, 1976.

16. Gill W, Da Costa J, Fraser I: The control and predictability of a cryolesion. Cryobiology 6:347–353, 1970.

17. Douglas WW, Malcolm JL: The effects of localized cooling on conduction in cat nerves. J Physiol (Lond) 130:53–71, 1955.

18. Mazur P: Physical and chemical factors underlying cell injury in cryosurgical freezing. In Rand RW (ed): Cryosurgery. Springfield, IL, Charles C Thomas, 1968.

19. Whittaker DK: Ice crystals formed in tissues during cryosurgery: I. Light microscopy. Cryobiology 2:192–201, 1974.

20. Whittaker DK: Ice crystals formed in tissues during cryosurgery: II. Electron microscopy. Cryobiology 2:202–217, 1974.

21. Denny-Brown D, Adams RD, Brenner C, Doherty MM: The pathology of injury to nerve induced by cold. J Neuropathol Exp Neurol 4:305–323, 1945.

22. Carter DC, Lee PW, Gill W, Johnston RI: The effect of cryosurgery on peripheral nerve function. J R Coll Surg Edinb 17:25–31, 1972.

23. Bogduk N, Macintosh J, Marsland A: Technical limitations to the efficacy of radiofrequency neurotomy for spinal pain. Neurosurgery 20:529–535, 1987.

24. Cosman ER, Nashold BS, Ovelman-Levitt I: Theoretical aspects of radiofrequency lesions in the dorsal root entry zone. Neurosurgery 15:945–950, 1984.

25. Smith HP, McWhorther JM, Challa VR: Radiofrequency neurolysis in a clinical model. J Neurosurg 55:246–253, 1981.

6

Trigeminal Ganglion Block and Neurolysis

HISTORY

The percutaneous trans–foramen ovale approach to the trigeminal (gasserian) ganglion using absolute alcohol was first described by Hartel in 1912.[1] In the evolution of the treatment, radiofrequency (RF) lesioning for this ganglion was described by Sweet and Wepsic in 1965,[2] retrogasserian glycerol injection by Hakanson in 1981,[3] and percutaneous balloon compression by Mullan and Lichtor in 1978 and published in 1983.[4]

ANATOMY

The trigeminal nerve is the largest among the cranial nerves. Sensation of the oral mucosa, anterior and middle cranial fossa, tooth pulp, surrounding gingiva, and periodontal membrane is innervated by the trigeminal nerve. The trigeminal ganglion is named after a Viennese anatomist, Johann Laurentius Gasser (Fig. 6–1A).

The ganglion lies within the cranium in an area called *Meckel's cave* or *Meckel's cavity*, close to the apex of

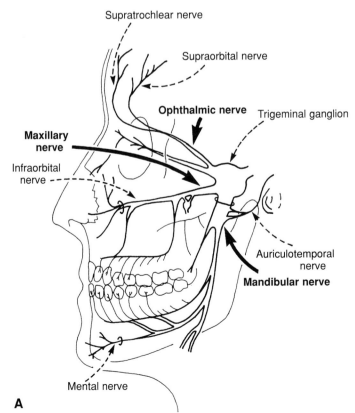

A

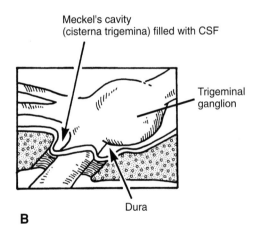

B

FIGURE 6–1

A, The figure shows the location of the trigeminal ganglion in the middle cranial fossa and the course of its three branches: (1) ophthalmic; (2) maxillary; and (3) mandibular. *B,* The relationship of the trigeminal ganglion in Meckel's cavity. CSF, cerebrospinal fluid.

the petrous part of the temporal bone (Fig. 6–1*B*). Medially, the trigeminal ganglion is bounded by the cavernous sinus; superiorly, by the inferior surface of the temporal lobe of the brain; and posteriorly, by the brain stem. Anteriorly, the ganglion gives off three branches intracranially: ophthalmic, maxillary, and mandibular. The two medial (ophthalmic and maxillary) are sensory, whereas the lateral most mandibular branch is partly motor. The trigeminal ganglion is somatotropically located. The ophthalmic branch is located dorsally, the maxillary branch is intermediate, and the mandibular branch is located ventrally.

These nerves and their branches provide the cutaneous and dermatomal innervation of the head and face as shown in Figure 6–2.

INDICATIONS

Approaches to the trigeminal ganglion by various methods aim to relieve the pain transmitted through the trigeminal nerve. In the past trigeminal ganglion block has been extensively used in the treatment of trigeminal neuralgia or tic douloureux. With the introduction of thermogangliolysis, the trigeminal ganglion block is rarely used, except for intraoperative or postoperative pain. In addition to idiopathic trigeminal neuralgia, secondary neuralgic pain due to facial pain resulting from terminal cancer or multiple sclerosis may also be treated with these approaches. These techniques are to be used

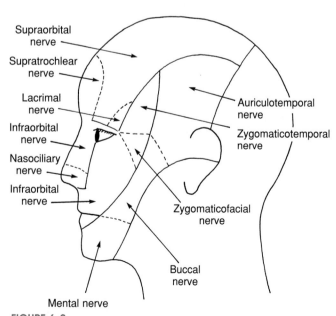

FIGURE 6–2

This drawing illustrates the innervation of the skin and the face by the peripheral branches of the trigeminal nerve.

▽ TABLE 6–1 Use of Trigeminal Ganglion Nerve Block	
Indications	**Contraindications**
Trigeminal neuralgia	Local infection
Cluster headaches	Sepsis
Intractable ocular pain	Coagulopathy
Cancer pain	
Surgical anesthesia	

only when conventional medical treatment is inadequate or causes undesirable side effects. Table 6–1 enumerates the indications and contraindications.

EQUIPMENT

Trigeminal Block
- 25-gauge needle (for skin infiltration)
- 5-mL syringe (for local anesthetic solution)
- 22-gauge, B-bevel, 8- to 10-cm needle (for injection of local anesthetic for a block)

Radiofrequency Lesioning
- RF thermocoagulation (RFTC) machine and cables
- 25-gauge needle (for skin infiltration)
- 5-mL syringe (for local anesthetic solution)
- 16-gauge intravenous catheter (for introducing the RF needle)
- RF needles—10 cm in length; 2 mm or 5 mm RF tip (depending on the branch to be lesioned)

Balloon Compression
- 25-gauge needle (for skin infiltration)
- 5-mL syringe (for local anesthetic solution)
- 2-mL syringe (for iohexol [Omnipaque] injection)
- 14-gauge, 10-mL needle (for initial insertion prior to Fogarty catheter)
- Fogarty catheter (4-French)

DRUGS

Block
- 1% lidocaine for infiltration
- 0.25% bupivacaine or 0.2% ropivacaine
- Methylprednisolone optional

Balloon Compression
- 1% lidocaine for infiltration
- Iohexol

Neurolytic Block
- Alcohol 97%—1-mL vial *or*
- Phenol in saline or glycerin 6%—1 mL *or*
- Phenol in iohexol 6% to 10%—1 mL
- Glycerol 40% to 50%—1 mL

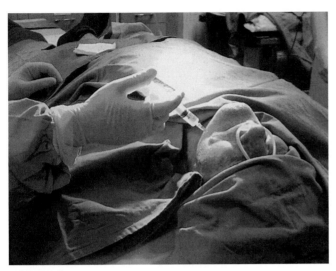

FIGURE 6–3

The needle entry point is 3 cm lateral to the corner of the mouth.

PROCEDURE

TECHNIQUE OF NEEDLE INSERTION FOR TRIGEMINAL GANGLION BLOCK

Analgesia and Sedation

Comfort should be provided to the patient during percutaneous procedures. The patient should be alert enough to respond to the testing, for example, with electrical stimulation. Generally, intravenous fentanyl, midazolam or methohexital is used. Propofol is also recommended.

Procedure

The procedure should be performed under fluoroscopic control.

The landmarks are the following:
1. The entry point is 2 to 3 cm lateral to the commissura labialis (angle of the mouth) (Fig. 6–3).
2. The needle should be directed 3 cm anterior to the external auditory meatus when seen from the side (Fig. 6–4B)
3. The needle should be directed toward the pupil when seen from the front of the face (Fig. 6–4A).

Position of the Patient

The patient is supine on the table with the head in an extended position. The C-arm is placed at the head of the table for posteroanterior (PA), lateral, and submental views. The direction of the needle is toward the pupil when one looks from the front and midpoint of the zygomatic arch when one looks from the side.

A finger may be placed inside the mouth. This helps guide the needle and prevents penetration of the oral mucosa (Fig. 6–5). There is a definite risk of meningitis if the needle enters the mucosa.

The direction of the needle should be verified under fluoroscopy in submental, lateral, and PA views (Fig. 6–6). To obtain the submental view, the C-arm of the fluoroscopy is first placed in the PA direction. In this view, the orbital line, the petrous ridge may be visualized through the orbits. The target site in this dimension is a point approximately 9 mm to 1 cm medial to the lateral rim of the internal auditory meatus. This usually coincides with the medial extent of a dip that occurs in the petrous ridge.

Then the C-arm is moved slightly lateral and oblique submentally to see the foramen ovale (Fig. 6–7). In many patients it is possible to see the foramen ovale. When the foramen ovale is seen, the needle is directed toward the foramen through the entrance point. The

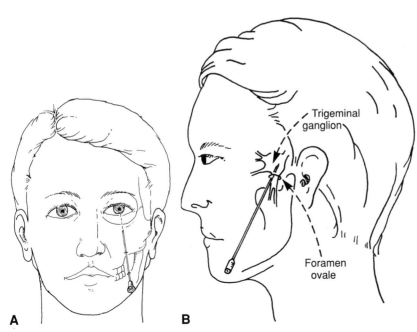

FIGURE 6–4

A, The drawing shows the needle penetration toward the pupil in the anterior view. *B*, This illustration shows the needle direction toward the external auditory meatus on the zygoma.

A   **B**

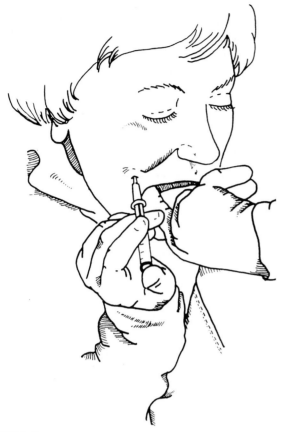

FIGURE 6–5

To prevent the needle from penetrating the cheek and the oral cavity, one can put a finger in the mouth, as the needle is advanced toward the foramen ovale.

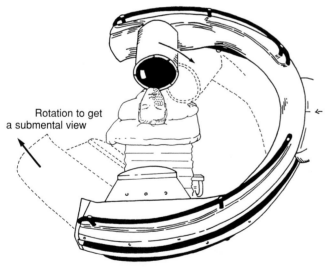

FIGURE 6–6

The fluoroscopic position to obtain the submental view of foramen ovale.

mandibular nerve is on the lateral part of the ovale, whereas the maxillary and ophthalmic divisions are more medial (Fig. 6–8).

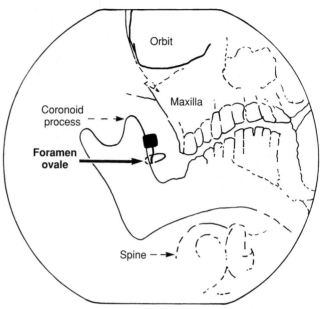

FIGURE 6–7

When the submental view is obtained, the foramen ovale is seen to appear medial to the medial edge of the mandible. Depending on the lateral rotation of the C-arm, the foramen ovale visualization can move more medially toward the maxilla.

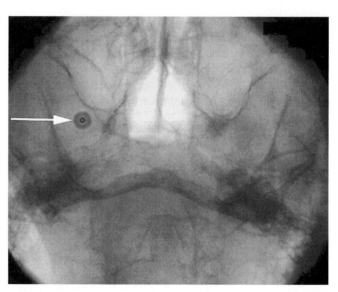

FIGURE 6–8

The submental view of the face with the needle in the foramen ovale. Note the "tunnel view" of the hub of the needle. The *arrow* indicates the rim of the foramen ovale.

When the needle enters the foramen ovale, the fluoroscope is turned laterally (Fig. 6–9). The lateral image should reveal that the needle is directed toward the direct angle produced by the clivus and the petrous ridge of the temporal bone (Figs. 6–10 to 6–12). The lateral view is important to verify the depth of the needle inside Meckel's cave. The aspiration test is mandatory. A 0.5-mL iohexol solution helps determine that the needle has not penetrated the dura.

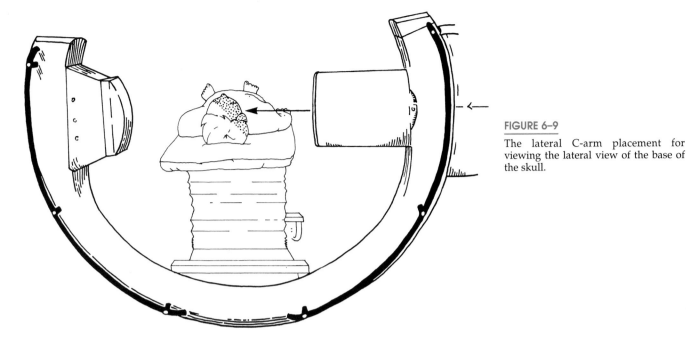

FIGURE 6–9

The lateral C-arm placement for viewing the lateral view of the base of the skull.

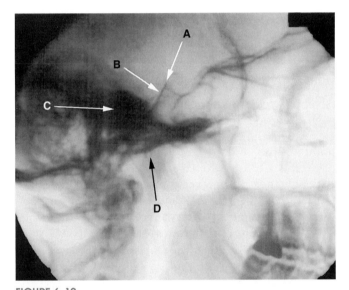

FIGURE 6–10

In the lateral view, one needs to identify the posterior clinoid process (A), the clivus (B), and the temporal bone (C) to locate the foramen ovale (D).

FIGURE 6–11

A line drawn perpendicularly (A—A) through where the intersection of the clivus and petrous part of the temporal bone meet identifies the foramen ovale at the base of the skull.

Diagnostic Block

For confirming that the pain generator is the trigeminal ganglion, after negative aspirations, up to 1 mL of local anesthetic (lidocaine, bupivacaine, or ropivacaine) is injected. The patient should have pain relief if the pain generator is present. The physician should monitor that the solution has not entered the cranial cerebrospinal fluid (CSF). The brain stem function should be evaluated to determine if the local anesthetic solution has not reached it. Brain stem function is affected if the patient complains of bilateral headache or fourth or sixth nerve palsy or if pupillary changes occur.

NEUROLYSIS OF THE TRIGEMINAL GANGLION

The amount of the neurolytic solution should not exceed 1 mL given in smaller aliquots. Otherwise, it may spread to the brain stem and cause severe complications. Phenol and alcohol have been used commonly in the past but are not recommended currently.

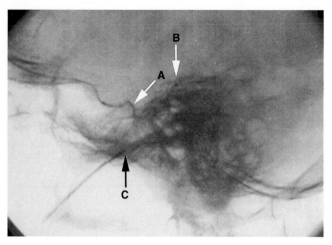

FIGURE 6–12

Another lateral view (see Fig. 6–10) of the cranium. A, clivus; B, petrous part of the temporal bone; and C, foramen ovale with needle entering it.

Technique for Glycerol Injection

After correct needle placement on the trigeminal ganglion, the patient is kept in a supine position. The needle should pierce the foramen ovale just anterior to its geometric center to place the needle into the trigeminal cistern. The needle is advanced until free flow of the CSF is observed. The patient is then placed in the semisitting position, and the neck is flexed. Contrast solution, iohexol 0.1 to 0.5 mL, is injected at this position in the cistern.

Failure of visualization or diffusion of the dye indicates a wrong placement of the needle and the needle should be repositioned. When the cistern is visualized, the contrast material is drawn back by free flow. The flow of the dye is slower than the CSF itself. The same amount of glycerol is injected in the cistern. The patient is kept at the same semisitting position for the next 2 hours.

During this injection, severe headache or dysesthesia may occur, and the patient should be warned about this result prior to the injection. Some patients may get benefit immediately, whereas some patients may experience relief within the next 2 weeks.

TECHNIQUE OF TRIGEMINAL GANGLION STIMULATION AND RADIOFREQUENCY LESIONING

Stimulation

The mandibular nerve has some motor fibers. If the nerve is stimulated at 2 Hz with 0.1 to 1.5 V, the muscle contraction of the lower mandible is observed. This is also a way of verifying that the needle is passed through the foramen ovale and is on the retrogasserian rootlets. If the first and second divisions are affected, there should be no motor response.

The second step is to seek paresthesia for proper localization. A stimulation at 50 to 100 Hz is given with 0.1 to 0.5 V. If the needle is properly located, there will be a tingling-like sensation or electric-like paresthesias in the innervation of that branch in the face. If this sensation is obtained after 0.5-V stimulation, then the needle should be redirected to get the same response at a lower voltage. However, it should be kept in mind that there might be residual sensorial deficits from a previous lesioning.

When the electrode is adjusted for localization, it should also be remembered that the gasserian ganglion and its retrogasserian rootlets lie on a plane running from a superomedial to inferolateral direction. If there is a motor response, it means that the needle is too lateral, and for a better response, it should be more medial.

After stimulation is completed, the physician should again rule out if the needle is in a vessel or not. If blood is aspirated, the needle position should be adjusted. If blood is still aspirated, the procedure should be terminated and a second attempt should be made another day. Impedance monitoring is not essential for trigeminal ganglion lesioning, but if used, it should be 150 to 350 Ω for rootlets bathing in the CSF and 1000 Ω if it is in a non-neural tissue.

Lesioning

Several types of electrodes may be used for lesioning, such as cordotomy-type electrodes and trigeminal electrodes with the Tew needle and the Racz-Finch curved-blunt needle.

If the needle is properly placed and stimulated, the patient is then ready for lesioning (Figs. 6–13 to 6–16).

First, 0.5 mL of 0.25% bupivacaine or 0.2% ropivacaine with 40 mg of triamcinolone acetate should be injected. One should wait at least for 30 seconds prior

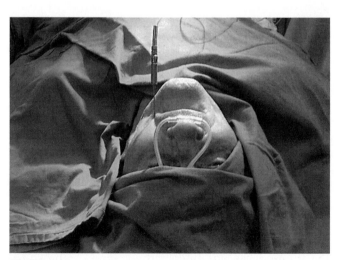

FIGURE 6–13

Radiofrequency needle entering the facial skin without a catheter. Note the draping of the patient with the area of entry exposed and an O$_2$ cannula in place for trigeminal ganglion radiofrequency.

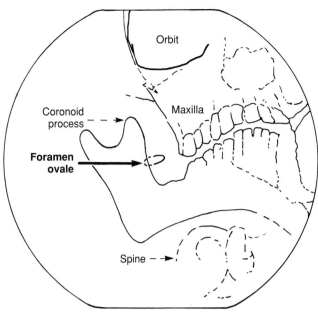

FIGURE 6–16

This drawing of the submental view of the face illustrates the relationship of the foramen ovale and the needle entry at the medial border of the mandible and maxilla. The needle entry is shown in the lateral aspect of the foramen ovale. (See Fig. 6–15.)

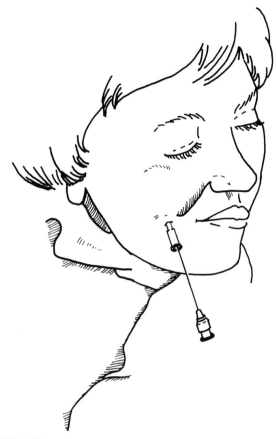

FIGURE 6–14

The alternative technique of introducing the curved-blunt Racz-Finch radiofrequency needle is shown in this drawing. Initially, an angiocatheter is introduced at the entry site toward the foramen ovale. Following that, the RF needle is inserted through the angiocatheter.

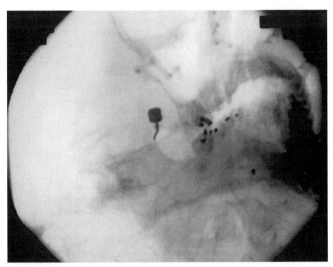

FIGURE 6–15

Submental view with a fluoroscope. Note the curved-blunt Racz-Finch radiofrequency needle entering the foramen ovale in its lateral aspect.

to RF lesioning. RF lesioning is done at 60°C for 90 seconds. If the patient cannot tolerate the lesioning, stop and wait another 30 seconds, and try again or add another 0.5 mL of local anesthetic prior to RF lesioning.

If more than one branch of the trigeminal nerve is affected, several lesions by repositioning of the needle should be performed. After each repositioning, the stimulation test should be repeated to seek paresthesia at the desired site.

For the first division lesioning, corneal reflex should be preserved at each lesion, and lesioning should begin at lesser degrees than 60°C to preserve the corneal reflex. After the lesioning is completed, the needle is removed. The patient is instructed to watch for swelling of the face and to put ice on the face to decrease any swelling that may occur.

FOLLOW-UP OF THE PATIENT AFTER RADIOFREQUENCY LESIONING

The immediate and late follow-up of the patient are important. Some authors prefer to do the lesioning on an outpatient basis, and some hospitalize the patient for a day. In some patients there is immediate pain relief, but the next day or within the first week the pain may return. In such patients, lesioning may be repeated. The patient should be monitored for an additional month to determine if side effects appear.

PERCUTANEOUS TRIGEMINAL GANGLION DECOMPRESSION

The percutaneous trigeminal ganglion decompression procedure is performed under light general anesthesia. The position of the patient is the same as it is with RF lesioning. The needle is introduced, as described earlier,

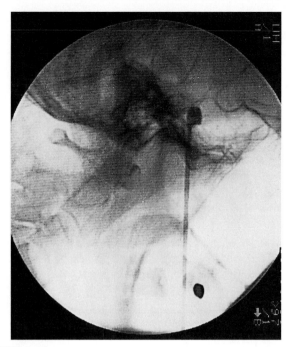

FIGURE 6–17

The lateral view of the balloon during trigeminal ganglion neurolysis.

through the foramen ovale. A 4-French Fogarty catheter is advanced through the needle to Meckel's cavity. The balloon of the catheter is advanced by injecting contrast solution. The shape of the balloon inside the cavity in the lateral position resembles a pear (Fig. 6–17). The inflated balloon is left there for 60 seconds or more, although there is no agreement on the duration.

The procedure should be done with vital sign monitoring because bradycardia and hypertension may be observed.

Complications of Balloon Lesioning

Significant masseter weakness is a common complication, especially in the initial period. This weakness generally disappears within the first 3 months. Hypesthesia, dysesthesia, anesthesia dolorosa, balloon failure, and hematoma on the cheek may also be observed (Table 6–2).

▽ TABLE 6–2 Complications of Trigeminal Ganglion Block or Neurolysis

- Annoying dysesthesia and anesthesia dolorosa, loss of corneal reflex
- Neurolytic keratitis
- Visual loss
- Retrobulbar hematoma
- Hematoma in the cheek
- Significant motor root deficit
- Carotid puncture
- Meningitis
- Inadvertent intracranial placement of the electrode resulting in intracranial hemorrhaging, penetration through the wrong foramen causing defects in the other cranial nerves

TRIAL STIMULATION

In the rare instance in patients with atypical facial pain, trial stimulation may relieve the pain. This trial can be done with a Stim catheter.[5]

PERMANENT ELECTRODE PLACEMENT

Following a successful trial, a compressed-quad electrode with an active soft tip can be steered to the appropriate segment of atypical facial pain (Figs. 6–18 and 6–19). The needle used for placing the soft-tip compressed-quad electrode is a curved-tipped Pyle's needle (Medtronic, Inc., Minneapolis, MN). Once the needle is at the foramen ovale, the electrode is passed through the foramen ovale using a curved stylet and lateral fluoroscopic visualization as well as sensory stimulation. When the approximate area is reached, the patient verifies that the stimulation covers the involved division of the trigeminal nerve. The technique calls for close cooperation between the anesthesiologist, who provides brief periods of intravenous sedation, and the interventionalist. The anchoring of the electrode is important (Figs. 6–20 to 6–23). We use a team of an

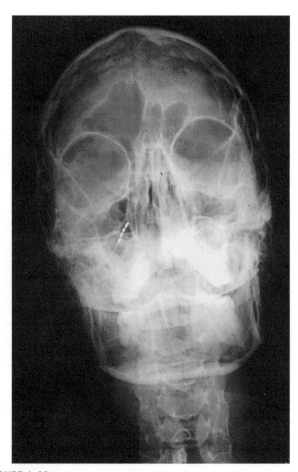

FIGURE 6–18

Anteroposterior view of the electrode in place.

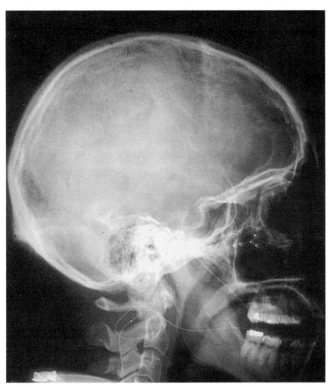

FIGURE 6–19

Lateral view of the electrode in place.

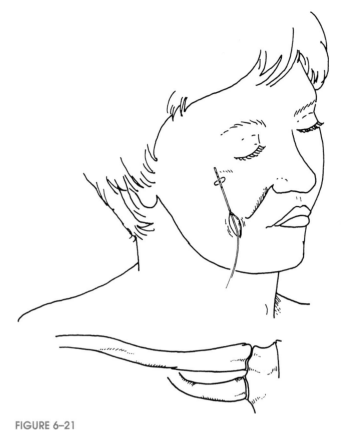

FIGURE 6–21

Step 2. Making the incision at the skin entry site. The needle is then removed, and the electrode interventionalist is anchored at this site.

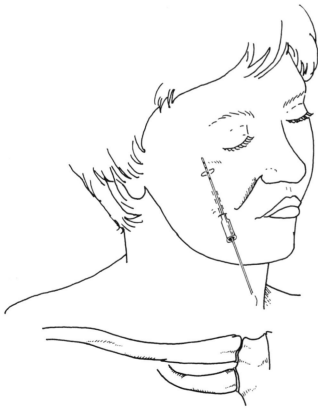

FIGURE 6–20

Step 1. Permanently placing the compact-quad electrode on the trigeminal ganglion.

interventionalist and a plastic surgeon, in which the plastic surgeon anchors the electrode to the cheek, subcutaneously 2 cm above the angle of the mandible and approximately 2 cm posteriorly; the second anchoring is then carried out, followed by a subcutaneous loop posterior to the mandibular ramus of the electrode to prevent pulling of the electrode during movement of the head during mastication.[6]

After tunneling and anchoring as described, the implantable pulse generator is placed in a pocket in the front of the chest or posteriorly in the back.

COMPLICATIONS

Percutaneous interventions of the trigeminal ganglion are not free of complications. In selected series, Taha and Tew compared the results and complications of percutaneous techniques. The total number of patients was 6205 for RF rhizotomy, 1217 for glycerol rhizotomy, and 759 for balloon compression.[7] Facial numbness occurred in 98% of the patients after RF rhizotomy, in 72% after balloon compression, and in 60% after glycerol injection. Taha and Tew, in their series, found that anesthesia dolorosa occurred in 1.5%, 1.8%, and 0.1%, respectively.[7] Anesthesia dolorosa occurred at a rate of 0.3% to 4% in RF lesioning.[8–10] For glycerol injection, anesthesia

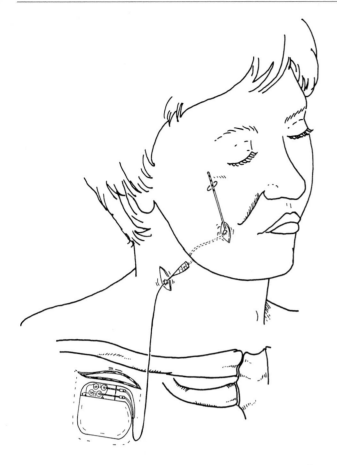

Inset in face

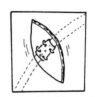

Inset in neck

FIGURE 6–22

Step 3. Anchoring the electrode (after the needle is removed) first in the face and second in the neck. A packet is also created below the clavicle subcutaneously to place the implantable pulse generator.

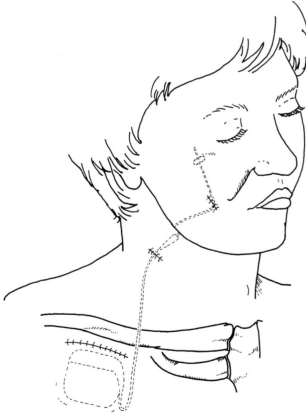

FIGURE 6–23

Step 4. Final subcutaneous positioning of the electrode and its extension connected to the implantable pulse generator sitting in the pocket.

dolorosa occurs in 0% to 2% of cases.[11–15] For balloon compression, ipsilateral masticatory weakness, hypoesthesia, dysesthesia, and anesthesia dolorosa may occur in 3% to 5% of the cases.[16–18]

LOSS OF CORNEAL REFLEX

The overall incidence of corneal reflex loss of neurolytic keratitis is 0.6% to 1.8%, depending on the technique used. Corneal anesthesia was the highest for RF rhizotomy at 7%; it was less for glycerol at 3.7% and 1.5% for balloon compression. It is zero for balloon compression and the highest for RF lesioning. This is not a desirable condition, but in some patients, because of the intolerable pain, it may be preferred.[7]

MOTOR DEFICIT

Motor deficit occurs during the lesioning of the third branch, the mandibular nerve. The incidence is the highest, 66%, with balloon compression. For RF rhizotomy it is 24%, and for glycerol injection it is 1.7%. The motor deficit improves within 1 year.

CAROTID ARTERY PUNCTURE

Carotid artery puncture occurs when the radiographic landmarks are not employed and the needle is too inferior and medial. Blunt technique is not recommended.

RETROBULBAR HEMATOMA AND HEMATOMA IN THE CHEEK

If the needle is advanced to the retrobulbar space, retrobulbar hematoma may develop. This is a dramatic complication to the patient, although it is relieved by conservative methods without any sequelae. The eyeball is pushed from the retrobulbar space and exophthalmus develops. Compression over the eye stops the bleeding, and the swelling subsides during the following days. Hematoma in the cheek may develop if the needle passes through a vessel while it is introduced. Compression over the cheek by cold pack after the needle is withdrawn may be helpful.

INFECTION

One of the main concerns is infection and the incidence of infection. In the series by Sweet, there were 24 cases of meningitis in 7000 cases. One of these patients died.[19] Ocular motor paralysis and cavernous sinus fistula[20] is a possibility. An intracranial hemorrhage[21] has been reported to be fatal. Misplacement of needles into incorrect skull base foramina can lead to vascular damage and secondary hypertension that, in turn, can lead to bleeding.[22] The most common problem from neurodestructive procedures is altered sensation or numbness that has been reported to range from 6% to 26% of patients undergoing RF-type procedures.

HELPFUL HINTS

With edentulous patients, the needle's point of introduction sometimes needs to be a little more posterior than for the patients with a full set of teeth; the needle will strike the foramen ovale at too acute an angle. This may be prevented if the procedure is done under fluoroscopy.

Because this is an uncomfortable procedure, some form of intravenous sedation such as fentanyl given immediately before the procedure often affords satisfactory analgesia for the procedure without obtunding the patient's ability to cooperate and provide necessary feedback.

The placement of the needle should be confirmed by the lateral view. In case of deep needle placement, one can enter the brain stem and cause hemorrhage.

The aspiration test is mandatory because the posterior part of the trigeminal ganglion is surrounded by an invagination of cranial dura mater containing CSF in Meckel's cavity. Inadvertent injection of therapeutic agents into this cul-de-sac can spread to other intracranial structures, producing profound and rapid loss of consciousness and collapse. This is obviously an emi-

nently reversible situation when local anesthetic agents are used, but in the event that such a catastrophe occurred with neurolytic agents, inadvertent neurolysis of adjacent cranial nerves could occur.

Irritation of the dura may cause persistent headache; in some patients, nausea and vomiting lasting for days may also be observed. If blood is aspirated, the needle should be replaced, and if bleeding continues, the procedure should be stopped.

During repeated lesioning if RFTC is applied, the aspiration test should be repeated and impedance should be monitored to verify the position of the needle. If the needle is in the nerve, the impedance is generally between 300 and 450 Ω.

To prevent hematoma in the cheek, ice compression after the needle is withdrawn should be done in every instance. Hemifacial numbness that develops after chemical neurolysis or extensive RF lesioning, especially if three branches of the trigeminal nerve are involved, is a distressing experience for patients.

Because of the subsequent analgesia of the conjunctiva, the eye must be protected from chronic inflammatory processes that would go undetected because of the altered sensation. Therefore, it is usually necessary to approximate the upper and lower eyelids surgically to reduce the area of conjunctiva exposed to dust and other environmental sources of contamination. Protective spectacles with side shields can also help reduce the introduction of foreign bodies into the numb eye.

Another difficulty with long-term hemifacial analgesia is saliva dribbling from the anesthetized half of the mouth; this can sometimes be alleviated by an antisialagogue such as diphenhydramine, 25 mg tid.

EFFICACY

The three most popular techniques are RF rhizotomy, retrogasserian glycerol injection, and percutaneous compression of the gasserian ganglion. All the techniques have several advantages and several disadvantages. The advantages of RF lesioning are a high pain relief rate, a low relapse rate, and a high degree of effectiveness.

There is a light sensory deficit after retrogasserian glycerol injection. Shorter duration of pain relief, higher recurrence rates, and development of fibrosis at the foramen ovale are the main disadvantages. Slight sensory deficit and moderate rate of recurrence may be the advantages of gasserian ganglion compression. However, it cannot be connected to a single branch, and the gauge of the needle entering the foramen ovale is larger than the ones used in previous methods, which may damage the nerve.

TECHNICAL SUCCESS

The technical success rate varies between 97.4% and 100% for RF lesioning at the initial phase. This success rate is 94% for glycerol and 99% for balloon compression. In another study, technical failure for glycerol was reported to be as high as 15%.[9, 14] However, there is no general agreement on these results.

INITIAL PAIN RELIEF

Initial pain relief had the highest success rate, with RF lesioning at 98%. For glycerol rhizotomy, it varied between 72% and 96%.[10] Balloon compression relieved pain in 89.9% to 100%.

PAIN RECURRENCE

To evaluate pain recurrence is not easy because of the heterogeneity of the follow-up reported. The highest rate of recurrence is 54% for glycerol rhizotomy, with a mean follow-up of 4 years.[10] In several series, this result varied.

Retrogasserian glycerol injection is also an effective method, but the initial pain relief and duration of pain relief are less than RF lesioning. It may easily be applied when RF facilities are absent. Partial sensorial loss may also develop with this technique. Fibrosis may develop at the entrance of foramen ovale, enhancing further injections.

Percutaneous balloon compression causes mild sensory loss in most cases. However, it is not possible to restrict compression to a single division. It is not as commonly used as other techniques.

All these techniques are less morbid and more cost effective than open surgical techniques. However, each technique must be applied in precise indications and in well-equipped centers with experienced hands.

Trigeminal nerve 64400; RFTC trigeminal 64600.

CONCLUSION

Procedures involving the trigeminal ganglion and its branches are occasionally carried out to facilitate acute facial pain relief during surgery. However, much more frequently the indications are chronic debilitating, painful conditions. Clearly, the use of fluoroscopy and additional training lead to better outcome and reduction of potentially devastating complications. All three percutaneous techniques may be used to block the trigeminal nerve in the treatment of neuralgic pain of the face. There are advantages and disadvantages of each of the techniques.

REFERENCES

1. Hartel F: Die Leitungsanesthesie und Injektionsbehandlung des Ganglion Gasseri und der Trigeminusaste. Arch Klin Chir 100:193–292, 1912.
2. Sweet WH, Wepsic JG: Controlled thermocoagulation of trigeminal ganglion and rootlets for differential destruction of pain fibers: I. Trigeminal neuralgia. J Neurosurg 40:43, 1974.
3. Hakanson S: Trigeminal neuralgia treated by the injection of glycerol into the trigeminal cistern. Neurosurgery 9:638–646, 1981.
4. Mullan S, Lichtor T: Percutaneous microcompression of the trigeminal ganglion for trigeminal neuralgia. J Neurosurg 59:1007–1012, 1983.
5. Tasker R: Percutaneous retrogasserian glycerol rhizotomy: Predictors of success and failure in the treatment of trigeminal neuralgia. J Neurosurg 72:851–856, 1990.
6. Steude U: Chronic trigeminal nerve stimulation for the relief of persistent pain. In Gildenberg PL, Tasker RR (eds): Textbook of Stereotactic and Functional Neurosurgery. New York, McGraw-Hill, 1998, pp 1557–1567.
7. Taha JM, Tew JM: Comparison of surgical treatments for trigeminal neuralgia: Reevaluation of radiofrequency rhizotomy. Neurosurgery 38:865–871, 1966.
8. Broggi G, Franzini A, Lasio G, et al: Long-term results of percutaneous retrogasserian thermorhizotomy for "essential" trigeminal neuralgia. Neurosurgery 26:783–787, 1990.
9. Burchiel K, Steege T, Howe J, Loeser J: Comparison of percutaneous radiofrequency gangliolysis and microvascular decompression for the surgical management of tic douloureux. Neurosurgery 9:111–119, 1981.
10. Fraoili B, Esposito V, Guidetti B, et al: Treatment of trigeminal neuralgia by thermocoagulation, glycerolization, and percutaneous compression of gasserian ganglion and/or retrogasserian rootlets: Long-term results and therapeutic protocol. Neurosurgery 24:239–245, 1989.
11. Fujimaki T, Fukushima T, Miyazaki S: Percutaneous retrogasserian glycerol injection in the management of trigeminal neuralgia: Long-term follow-up results. J Neurosurg 73:212–216, 1990.
12. Burchiel K: Percutaneous retrogasserian glycerol rhizolysis in the management of trigeminal neuralgia. J Neurosurg 69:361–366, 1988.
13. Wilkinson H: Trigeminal nerve peripheral branch phenol/glycerol injections for tic douloureux. J Neurosurg 90:828–832, 1999.
14. North RB, Kidd DH, Piantadosi S, Carson BS: Percutaneous retrogasserian glycerol rhizotomy: Predictors of success and failure in treatment of trigeminal neuralgia. J Neurosurg 72:851–856, 1990.
15. Sweet WH, Poletti CE, Macon JB: Treatment of trigeminal neuralgia and other facial pains by retrogasserian injection of glycerol. Neurosurgery 9:647–654, 1981.
16. Lobato RD, Rivas JJ, Rosario S, Lamas E: Percutaneous microcompression of the gasserian ganglion for trigeminal neuralgia. J Neurosurg 72:546–553, 1990.
17. Belber CJ, Rak RA: Balloon compression rhizolysis in the surgical management of trigeminal neuralgia. Neurosurgery 20:908–913, 1987.
18. Brown JA, McDaniel M, Weaver MT: Percutaneous trigeminal nerve compression for treatment of trigeminal neuralgia: Results in 50 patients. Neurosurgery 32:570–573, 1993.
19. Sweet WH: Complications of treating trigeminal neuralgia: An analysis of the literature and response to questionnaire. In Rovit RL, Murali R, Jannetta PJ (eds): Trigeminal Neuralgia. Baltimore, Williams & Wilkins, 1990, pp 251–279.
20. Sekhar LN, Heros RG, Kerber CW: Carotid-cavernous fistula following retrogasserian procedures. J Neurosurg 51:700–706, 1979.
21. Rish BL: Cerebrovascular accident after percutaneous radiofrequency thermocoagulation of the trigeminal ganglion. J Neurosurg 44:376–377, 1976.
22. Sweet WH, Poletti CE, Roberts JT: Dangerous rises in blood pressure upon heating of trigeminal rootlets: Increased bleeding time in patients with trigeminal neuralgia. Neurosurgery 17:843–844, 1985.

C H A P T E R

7

Maxillary Nerve Block

HISTORY

There are four different approaches to the maxillary nerve. Of these approaches, an oral approach is commonly used by dentists. An orbital approach described originally by Rudolph Matas involves inserting a needle through the orbital cavity and exiting the infraorbital fissure.[1] Schlosser[2] described an anterolateral approach with skin entry anterior to the coronoid process of the mandible and inferior to the zygomatic arch. The more commonly used lateral approach by Levy and Baudoin[3] is described in this chapter. With the two lateral approaches, the sphenopalatine ganglion is commonly blocked with the maxillary nerve.

ANATOMY

The main part of the maxillary nerve, which constitutes the second division of the trigeminal nerve, can be anesthetized in the pterygopalatine fossa. Its branches can be anesthetized at the posterior and lateral borders of the maxilla, and its terminal branch can be anesthetized as it emerges through the infraorbital foramen on the front of the face 1 cm below the orbital margin in the same vertical plane as the pupil (Fig. 7–1).

The maxillary nerve is a purely sensory nerve that begins at the gasserian ganglion and travels anteriorly and inferiorly along the cavernous sinus through the foramen rotundum. It extends to the superior aspect of the pterygopalatine fossa along the inferior portion of the orbit in the infraorbital fissure and exits through the infraorbital foramen. The 10 branches of the maxillary nerve supply sensation to the dura, upper jaw, teeth, gums, hard and soft palates, and cheek as well as parasympathetic fibers. The maxillary artery and five terminal branches are also contained with the ptery-

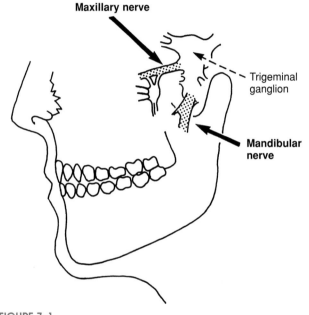

FIGURE 7–1
Maxillary nerve anatomy.

gopalatine fossa. Also within this space are emissary veins from the orbit.

INDICATIONS

The maxillary nerve block is usually performed for regional analgesia of the upper jaw and can be used for acute intraoperative pain during maxillofacial surgery. It provides excellent postoperative pain relief for such surgical maneuvers, and it is also used to treat chronic pain, most frequently for diagnostic and therapeutic blocks involving painful tumors of the maxillary antrum that are unresponsive to more conventional methods.

49

CONTRAINDICATIONS

Absolute
- Local infection
- Coagulopathies

Relative
- Altered anatomy

EQUIPMENT

Nerve Block
- 25-gauge, ¾-inch needle
- 22-gauge, 3½-inch spinal needle
- 3-mL syringe
- 5-mL syringe
- IV T-piece extension

Neurolytic Block/Pulse Electrode Magnetic Field
- 16-gauge, 1½-inch angiocatheter
- 10-cm curved radiofrequency thermocoagulation needle with 5-mm active tip

DRUGS

Block
- 1.5% lidocaine for skin infiltration
- 2% lidocaine
- 0.5% bupivacaine/ropivacaine
- Steroids (optional)

Neurolytics
- 6% phenol with or without contrast agent

- 40% to 50% glycerol with or without contrast agent

PREPARATION OF THE PATIENT

For preoperative medication, use the standard American Society of Anesthesiologists' recommendations for conscious sedation.

PROCEDURE

POSITION OF THE PATIENT

The patient is placed supine with the head straight (Fig. 7–2).

TECHNIQUE

The mandibular notch is identified, which is most easily done by having the patient open and close the mouth. A 22-gauge, 7.5- to 8-cm needle is then placed perpendicular to the skin at the posterior and inferior aspects of the notch, which should be close to the middle of the zygoma (Fig. 7–3). The needle is advanced until it encounters the lateral pterygoid plate (4 to 5 cm). The needle is then withdrawn and redirected anteriorly and superiorly at about a 45-degree angle toward the upper root of the nose. The needle is again advanced with the pterygopalatine fossa until a paresthesia is obtained. It is important to obtain a paresthesia or else the block will have a high rate of failure. To minimize a cerebrospinal fluid (CSF) injection, the needle should not be advanced

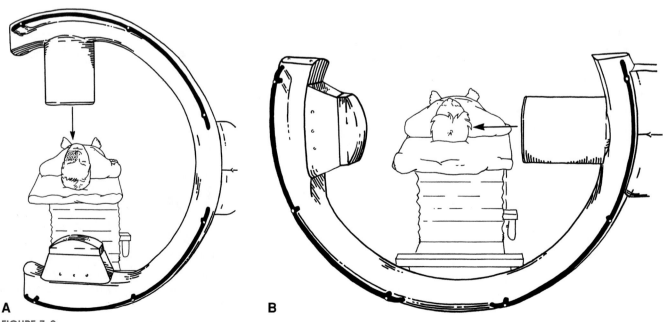

A   **B**

FIGURE 7–2

The patient is supine with the C-arm positioned for the AP view (*A*) and lateral view (*B*).

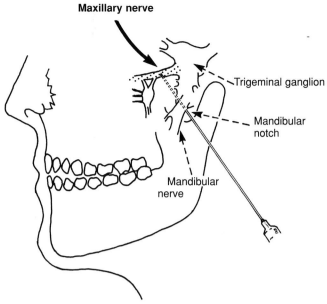

Maxillary nerve

Trigeminal ganglion

Mandibular notch

Mandibular nerve

FIGURE 7–3

A patient with the needle on the maxillary nerve entering through the mandibular notch.

farther than 1.5 cm past the lateral pterygoid plate (see Fig. 7–3).

From 3 to 5 mL of local anesthetic is injected, although some authors advocate the use of as much as 10 mL. Neurolytic procedures can be done with 6% phenol or absolute alcohol. A maximum volume of 1 to 1.5 mL delivered in 0.1-mL divided doses is recommended.

Final Injection of Test Solution or Technique of Neurolysis

Local Anesthetic Nerve Block
- Diagnostic—1 to 3 mL
- Therapeutic—3 to 5 mL

Neurolytic
- 6% phenol—1 to 1.5 mL after negative aspiration
- 40% to 50% glycerol—1 to 1.5 mL after negative aspiration (Fig. 7–4)

Pulsed Electrode Magnetic Field

Placement of the radiofrequency (RF) needle is the same as described previously (Fig. 7–4). Confirmation of proper needle placement is with sensory stimulation (50 Hz, 0.3 to 0.6 V) and motor stimulation (2 Hz, 0.6 to 1.2 V). Once satisfactory placement is obtained, pulsed electrode magnetic field technique for 120 to 180 seconds at 42°C for two cycles is performed. A local anesthetic does not need to be injected prior to removal of the needle.

COMPLICATIONS

It is essential that the needle be introduced in a horizontal fashion, and it certainly should not enter the pterygomaxillary fissure in a cephalad direction or advance too deeply, because anesthetic injections here are rapidly spread to the posterior aspect of the orbit and the optic nerve, producing temporary blindness with reversible agents or, more seriously, permanent blindness with neurolytic agents. Because of the exceedingly vascular nature of the compartment in which the maxillary nerve lies (the pterygomaxillary fissure is a veritable network of small vessels), intravascular injection is quite possible, and meticulous aspiration tests are essential.

HELPFUL HINTS

Injection into the CSF with the complication noted previously can occur. Careful aspiration can help prevent

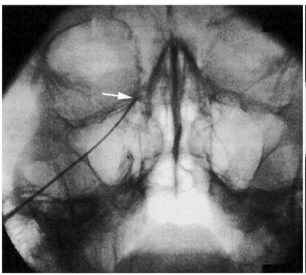

A

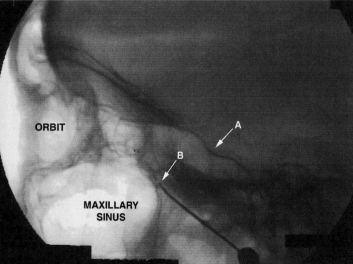

ORBIT

A

B

MAXILLARY SINUS

B

FIGURE 7–4

A, The needle is in the pterygopalatine fossa *(arrow)*. *B*, Confirmation of the needle in the lateral view.

vascular and subarachnoid injection. The close proximity of the orbit to this nerve makes it likely to be involved in a complication. Orbital swelling, anesthesia of the orbital tissues, ophthalmoplegia, loss of visual acuity, or diplopia can occur if the local anesthetic or neurolytic solution enters the infraorbital fissure. Damage to vascular structures can cause hemorrhage into the orbit, and blindness can occur.

Because the maxillary nerve injection site is quite vascular, hematoma formation is common. An intravascular injection can also occur despite negative aspiration if the maxillary or mandibular artery or vein is injured during the performance of the block. Aspiration of air usually indicates that the needle has been placed too far posteriorly and the pharynx has been entered. If this occurs, it is prudent to change the needle before proceeding.

Other peripheral nerve/myoneurals 64450.

EFFICACY

On an individual patient basis, maxillary nerve block has been helpful in managing maxillary facial pain, but no reliable data can be found for efficacy.

FURTHER READINGS

Bonica JJ (ed): The Management of Pain, 2nd ed. Philadelphia, Lea & Febiger, 1990.

Cousins MJ, Bridenbaugh PO (eds): Neural Blockade in Clinical Anesthesia and Management of Pain, 3rd ed. Philadelphia, Lippincott Williams & Wilkins, 1998.

Raj PP (ed): Practical Management of Pain, 3rd ed. St. Louis, Mosby, 2000.

REFERENCES

1. Allen CW: Local and Regional Anesthesia. Philadelphia, WB Saunders, 1915.
2. Schlosser H: Erfahrungen in der Neuralgiebehandlung mit Alkoholeinspritungen: Verhandl. D Cong Finnere Med 24:49, 1907.
3. Levy F, Baudoin A: Les Injections Profondes dans le Traitement de la Neuralgie. Presse Med 13:108, 1906.

Mandibular Nerve Block

HISTORY

Mandibular nerve blocks were performed after the trigeminal ganglion block was described (see Chapter 6). There is no other specific history on this block.

ANATOMY

The mandibular nerve is the third and only mixed division of the trigeminal ganglion, being formed by the union of a large sensory root and a small motor root (Fig. 8–1). The former arises from the anterolateral

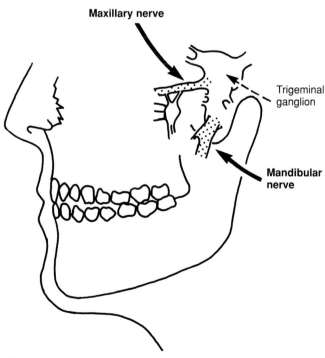

Maxillary nerve

Trigeminal ganglion

Mandibular nerve

FIGURE 8–1

The drawing shows the anatomic location of the trigeminal ganglion and its mandibular and maxillary branches (lateral view).

portion of the gasserian ganglion, whereas the latter is the same motor nerve mentioned in connection with the trigeminal ganglion (see Chapter 6), which arises from the pons and passes beneath the gasserian ganglion to reach the foramen ovale, through which, together with the sensory root, it leaves the cranial cavity. Within or immediately outside the foramen, the two roots fuse into a single trunk. The formed nerve then progresses anteriorly and inferiorly deep in the infratemporal fossa just anterior to the middle meningeal artery, lateral to the otic ganglion and internal pterygoid muscle, and medial to the external pterygoid, the masseter and the temporal muscles, and the ramus of the mandible.

Soon after it is formed, the mandibular nerve gives off two small branches: the nervus spinosus, which enters the cranial cavity with the middle meningeal artery to supply the dura, and the nerve to the internal pterygoid muscle. It then divides into a small anterior and large posterior trunk. The small anterior trunk, which is composed mostly of motor fibers, then promptly divides into the masseteric, the anterior and posterior deep temporal, and the external pterygoid nerves that supply the muscles of mastication and also gives off a small sensory branch, the buccinator, which supplies the mucous membrane and skin over this muscle. The large posterior trunk, on the other hand, is composed mostly of sensory fibers; after a short course it also divides into the auriculotemporal, the lingual, and inferior alveolar nerves. The auriculotemporal nerve arises from the posterior aspect of this trunk and immediately runs posterolaterally beneath the external pterygoid muscle to reach the medial side of the neck of the mandible, where it turns sharply cephalad to ascend between the anterior border of the auricle and the condyle of the mandible under cover of the parotid gland, finally reaching the subcutaneous tissue overlying the zygomatic arch, where it divides into the anterior auricular, the external meatal, articular, parotid, and superficial temporal branches. The lingual and inferior alveolar nerves proceed in an inferolateral direction to reach the medial side of the ramus of the mandible and to be distributed to the anterior two thirds of the tongue and inferior jaw, respectively.

INDICATIONS

The mandibular nerve block is excellent for intraoperative or postoperative pain control after surgical reduction of a fractured mandible. It is also useful for chronic pain states, such as carcinoma of the tongue, lower jaw, or floor of the mouth.

CONTRAINDICATIONS

Absolute
- Local infection
- Coagulopathies

Relative
- Distorted normal anatomy

EQUIPMENT

Nerve Block
- 22-gauge, 3½-inch spinal needle
- 25-gauge, ¾-inch infiltration needle
- 3-mL syringe
- 5-mL syringe
- IV T-piece extension

Pulsed Electrode Magnetic Field
- 10-cm Racz-Finch radiofrequency thermocoagulation (RFTC) needle
- 5-cm RFTC needle may be acceptable
- 16-gauge, 1¼-inch angiocatheter

DRUGS

Nerve Block
- 1.5% lidocaine for skin infiltration
- 0.5% bupivacaine/ropivacaine
- 2% lidocaine
- Steroids (optional)
- Iohexol (Omnipaque 240) contrast medium

Neurolytics
- 6% phenol
- Absolute alcohol
- 50% glycerol

PREPARATION OF THE PATIENT

PHYSICAL EXAMINATION

Examine for anatomic anomalies and local infections that may interfere with performance of the block. Also confirm that the jaw can be opened and closed.

PREOPERATIVE MEDICATION

For preoperative medication, use the standard American Society of Anesthesiologists' recommendations for conscious sedation.

PROCEDURE

POSITION OF THE PATIENT

The patient is placed supine on the table, and the C-arm is placed in an anteroposterior and lateral position at the mandibular notch level (Fig. 8–2).

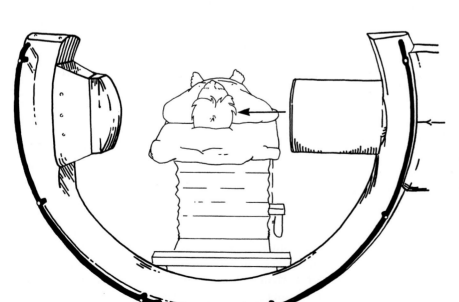

FIGURE 8–2

The position of the patient and C-arm for an external approach to a mandibular nerve block (lateral view).

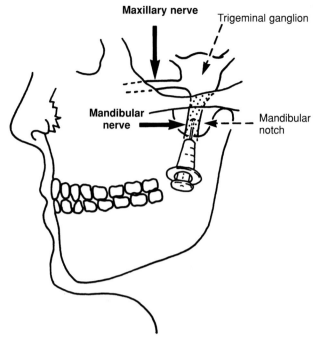

FIGURE 8–3

Point of needle entry in the mandibular notch for extraoral mandibular nerve block.

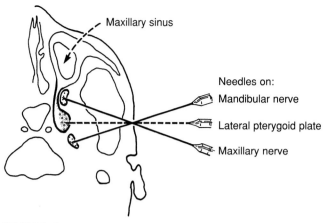

FIGURE 8–4

Transverse section of the head and face at the level of the mandibular notch showing needle placement on the mandibular nerve, on the lateral pterygoid plate, and on the maxillary nerve. After the pterygoid plate is touched, the needle is slightly withdrawn and pushed posterior until it slips off the pterygoid plate.

TECHNIQUE

The approach for blocking this nerve is identical to that for blocking the maxillary nerve, that is, the needle is introduced through the mandibular notch of the mandible and advanced through the infratemporal fossa, with the lateral pterygoid plate serving as a bony end point (Figs. 8–3 and 8–4). However, in this instance, the needle is walked backward off the lateral pterygoid plate, maintaining the same depth as the plate until paresthesia of the lower lip, lower jaw, or ipsilateral tongue or ear is obtained.

For best results, paresthesia should be elicited before 2 to 4 mL of anesthetic solution is injected.

COMPLICATIONS

Mandibular nerve block is a relatively straightforward block, associated with a high degree of success. However, there is always the risk of complications. As the needle is walked posteriorly off the lateral pterygoid plate, it comes to lie on the superior constrictor muscle of the pharynx, which is attached to the border of the lateral pterygoid plate. If the needle is advanced deeper at this stage, it can enter the pharynx. A very close pos-

terolateral relation of the mandibular nerve at this site is the middle meningeal artery, which enters the cranial cavity through the spinous foramen, thus making meticulous aspiration tests necessary.

Hemorrhage in the cheek often occurs during and following block by the anterolateral extraoral route.

HELPFUL HINTS

It should never be necessary to advance the needle more than 5.5 cm beyond the skin. If paresthesia is not obtained at this depth, the needle should be withdrawn and the landmarks reconsidered before it is again introduced.

EFFICACY

No efficacy studies are available. The efficacy is determined by the patient's successful pain relief from the nerve block.

Other peripheral nerve/myoneurals 64450.

FURTHER READINGS

Katz J: Somatic nerve blocks: Head and neck. In Raj PP (ed): Practical Management of Pain, 2nd ed. St. Louis, Mosby–Year Book, 1992, pp 718–719.

Romanoff M: Somatic nerve blocks of the head and neck. In Raj PP (ed): Practical Management of Pain, 3rd ed. St. Louis, Mosby, 2000, pp 579–596.

CHAPTER 9

Glossopharyngeal Nerve Block

HISTORY

The early use of glossopharyngeal nerve block in pain management centered around two applications: (1) the treatment of glossopharyngeal neuralgia and (2) the palliation of pain secondary to head and neck malignancies. In the late 1950s, the clinical use of the glossopharyngeal nerve block as an adjunct to awake endotracheal intubation was documented.

Weisenburg first described pain in the distribution of the glossopharyngeal nerve in a patient with a cerebellopontine angle tumor in 1910.[1] In 1921, Harris reported the first idiopathic case and coined the term *glossopharyngeal neuralgia*.[2] He suggested that blockade of the glossopharyngeal nerve might be useful in palliating this painful condition.

Early attempts at permanent treatment of glossopharyngeal neuralgia and cancer pain in the distribution of the glossopharyngeal nerve consisted principally of extracranial surgical section or alcohol neurolysis of the glossopharyngeal nerve.[3] These approaches met with limited success in the treatment of glossopharyngeal neuralgia but were useful in some patients suffering from cancer pain mediated by the glossopharyngeal nerve. Intracranial section of the glossopharyngeal nerve was first performed by Adson in 1925 and was subsequently refined by Dandy. The intracranial approach to section of the glossopharyngeal nerve appeared to yield better results for both glossopharyngeal neuralgia and cancer pain but was a much riskier procedure.[4] Recently, interest in extracranial destruction of the glossopharyngeal nerve by glycerol or by creation of a radiofrequency lesion has been renewed.

ANATOMY

The glossopharyngeal nerve contains both motor and sensory fibers.[5] The motor fibers innervate the stylopharyngeus muscle. The sensory portion of the nerve innervates the posterior third of the tongue, the palatine tonsil, and the mucous membranes of the mouth and pharynx. Special visceral afferent sensory fibers transmit information from the taste buds of the posterior third of the tongue. Information from the carotid sinus and body, which help control blood pressure, pulse, and respiration, are carried via the carotid sinus nerve, a branch of the glossopharyngeal nerve.[5] Parasympathetic fibers pass via the glossopharyngeal nerve to the otic ganglion. Postganglionic fibers from the ganglion carry secretory information to the parotid gland (Fig. 9–1).[6]

The glossopharyngeal nerve exits the jugular foramen near the vagus and accessory nerves and the internal jugular vein.[7] All three nerves lie in the groove between the internal jugular vein and internal carotid artery. Inadvertent puncture of either vessel during

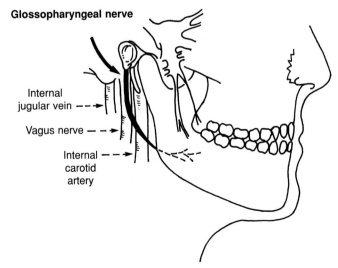

Glossopharyngeal nerve

Internal jugular vein

Vagus nerve

Internal carotid artery

FIGURE 9–1

The anatomy of the glossopharyngeal nerve as it exits the jugular vein area. Note the close relationship of the vagus nerve.

glossopharyngeal nerve block can result in intravascular injection or hematoma formation. Even small amounts of local anesthetic injected into the carotid artery at this site can produce profound local anesthetic toxicity.[8]

One landmark for glossopharyngeal nerve block is the styloid process of the temporal bone. This structure is the calcification of the cephalad end of the stylohyoid ligament. Although usually easy to identify, when ossification is limited, it may be difficult to locate with the exploring needle.

INDICATIONS

Indications for glossopharyngeal nerve block are summarized in Table 9–1. In addition to application for surgical anesthesia, glossopharyngeal nerve block with local anesthetics can be used as a diagnostic tool when performing differential neural blockade on an anatomic basis in the evaluation of head and facial pain.[9] Glossopharyngeal nerve block is used to help differentiate geniculate ganglion neuralgia from glossopharyngeal neuralgia. If destruction of glossopharyngeal nerve is being considered, this technique is useful as an indicator of the extent of motor and sensory impairment that the patient will likely experience.[10] Glossopharyngeal nerve block with local anesthetic may be used to palliate acute pain emergencies, including glossopharyngeal neuralgia and cancer pain until pharmacologic, surgical, and antiblastic methods take effect.[11] This technique is also useful for atypical facial pain in the distribution of the glossopharyngeal nerve[12] and as an adjunct for awake endotracheal intubation.[13]

Destruction of the glossopharyngeal nerve is indicated in the palliation of cancer pain, including invasive tumors of the posterior tongue, hypopharynx, and tonsils.[5] This technique is useful in the management of the pain of glossopharyngeal neuralgia for those patients who have failed to respond to medical management or who are not candidates for surgical microvascular decompression.[8]

CONTRAINDICATIONS

Contraindications to blockade of the glossopharyngeal nerve are summarized in Table 9–2. Local infection and sepsis are absolute contraindications to all procedures. Coagulopathy is a strong contraindication to glossopharyngeal nerve block, but owing to the desperate nature of many patients' suffering from invasive head and face malignancies, ethical and humanitarian considerations dictate its use, despite the risk of bleeding.

When clinical indications are compelling, blockade of the glossopharyngeal nerve using a 25-gauge needle may be carried out in the presence of coagulopathy, albeit with increased risk of ecchymosis and hematoma formation.

EQUIPMENT

Local Nerve Block
- 25-gauge, ¾-inch needle
- 22-gauge, 1½-inch needle
- 3-mL syringe
- IV T-piece extension

Pulsed Electrode Magnetic Field—Racz-Finch Kit Needle
- 16-gauge, 1¼-inch angiocatheter
- 5 cm with 5-mm active-tip radiofrequency thermocoagulation (RFTC) needle

DRUGS

Local Nerve Block
- 1.5% lidocaine for skin infiltration
- 0.5% ropivacaine/bupivacaine
- 2% lidocaine
- Steroids (optional)
- Iohexol (Omnipaque 240)

Neurolysis
- 6% phenol in glycerin/iohexol
- Absolute alcohol (97%)

▽ TABLE 9–1 Indications for Glossopharyngeal Nerve Block

Local Anesthetic Block
  Surgical anesthesia
  Anatomic differential neural blockade
  Prognostic nerve block prior to neurodestructive procedures
  Acute pain emergencies (palliation)
  Adjunct to awake intubation
Neurolytic block or neurodestructive procedure
  Cancer pain (palliation)
  Management of glossopharyngeal neuralgia

▽ TABLE 9–2 Contraindications to Glossopharyngeal Nerve Block

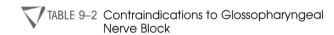

Local infection
Sepsis
Coagulopathy
Disulfiram therapy (if alcohol is used)
Significant behavioral abnormalities

PREPARATION OF THE PATIENT

PHYSICAL EXAMINATION

The physical examination should include an assessment of the ability to move the neck and inspection for normal landmarks at the site of the needle insertion.

PREOPERATIVE MEDICATION

For preoperative medication, use the standard American Society of Anesthesiologists' recommendations for conscious sedation.

PROCEDURE

POSITION OF THE PATIENT AND PHYSICIAN

The patient is placed in the supine position. An imaginary line is visualized running from the mastoid process to the angle of the mandible.[14] The fluoroscope should be placed in an oblique position and directed toward the area of the mandible and the mastoid process (Fig. 9–2). The styloid process should lie just below the midpoint of this line.

TECHNIQUE

The skin is prepared with antiseptic solution. A 22-gauge, 1.5-inch needle attached to a 10-mL syringe is advanced at this midpoint location in a plane perpen-

dicular to the skin. The styloid process should be encountered within 3 cm. After contact is made, the needle is withdrawn and walked off the styloid process posteriorly. As soon as bony contact is lost and careful aspiration reveals no blood or cerebrospinal fluid, 7 mL of 0.5% preservative-free lidocaine combined with 80 mg of methylprednisolone is injected in incremental doses.

Subsequently, daily nerve blocks are performed in the same manner but substituting 40 mg of methylprednisolone for the first 80-mg dose. This approach may also be used for breakthrough pain in patients who previously experienced adequate pain control with oral medications (Figs. 9–3 and 9–4).[8]

Neurolytic Block
- 1 mL of alcohol or phenol after negative aspiration

Pulsed Electrode Magnetic Fields
- Angiocatheter inserted at the styloid process under fluoroscopy
- Blunt RFTC needle is inserted until bone contacted and walked off bone posteriorly. Sensory and motor stimulation is done as per routine, pulsed electrode magnetic fields (pEMF) is done at 42°C with three cycles of 120 seconds.

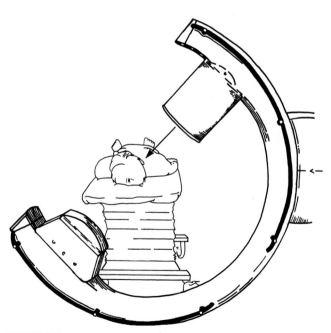

FIGURE 9–2

The C-arm is turned obliquely toward the mandible to visualize the styloid process.

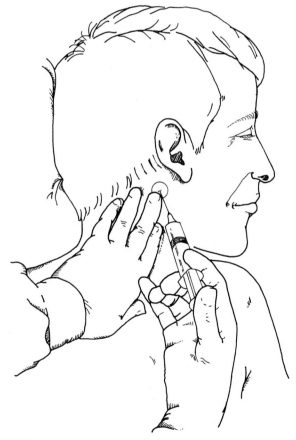

FIGURE 9–3

The site of entry for a glossopharyngeal nerve block between the mastoid process and the angle of the mandible.

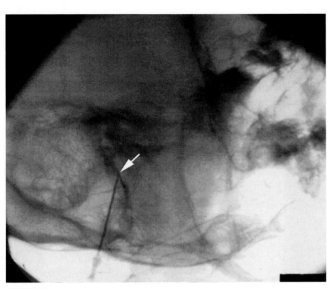

FIGURE 9–4

The lateral radiographic view shows the rim of the needle on the styloid process *(arrow)*. This position ensures that the needle tip is close to the glossopharyngeal nerve.

COMPLICATIONS

Because extraoral blocks of the glossopharyngeal nerve can readily spread to the vagus and accessory nerves, neurolytic blocks often produce analgesia of the hemilarynx and/or trapezius muscle, and sternocleidomastoid paralysis on the ipsilateral side. Both these complications may be well tolerated by patients with terminal cancer pain. Glossopharyngeal nerve block is occasionally used in the exceedingly rare condition of idiopathic glossopharyngeal neuralgia.

The major complications associated with glossopharyngeal nerve block are related to trauma to the internal jugular vein and carotid artery.[5] Hematoma formation and intravascular injection of local anesthetic with subsequent toxicity are significant problems for the patient. Blockade of the motor portion of the glossopharyngeal nerve can result in dysphagia secondary to weakness of the stylopharyngeus muscle.[9] If the vagus nerve is inadvertently blocked, as it often is during glossopharyngeal nerve block, dysphonia secondary to paralysis of the ipsilateral vocal cord may occur. Reflex tachycardia secondary to vagal nerve block is also observed in some patients.[5] Inadvertent block of the hypoglossal and spinal accessory nerves during glossopharyngeal nerve block results in weakness of the tongue and trapezius muscle.[15]

A small percentage of patients who undergo chemical neurolysis or neurodestructive procedures of the glossopharyngeal nerve experience postprocedure dysesthesias in the area of anesthesia.[16] These symptoms range from a mildly uncomfortable burning or pulling sensation to severe pain. Such severe postprocedure pain is called *anesthesia dolorosa*. Anesthesia dolorosa can be worse than the patient's original pain and is often times harder to treat. Sloughing of skin and subcutaneous tissue has been associated with anesthesia dolorosa.

The glossopharyngeal nerve is susceptible to trauma from needle, hematoma, or compression during injection procedures. Such complications, although usually transitory, can be quite upsetting to the patient.

Even though risk of infection is uncommon, it is ever present, especially in patients with cancer who are immunocompromised.[10] Early detection of infection is crucial to avoiding potentially life-threatening sequelae.

HELPFUL HINTS

Often, patients with pharyngeal cancer will have undergone radical neck dissection and the sternocleidomastoid muscle will have been removed. This makes identification of the styloid process much easier, since this particular bony landmark is now almost subcutaneous, allowing this block to be performed easily.

Because of the proximity of the large vascular conduits of the internal carotid artery and the internal jugular vein, the risks of intravascular injection are always significant, demanding meticulous aspiration tests. With the temporary and perhaps permanent analgesia produced by this block, a degree of incoordination of swallowing, with the accompanying potential risk of aspiration, must be appreciated by patients and attendants alike. With numbness of half of the pharynx and the larynx, ingestion and swallowing are often severely compromised.

EFFICACY

No data are available to establish the efficacy of the block. Pain relief by the patient is a good indication of success.

Other peripheral nerve/myoneurals 64450.

REFERENCES

1. Weisenburg TH: Cerebellopontine tumour diagnosed for six years as tic douloureux. JAMA 54:1600–1604, 1910.
2. Harris W: Persistent pain in lesions of the peripheral and central nervous system. Brain 44:557–571, 1921.
3. Doyle JB: A study of four cases of glossopharyngeal neuralgia. Arch Neurol Psychiatry 9:34–36, 1923.
4. Dandy WE: Glossopharyngeal neuralgia: Its diagnosis and treatment. Arch Surg 15:198–215, 1927.
5. Bonica JJ: Neurolytic blockade and hypophysectomy. In Bonica JJ (ed): The Management of Pain, 2nd ed. Philadelphia, Lea & Febiger, 1990, pp 1996–1999.
6. Pitkin GP: The glossopharyngeal nerve. In Southworth JL, Hingson RA (eds): Conduction Anesthesia. Philadelphia, JB Lippincott, 1946, pp 46–49.

7. Bajaj P, Gemavat M, Singh DP: Ninth cranial nerve block in the management of malignant pain in its territory. Pain Clin 6:153–208, 1993.

8. Waldman SD, Waldman KA: The diagnosis and treatment of glossopharyngeal neuralgia. Am J Pain Manage 5:19–24, 1995.

9. Waldman SD: The role of neural blockade in the management of headaches and facial pain. Curr Rev Pain 1:346–352, 1997.

10. Waldman SD: The role of nerve blocks in pain management. In Weiner R (ed): Comprehensive Guides to Pain Management. Orlando, PMD Press, 1990, pp 10-1–10-33.

11. Waldman SD: Management of acute pain. Postgrad Med 87:15–17, 1992.

12. Waldman SD: The role of nerve blocks in the management of headache and facial pain. In Diamond S (ed): Practical Headache Management. Boston, Kluwer, 1993, pp 99–118.

13. Brown DL: Glossopharyngeal nerve block. In Brown DL (ed): Atlas of Regional Anesthesia, 2nd ed. Philadelphia, WB Saunders, 1999, pp 203–208.

14. Murphy TM: Somatic blockade of the head and neck. In Cousins MJ, Bridenbaugh PO (eds): Neural Blockade in Clinical Anesthesia and Management of Pain, 2nd ed. Philadelphia, JB Lippincott, 1988, pp 546–548.

15. Katz J: Glossopharyngeal nerve block. In Katz J (ed): Atlas of Regional Anesthesia, 2nd ed. Norwalk, CT, Appleton & Lange, 1994, p 52.

16. Brisman R: Retrogasserian glycerol injection. In Brisman R (ed): Neurosurgical and Medical Management of Pain. Boston, Kluwer, 1989, pp 51–56.

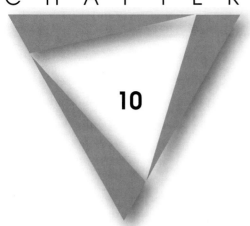

CHAPTER

10

Cervical (C3–C7) Nerve Root Block and Radiofrequency Thermocoagulation

HISTORY

No clear report of selective sleeve root injection can be found. Clinically, this block has been used frequently for diagnostic and therapeutic purposes.

ANATOMY

The anterior and posterior roots of cervical nerves C2–C4 emerge from the spinal canal through their respective intervertebral foramina. The first cervical nerve—the suboccipital nerve—emerges between the occipital bone and the posterior arch of the atlas. The posterior sensory root of this nerve is much smaller than the anterior motor root and may be much smaller than the anterior motor root and may be entirely absent.[1]

After the mixed nerves are formed by the union of the anterior and posterior roots, they divide into anterior and posterior primary divisions. The exception is the first cervical nerve, which seldom has an anterior division. Because the first cervical nerve is composed almost exclusively of motor fibers to the muscles of the suboccipital triangle and only rarely has any significant sensory component, it is usually unnecessary to block this nerve.

After exiting the intervertebral foramina, the anterior primary rami of C2–C4 pass in an anterior-caudal lateral direction behind the vertebral artery and vein, in the gutter formed by the anterior and posterior tubercles of the corresponding transverse processes of the cervical vertebrae (Fig. 10–1A).[2, 3] The tubercles of the transverse processes lie 0.5 inch (1.3 cm) to 1.25 inches (3.2 cm) below the skin, depending on the size of the patient and the cervical level. The lower cervical tubercles are more superficial than the tubercles of the upper cervical transverse processes.[4] The anterior tubercles are located farther cephalad and medial than the posterior tubercles.[1]

The first cervical nerve passes under the vertebral artery in its relationship to the posterior arch of the atlas and is held in place by a fibrous tunnel.[1] The anterior primary rami of C2–C4 are also held firmly on the transverse process by a fibrous tunnel. After leaving the transverse processes, these nerves are enclosed in a perineural space formed by the muscles and tendons attached to the anterior and posterior tubercles of their respective cervical vertebrae. The muscles and tendons of the anterior tubercles are the longus colli, the longus capitis, and the scalenus anterior. Those attached to the posterior tubercles are the scalenus medius, the scalenus cervicis, and the longissimus cervicis.[1-3]

The ascending branches (small occipital and great auricular nerves) supply the occipitomastoid region of the head, the auricle of the ear, and the parotid gland; the transverse branch (superficial cervical) innervates the anterior part of the neck between the lower border of the jaw and the sternum; and the descending branches (suprarenal, supraclavicular, and superacromial) supply the shoulder and upper pectoral region (Fig. 10–1B).[5-8]

The deep cervical plexus supplies mainly the deep structures of the anterior and lateral neck and sends branches to the phrenic nerve. It also contributes to the hypoglossal loop.[8] One group of nerve branches—the lateral (external) group—proceeds from beneath the sternocleidomastoid muscle in a posterolateral direction toward the posterior triangle. This group provides muscular branches to the scalenus medius, sternocleidomastoid, trapezius, and levator scapulae muscles. The medial (ventral) group runs medially and forward to the anterior triangle. It provides muscular branches to the rectus capitis lateralis and rectus capitis anterior, longus capitis, and longus colli muscles and to the diaphragm via the phrenic nerve. By means of the ansa hypoglossi, it also innervates the thyrohyoid, geniohyoid, omohyoid, sternothyroid, and sternohyoid muscles.[2, 5, 8]

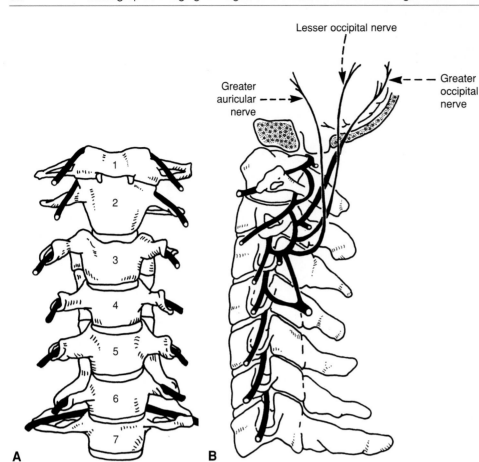

Lesser occipital nerve

Greater auricular nerve

Greater occipital nerve

FIGURE 10–1

A, Drawing of the anteroposterior view of the cervical spine showing C3–C7 nerve root exiting. *B,* Drawing of the lateral view of the cervical spine showing C1–C8 nerve roots.

The cervical plexus also communicates with the vagus, hypoglossal, and accessory cervical nerves.[8] These communications may explain some of the side effects often seen with cervical plexus blockade.

INDICATIONS

- Atlanto-occipital and atlantoaxial joint pain
- Occipital headaches
- Upper cervical pain
- Occipital neuralgia

CONTRAINDICATIONS

- Local infections
- Coagulopathies
- Suboccipital craniotomy with no bone and/or distorted anatomy
- Vertical metastasis

EQUIPMENT

Local Block
- 25-gauge, ¾-inch infiltration needle
- 22-gauge, 3½-inch spinal needle
- 3-mL syringe

- 5-mL syringe
- IV T-piece extension set

Pulsed Electrode Magnetic Fields and Radiofrequency Thermocoagulation
- 16-gauge, 1¼-inch angiocatheter
- 10 cm with 10-mm active-tip radiofrequency thermocoagulation (RFTC) needle
- RFTC set with cables

Cryoneurolysis
- 12-gauge, 1½-inch angiocatheter
- Cryoneurolysis probe set

DRUGS

- 1.5% lidocaine
- 0.5% bupivacaine/ropivacaine
- 2% lidocaine
- Steroids (optional)
- Iohexol (Omnipaque 240) contrast medium

PREPARATION OF THE PATIENT

PHYSICAL EXAMINATION

Active range of motion of the cervical spine is generally performed to provoke the patient's symptoms and to assess limitation of motion. Pain provocation can be isolated to, or emphasized in, the upper cervical spine by means of testing rotation or lateral bending from a position of protraction and retraction. The flexion and extension of the C–C2 segment are greatest during retraction and protraction, respectively.[6] Thus, an affliction of these segments is more accurately elicited by protraction or retraction rather than by general extension or flexion of the entire cervical spine.

PREOPERATIVE MEDICATION

For preoperative medication, use the standard American Society of Anesthesiologists' recommendations for conscious sedation.

PROCEDURE

POSITION OF THE PATIENT

Figure 10–2 shows an anteroposterior view of the head in supine position with the fluoroscope.

TECHNIQUE

The patient is placed supine on the fluoroscopy table with the head and neck slightly extended. The neck, submandibular, and retroauricular regions are prepared. The fluoroscopic unit is brought in from the head. Lateral fluoroscopic images are obtained, and the "lateral mass" of C2 (including the C2 transverse process and inferior articular pillar) and the ventral aspect of the C2 vertebral body are identified. Parallax is eliminated with lateral rotation and cephalad or caudad angulation of the x-ray beam as needed. A skin entry site is marked and anesthetized below the angle of the mandible. Anterior oblique angulation of the fluoroscopic unit is used initially; after the electrode has been introduced through the skin, lateral images are used to guide placement, because no clear radiographic landmarks are present on anterior oblique fluoroscopic images (see Fig. 10–2). (A coaxial, or "tunnel vision" approach is not feasible.) A 10-cm, 5-mm active-tip 20-gauge RF electrode with a small distal curve (10 to 15 degrees) is introduced under lateral fluoroscopic guidance and directed medially and cephalad under lateral fluoroscopic imaging toward the ventral lateral aspect of the C2 vertebral body at its junction with the ipsilateral ventral inferior medial C2 transverse process. The path of the electrode passes lateral and dorsal to the carotid sheath. Care is taken to stay ventral to the existing C3 nerve root and ventral to the vertebral artery yet dorsal to the pharyngeal structures. Bony contact may be made at the ventrolateral aspect of the lateral inferior end plate of the C2 vertebral body at its junction with the C2–C3 intervertebral disc. The electrode is then rotated and directed cephalad, hugging bone, into the sulcus

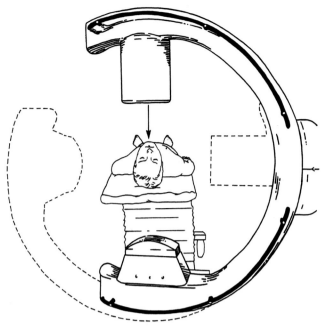

FIGURE 10–2

Drawing of the fluoroscope with the patient in the supine position. The fluoroscope is in an anteroposterior and oblique view.

along the ventral lateral aspect of the C2 vertebral body, medial to the ventral aspect of the C2 transverse process (Fig. 10–3).

Careful aspiration is performed—no blood or other body fluid should be aspirated. A small-volume contrast study is then performed, using 0.2 to 0.4 mL of nonionic contrast medium, such as iohexol, 240 mg/mL. Contrast spread should be limited to the immediate perivertebral region, outlining the sulcus on anteroposterior fluoroscopic imaging (Fig. 10–4). In lateral radiographs, the contrast should appear to silhouette the ventral aspect of the transverse process of C2.

RADIOFREQUENCY THERMOCOAGULATION TECHNIQUE

Sensory stereotaxy is performed next, using 0.15 to 0.2 V at 50 Hz, 1-msec pulse duration. The electrode is manipulated with very small movements along the ventral sulcus of C2 until concordant suboccipital pain is reproduced in a patient-blinded fashion. Elicitation of sharp, radiating infra-auricular/neck pain indicates stimulation of the ventral C3 nerve root and is unacceptable. Elicitation of deep or superficial infra-auricular pain or anterior cervical/submandibular pain may indicate possible stimulation of the chorda tympani and is unacceptable. There are no motor branches associated with the ramus communicans nerve; motor stimulation generally is not performed. Once concordant suboccipital pain has been elicited in a reproducible, patient-blinded fashion, 0.5 to 1 mL 2% lidocaine is injected before RF lesioning.

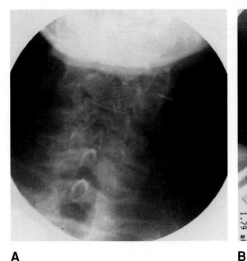
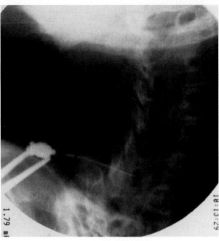

A   B

FIGURE 10–3

Radiographic anteroposterior *(A)* and oblique *(B)* images of a cervical sleeve root injection with needle in place. Shown at C3 in AP view, and C7 in lateral view.

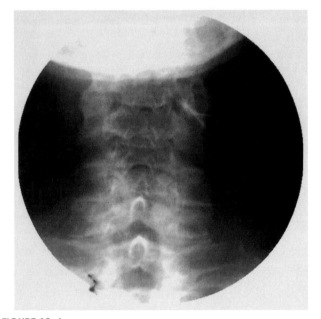

FIGURE 10–4

Radiographic anteroposterior image of a cervical sleeve root injection that shows contrast agent along the C3 nerve root.

The RF lesion is performed at 80°C for a period of 60 seconds and repeated once the electrode tip has returned to ambient body temperature. The size of the lesion created by the 2-mm active tip is small, but this approach reduced the risk of inadvertent C3 or chorda tympani lesion that could occur with a 5-mm active tip. After the lesioning, a small amount of corticosteroid, with or without local anesthetic, may be injected and the electrode removed. The patient may be discharged after a 1- to 2-hour postprocedure observation period. Patients frequently complain of some deep neck soreness, which may last 2 to 3 days, and occasionally of pain with swallowing, which is similarly self-limited. Occasionally, despite negative stimulation, patients may complain of some temporary pain in the infra-auricular region radiating down the ipsi-

lateral neck. This may be a result of localized inflammation irritating the chorda tympani or ventral C2 nerve root after the thermal lesion and is generally self-limited.

COMPLICATIONS

The complications of the cervical root block are similar to those of the blocks performed in the atlantoaxial and atlanto-occipital joints (see Chapters 13 and 14).

HELPFUL HINTS

It must be emphasized that, like C2 cervical dorsal root ganglion lesioning and percutaneous cordotomy, the technique of C2 ramus communicans lesion is technically demanding. A considerable potential for patient morbidity exists if the procedure is performed by inexperienced practitioners unfamiliar with advanced fluoroscopy-guided procedures and upper cervical bony and soft tissue anatomy.

EFFICACY

No reliable statistical data are available for the efficacy of cervical nerve root block. Efficacy can be determined only on a case-by-case basis, depending on the patient's pain relief.

Paracervical nerve 64435; cervical plexus 64413; RFTC other nerve 64640.

FURTHER READINGS

Bovim G, Berg R, Dale LG: Cervicogenic headache: Anesthetic blockades of cervical nerves (C2–C5) and facet joint (C2–C3). Pain 49:315–320, 1992.

Sluijter M: C1 dorsal nerve root lesion in the treatment of suboccipital headache. Personal communication, 1998.

REFERENCES

1. Wertheim HM, Rovenstine EA: Cervical plexus block. NY State J Med 39:1311–1315, 1939.
2. Collins VJ: Blocks of cervical spinal nerves. In Fundamentals of Nerve Blocks. Philadelphia, Lea & Febiger, 1960, pp 234–248.
3. Winnie AP, Ramamurthy S, Durrani Z, Radonjic R: Interscalene cervical plexus block: A single-injection technique. Anesth Analg 54:370–375, 1975.
4. Moore DC: Regional block. In A Handbook for Use in the Clinical Practice of Medicine and Surgery, 2nd ed. Springfield, IL, Charles C Thomas, 1937, pp 88–98.
5. Adriani J: Labat's Regional Anesthesia: Techniques and Clinical Applications, 3rd ed. Philadelphia, WB Saunders, 1967, pp 180–195.
6. Pai U, Raj P: Peripheral nerve blocks: Cervical plexus. In Raj P (ed): Handbook of Regional Anesthesia. New York, Churchill Livingstone, 1985, pp 163–167.
7. Cousins MJ, Bridenbaugh PO (eds): Neural Blockade in Clinical Anesthesia and Management of Pain, 2nd ed. Philadelphia, JB Lippincott, 1988.
8. Bonica JJ: General considerations of pain in the neck and upper limb. In Bonica JJ (ed): The Management of Pain, 2nd ed. Philadelphia, Lea & Febiger, 1990, pp 823–825.

Sphenopalatine Ganglion Block and Neurolysis

HISTORY

The sphenopalatine ganglion (SPG) has been involved in the pathogenesis of pain since Sluder first described sphenopalatine neuralgia in 1908 and treated it with an SPG block (SPGB).[1] Over the past century, physicians have performed SPGB for pain syndromes ranging from headache and facial pain to sciatica and dysmenorrhea.[1] In the medical literature on SPGB, large gaps—spanning decades—reflect physicians' varying interest in and skepticism about the efficacy of SPGB.

ANATOMY

The SPG is the largest group of neurons outside the cranial cavity (Fig. 11–1). It lies in the pterygopalatine fossa, which is approximately 1 cm wide and 2 cm high and resembles a "vase" on a lateral fluoroscopic view. The pterygopalatine fossa is bordered anteriorly by the posterior wall of the maxillary sinus, posteriorly by the medial plate of the pterygoid process, medially by the perpendicular plate of the palatine bone, and superiorly by the sphenoid sinus, and laterally it communicates with the infratemporal fossa.[2]

The foramen rotundum, through which the maxillary branch of the trigeminal nerve passes, is located on the superolateral aspect of the pterygopalatine fossa; the opening to the pterygoid canal, which houses the vidian nerve, is located on the inferomedial portion of the fossa.

The ganglion within the fossa is located posterior to the middle turbinate of the nose and lies a few millimeters deep to the lateral nasal mucosa. Also contained in the fossa is the maxillary artery and its multiple branches.

The SPG has a complex neural center and has multiple connections. It is "suspended" from the maxillary branch of the trigeminal nerve at the pterygopalatine

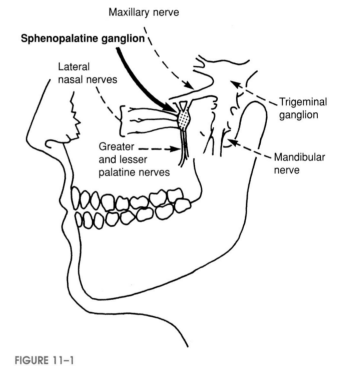

FIGURE 11–1

Anatomy of the sphenopalatine ganglion and its immediate connections.

fossa via the pterygopalatine nerves and lies medial to the maxillary branch when viewed in the sagittal plane. Posteriorly, it is connected to the vidian nerve, also known as the *nerve of the pterygoid canal*, which is formed by the greater petrosal and the deep petrosal nerves. The ganglion itself has efferent branches and forms the superior posterior lateral nasal and pharyngeal nerves. Caudally, the ganglion is in direct connection with the greater and lesser palatine nerves.

As a neural center, the ganglion has sensory, motor, and autonomic components. The sensory fibers arise from the maxillary nerve, pass through the SPG, and are distributed to the nasal membranes, the soft palate, and some parts of the pharynx.[3] A few motor nerves are also believed to be carried with the sensory trunks.

The autonomic innervation is more complex. The sympathetic component begins with preganglionic sympathetic fibers originating in the upper thoracic spinal cord, forming the white rami communicantes, coursing through the sympathetic ganglion, where the preganglionic fibers synapse with the postganglionic ones. The postganglionic fibers then join the carotid nerves before branching off and traveling through the deep petrosal and vidian nerves. The postganglionic sympathetic nerves continue their path through the SPG on their way to the lacrimal gland and the nasal and palatine mucosa.

The parasympathetic component has its preganglionic origin in the superior salivatory nucleus then travels through a portion of the facial nerve (cranial nerve VII) before forming the greater petrosal nerve. The greater petrosal nerve in turn joins the deep petrosal nerve to form the vidian nerve, which ends in the SPG.

Within the ganglion, the preganglionic fibers synapse with their postganglionic cells and continue on to the nasal mucosa, and one branch travels with the maxillary nerve to the lacrimal gland.

INDICATIONS

Currently, SPGB is used for relief of facial pain and headache (Table 11–1).

The indications supported by current literature include sphenopalatine and trigeminal neuralgia, cluster and migraine headaches, and atypical facial pain. SPGB has been used to treat many painful medical syndromes.

Sluder, who is credited as the first physician to describe SPGB for the treatment of sphenopalatine neuralgia, described a unilateral facial pain at the root of the nose that sometimes spread toward the zygoma and extended back to the mastoid and occiput.[1] This pain is typically associated with the parasympathetic features such as lacrimation, rhinorrhea, or mucosal congestion.[14] Sluder believed the cause of this pain was the

▽ TABLE 11–1   Use of Sphenopalatine Ganglion Block

Indications
Sphenopalatine neuralgia
Trigeminal neuralgia
Headaches
  Cluster
  Migraine
Atypical facial pain
Herpes zoster ophthalmicus

Not recommended for
Back pain
Sciatica
Angina
Arthritis

spread of infection from the paranasal sinuses that irritated the SPG. This was initially accepted as a possible cause but came into question when other syndromes, such as low back pain, sciatica, and dysmenorrhea, were attributed to irritation of the SPG.

Eagle, in the early 1940s, sought to revive interest in sphenopalatine neuralgia when he presented his thesis to the American Laryngological, Rhinological, and Otological Society. He agreed with Sluder on the existence of sphenopalatine neuralgia but disagreed on its cause.[3] Eagle believed that intranasal deformities, such as deviated septum, septal spurs or ledges, and prominent turbinates, were responsible for irritation of the ganglion, which caused the pain.

Others attribute it to a reflex vasomotor change or possibly a vasomotor syndrome.[5] Regardless of the cause, sphenopalatine neuralgia is an indication for SPGB.

Trigeminal neuralgia is also an indication for SPGB. In 1925, Ruskin disagreed with Sluder on the indication for SPGB and suggested involvement of the SPG in the pathogenesis of trigeminal neuralgia.[6] The SPG is directly connected to the maxillary branch of the trigeminal nerve via the pterygopalatine nerves. He believed that blockade of the SPG would in turn relieve the symptoms associated with trigeminal neuralgia. Few case reports in the current literature support this theory.[7]

Although new medications for the treatment of migraine and cluster headache are introduced every year, a certain small subset of patients fails to respond to oral and parenteral dosing and are forced to seek alternative methods for pain control. In recent years, blockade of the SPG has been used in such cases, with varying success.[8–10]

Another indication for SPGB is atypical facial pain. Such pain is usually unilateral; is described as constant, aching, and burning; and is not confined to the distribution of a cranial nerve.[11] It may involve the entire face, scalp, and neck. The pain may have a sympathetic component, which makes the SPGB ideal, because the postganglionic sympathetic nerves pass through the ganglion.

Other reported indications for SPGB include back pain, sciatica, angina, arthritis, herpes zoster ophthalmicus, and pain from cancer of the tongue and floor of the mouth.[12–14] These are not "true" indications for SPGB; instead, they reveal its broad applications in situations when conventional therapies are ineffective.

CONTRAINDICATIONS

Absolute
- Local infection
- Coagulopathy

Relative
- Where anatomy has been altered secondary to surgery, infection, or genetic variations

EQUIPMENT

- 25-gauge, ¾-inch infiltration needle
- 18-gauge needle for drug aspiration
- 16-gauge, 1¼-inch angiocatheter
- 22-gauge, 3½-inch spinal needle for ganglion block
- 10-cm curved-blunt radiofrequency thermocoagulation (RFTC) needle with a 10-mm active tip for RF lesioning

DRUGS

- Iohexol (Omnipaque) contrast solution
- Preservative-free normal saline (0.9%)
- 1.5% lidocaine for infiltration
- 0.5% bupivacaine or ropivacaine, preservative free, for diagnostic block
- 2% lidocaine, preservative free, for diagnostic block
- Water-soluble steroids: methylprednisolone or triamcinolone diacetate
- Triple-antibiotic ointment for skin after procedure

PREPARATION OF THE PATIENT

Rule out paranasal sinus infections, which can cause irritation of the ganglion resulting in pain. Nasal deformities can be responsible for the irritation of the ganglion and thus the pain.[3, 4] Trigeminal neuralgia may be the cause of this disorder.[6] There may be dysequilibrium between sympathetic and parasympathetic tone in the ganglion that results in release of substance P or blockade of local enkephalins.[15]

PREOPERATIVE MEDICATION

For preoperative medication, use the standard American Society of Anesthesiologists' (ASA) recommended conscious sedation.

MONITORING

For monitoring, use the standard ASA recommended monitors, such as electrocardiograph, sphygmomanometer, and pulse oximetry.

PROCEDURE

POSITION OF THE PATIENT

The patient lies supine with the head inside the C-arm (Fig. 11–2A). The anterior position view is then taken (Fig. 11–2B).

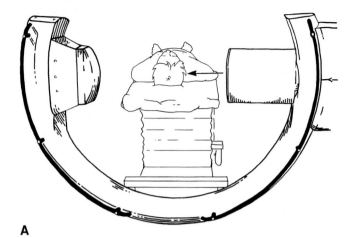

A

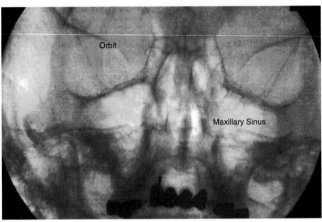

B

FIGURE 11–2

A, The patient lies supine with the head inside the C-arm. The beam of the C-arm is directed toward one side of the face just below the orbit. *B,* This radiographic image shows the posteroanterior view of the front of the face, identifying the orbit and maxillary sinus.

SITE OF NEEDLE ENTRY

The needle is inserted under the zygoma in the coronoid notch. A lateral view of the upper cervical spine and the mandible is obtained and the head is rotated until the rami of the mandible are superimposed one on the other (Fig. 11–3). The C-arm is moved slightly cephalad until the pterygopalatine fossa is visualized. It should resemble a vase when the two pterygopalatine plates are superimposed on one another and are located just posterior to the posterior aspect of the maxillary sinus.

TECHNIQUE OF NEEDLE ENTRY

When a blunt needle is used, a 1.25-inch angiocatheter four sizes larger than the blunt needle must be inserted first. The needle is directed medial, cephalad, and slightly posterior toward the pterygopalatine fossa. An anteroposterior view confirms the proper direction and positioning of the needle (Fig. 11–4). The tip of the needle should be advanced until it is adjacent to the lateral nasal mucosa. If resistance is felt at any time, the

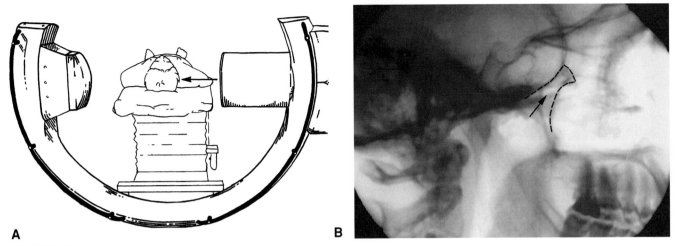

FIGURE 11–3

A, The C-arm position to obtain the lateral view of pterygopalatine fossa. The beam of the C-arm should be directed toward the root of the nose *(arrow)*. *B,* This radiographic view identifies the "inverted flower vase" image of the pterygopalatine fossa.

needle must be slightly withdrawn and redirected. The operator takes care to avoid advancing the needle through the lateral nasal wall.

In the lateral view, note that the needle is residing in the inverted vase. Figures 11–5 and 11–6 show the landmarks needed to confirm the correct placement of the needle.

INJECTION OF LOCAL ANESTHETIC

Once it is properly positioned, 1 to 2 mL of local anesthetic is injected, with or without steroid. As much as 5 mL of local anesthetic can be injected for a diagnostic block.

TECHNIQUE OF NEUROLYSIS

Radiofrequency Thermocoagulation Lesioning

Lesioning of the SPG can be performed with either RFTC or pulsed electrode magnetic fields (pEMF). With radiofrequency (RF), RFTC sensory testing is done after the needle is correctly placed radiographically. Paresthesia should be felt at 0.5 to 0.7 V at 50 Hz when the needle is correctly situated on the ganglion. If the paresthesia is felt in the upper teeth, the maxillary branch of the trigeminal nerve is being stimulated and the needle must be redirected more caudal. Stimulation of the greater and lesser palatine nerves results in paresthesias of the hard palate. In this case, the needle is anterior and

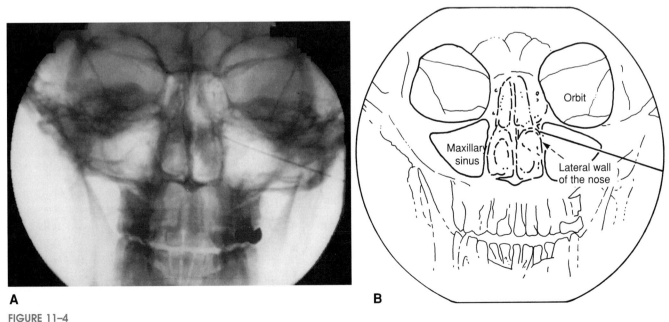

FIGURE 11–4

A, The radiographic anteroposterior view of the face shows the needle tip at the lateral wall of nose at the superomedial angle of the maxillary sinus. *B,* The drawing of the posteroanterior view of the radiograph shows the needle tip at the lateral wall of the nose.

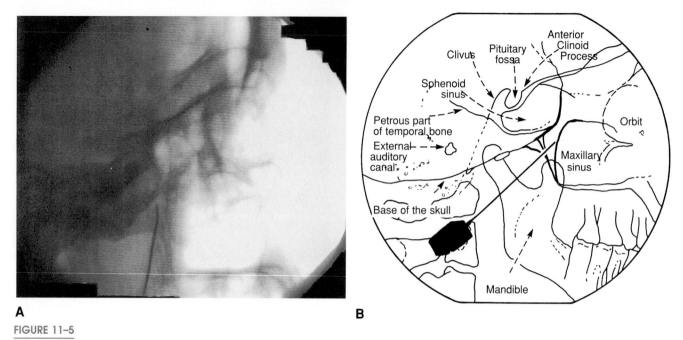

A   **B**

FIGURE 11–5

A, The radiographic lateral view of face shows the radiofrequency needle in the "inverted vase" of the pterygopalatine fossa. *B,* A drawing of the lateral view of the face identifies correct needle placement on the sphenopalatine ganglion.

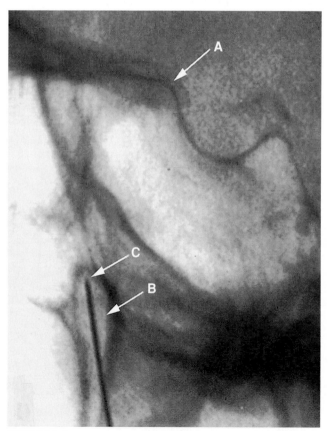

FIGURE 11–6

Close-up radiograph of the lateral view of the pterygopalatine fossa. The following is a key to the letters shown on the figure: A, anterior clinoid process; B, pterygopalatine fossa; C, needle tip in the pterygopalatine fossa. Correct placement of the needle is seen in the lateral oblique view.

lateral and should be redirected in a more posterior and medial direction. An insulated 20- or 22-gauge, 10-cm, curved, blunt-tipped RFK (Racz-Finch Kit [Radionics, Inc., Burlington, VT]) needle with a 5- to 10-mm active tip is used. After proper placement and stimulation as described in the technique section, RF lesioning is performed for 70 to 90 seconds at 80°C. Two lesions are usually made. Before lesioning, 1 to 2 mL of local anesthetic is injected. PEMF lesioning is performed at 42°C for 120 seconds. Two or three lesions (120 seconds) can be made without local anesthetic, since the temperature of the lesioning is barely above the normal body temperature. Expected effect after local anesthetic block is numbness of the root of the nose and palate. There may be lacrimation from the ipsilateral side of the eye.

COMPLICATIONS

A reflex bradycardia can occur in some patients during RF and pEMF lesioning of the SPG.

When the lesioning is halted, the bradycardia is resolved. In some patients, atropine may need to be given to complete the lesioning. A reflex resembling the oculocardiac reflex may be the cause. The afferent information may travel back through the vidian nerve, geniculate ganglion, and nervus intermedius to reach the solitary tract nucleus, which has interconnections to the dorsal vagal nucleus.[16]

Infection can occur if proper aseptic technique is breached. Epistaxis can occur if too much pressure is applied to the needle and it is pushed through the lateral nasal wall. Hematoma formation is possible if the large venous plexus overlying the pterygopalatine fossa or the maxillary artery is punctured.

RF lesioning of the SPG can result in hypesthesia or numbness of the palate, maxilla, or the posterior pharynx but is usually transient.[2, 9]

EFFICACY

Current literature on the efficacy of SPGB for various medical conditions is scant and patient populations rather small. One study by Sanders and Zuurmond examined the efficacy of SPGB in 66 patients suffering from episodic and chronic cluster headaches.[9] All had previously been treated with various pharmacologic and/or surgical therapies, without significant pain relief. The patients were divided into two groups, those with episodic pain and those with chronic pain, with sample sizes of 56 and 10 patients, respectively. All received three RF lesions at 70°C for 60 seconds. Thirty-four (60.7%) of 56 patients with episodic cluster headaches and 3 (30%) of the 10 with the chronic type received complete pain relief during a mean follow-up period of 29 months.

Salar and associates reported using percutaneous RFTC of the SPG for sphenopalatine neuralgia in seven patients.[2] Each received two lesions at 60°C and 65°C, respectively, for 60 seconds. One patient required repeat lesioning, and two underwent repeat lesioning, and another two underwent two additional RF procedures. All the patients were pain free over a follow-up period ranging from 6 to 34 months.

Prasanna and Murthy reported complete pain relief for at least 12 months in a patient suffering from herpes zoster ophthalmicus who was treated with SPGB for residual ear pain that had not been alleviated with previous stellate ganglion blocks.[13] The same authors also reported immediate short-term pain relief with intranasal blockade of the SPG in 10 patients suffering intractable pain from cancer of the tongue and the floor of the mouth.[14] Further studies are needed.

Sphenopalatine ganglion 64505; RFTC other nerve 64640.

REFERENCES

1. Waldman S: Sphenopalatine ganglion block—80 years later. Reg Anesth 18:274–276, 1993.
2. Salar G, Ori C, Iob I: Percutaneous thermocoagulation for sphenopalatine ganglion neuralgia. Acta Neurochir (Wien) 84:24–28, 1987.
3. Eagle W: Sphenopalatine neuralgia. Arch Otolaryngol 35:66–84, 1942.
4. Sluder C: Etiology, diagnosis, prognosis, and treatment of sphenopalatine neuralgia. JAMA 61:1201–1216, 1913.
5. Bonica JJ: Pain in the head. The Management of Pain, 2nd ed. Philadelphia, Lea & Febiger 1992, pp 651–675.
6. Ruskin S: Contributions to the study of the sphenopalatine ganglion. Laryngoscope 35:87–108, 1925.
7. Manahan A, Maleska M, Malone P: Sphenopalatine ganglion block relieves symptoms of trigeminal neuralgia: A case report. Nebr Med J 81:306–309, 1996.
8. Cepero R, Miller R, Bressler K: Long-term results of sphenopalatine ganglioneurectomy for facial pain. Am J Otolaryngol 8:171–174, 1987.
9. Sanders M, Zuurmond W: Efficacy of sphenopalatine ganglion blockade in 66 patients suffering from cluster headaches: A 12- to 70-month follow-up evaluation. J Neurosurg 87:876–880, 1997.
10. Ryan R, Facer G: Sphenopalatine ganglion neuralgia and cluster headache: Comparisons, contrasts, and treatment. Headache 17:7–8, 1977.
11. Phero JC, McDonald JS, Green DB, Robins GS: Orofacial pain and other related syndromes. In Raj PP (ed): Practical Management of Pain, 2nd ed. St. Louis, Mosby–Year Book, 1992.
12. Lebovits A, Alfred H, Lefkowitz M: Sphenopalatine ganglion block: Clinical use in the pain management clinic. Clin J Pain 6:131–136, 1990.
13. Prasanna A, Murthy P: Combined stellate ganglion and sphenopalatine ganglion block in acute herpes infection. Clin J Pain 9:135–137, 1993.
14. Prasanna A, Murthy S: Sphenopalatine ganglion block and pain of cancer. J Pain 8:125, 1993.
15. Pollock B, Kondziolka D: Stereotactic radiosurgical treatment of sphenopalatine neuralgia. J Neurosurg 87:450–453, 1997.
16. Konen A: Unexpected effects due to radiofrequency thermocoagulation of the sphenopalatine ganglion: Two case reports. Pain Digest 10:30–33, 2000.

C H A P T E R

12

Stellate Ganglion Block

HISTORY

Selective block of the sympathetic trunk was first reported by Sellheim and, shortly thereafter, by Kappis in 1923[1] and Brumm and Mandl[2] in 1924. After 1930, the technique and the indications were established by White and Sweet[3] in the United States and Leriche and Fontaine[4] in Europe.

ANATOMY

Cell bodies for preganglionic nerves originate in the anterolateral horn of the spinal cord; fibers destined for the head and neck originate in the first and second thoracic spinal cord segments, whereas preganglionic nerves to the upper extremity originate at segments T2–T8, and occasionally T9. Preganglionic axons to the head and neck exit with the ventral roots of T1 and T2, then travel as white communicating rami before joining the sympathetic chain and passing cephalad to synapse at either the inferior (stellate), middle, or superior cervical ganglion. Postganglionic nerves either follow the carotid arteries (external or internal) to the head or integrate as the gray communicating rami before joining the cervical plexus or upper cervical nerves to innervate structures of the neck.

To achieve successful sympathetic denervation of the head and neck, the stellate ganglion should be blocked, because all preganglionic nerves either synapse here or pass through on their way to more cephalad ganglia. Blockade of the middle or superior ganglion would miss the contribution of sympathetic fibers traveling from the stellate ganglion to the vertebral plexus and, ultimately, to the corresponding areas of the cranial vault supplied by the vertebral artery.[5]

Sympathetic nerves to the upper extremity exit T2–T8 through ventral spinal routes, travel as white communicating rami to the sympathetic chain, then

pass cephalad to synapse at the second thoracic ganglion, first thoracic or inferior cervical (stellate) ganglion, and, occasionally, the middle cervical ganglion. Most postganglionic nerves leave the chain as gray communicating rami to join the anterior divisions at C5–T1, nerves that form the brachial plexus. Some postganglionic nerves pass directly from the chain to form the subclavian perivascular plexus and innervate the subclavian, axillary, and upper part of the brachial arteries.[6]

In most humans, the inferior cervical ganglion is fused to the first thoracic ganglion, forming the stellate ganglion. Although the ganglion itself is inconstant, it commonly measures 2.5-cm long, 1.0-cm wide, and 0.5 cm thick. It usually lies in front of the neck of the first rib and extends to the interspace between C7 and T1. When elongated, it may lie over the anterior tubercle of C7; in persons with unfused ganglia, the inferior cervical ganglion rests over C7, and the first thoracic ganglion over the neck of the first rib. From a three-dimensional perspective, the stellate ganglion is limited medially by the longus colli muscle, laterally by the scalene muscles, anteriorly by the subclavian artery, posteriorly by the transverse processes and prevertebral fascia, and inferiorly by the posterior aspect of the pleura. At the level of the stellate ganglion, the vertebral artery lies anterior, having originated from the subclavian artery. After passing over the ganglion, the artery enters the vertebral foramen and is located posterior to the anterior tubercle of C6 (Fig. 12–1).

Because the classic approach to blockade of the stellate ganglion is at the level of C6 (Chassaignac's tubercle), the needle is positioned anterior to the artery. Other structures posterior to the stellate ganglion are the anterior divisions of the C8 and T1 nerves (inferior aspects of the brachial plexus). The stellate ganglion supplies sympathetic innervation to the upper extremity through gray communicating rami of C7, C8, T1, and, occasionally, C5 and C6. Other inconstant contributions to the

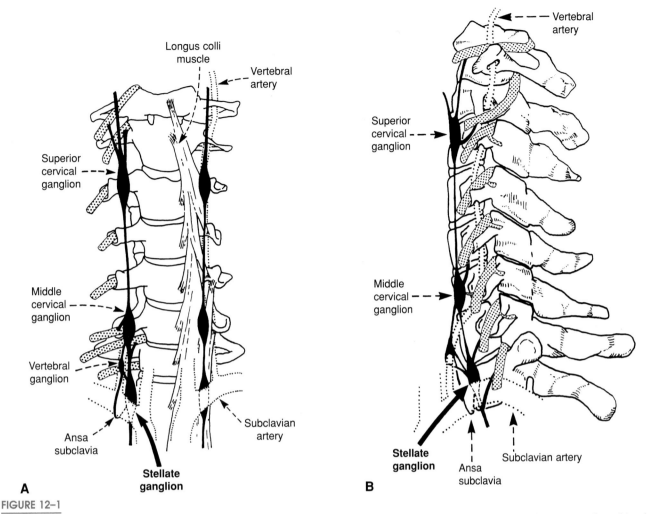

FIGURE 12–1

A, The anterior view of the anatomy and relations of the stellate ganglion. Note the connections of the stellate ganglion superiorly and its close relation to longus colli muscle. *B,* The lateral view of the anatomy of the stellate ganglion. Note the vertebral artery is anterior to the stellate ganglion at C7 and becomes posterior at C6.

upper extremity are from the T2 and T3 gray communicating rami, which do not pass through the stellate ganglion but join the brachial plexus and ultimately innervate distal structures of the upper extremity. These fibers have some times been implicated when relief of sympathetically mediated pain is inadequate despite evidence of a satisfactory stellate block.[7]

INDICATIONS

Stellate ganglion block is useful in the treatment of a variety of painful conditions, including Raynaud's disease, arterial embolism in the area of the arm, accidental intra-arterial injection of drugs, and Meniere's disease. Although stellate ganglion block for treatment of Meniere's disease is controversial, several clinicians have had success with it. Stellate ganglion block is beneficial in the treatment of acute herpes zoster of the face and lower cervical and upper thoracic dermatomes. The technique may also be used for palliation of postherpetic neuralgia involving this anatomic area.

The post-traumatic syndrome, which is often accompanied by swelling, cold sweat, and cyanosis, is an ideal indication for stellate ganglion block. Several clinical syndromes fall into this category, including complex regional pain syndromes types I (reflex sympathetic dystrophy) and II (causalgia), and Sudeck's disease. Stellate ganglion block is also useful in the treatment of facial reflex sympathetic dystrophy.

For patients requiring vascular surgery on the upper extremities, stellate ganglion block has diagnostic, prognostic, and, in some cases, prophylactic value.

Simultaneous bilateral blocks are not advisable. Nevertheless, in cases of pulmonary embolism, bilateral stellate ganglion block is absolutely indicated as immediate therapy.

CONTRAINDICATIONS

Absolute contraindications of stellate ganglion block are as follows:

- Anticoagulant therapy, because of the possibility of bleeding if there is vascular damage during insertion of the needle
- Pneumothorax and pneumonectomy on the contralateral side, because of the danger of additional pneumothorax on the ipsilateral side
- Recent cardiac infarction, because stellate ganglion block cuts off the cardiac sympathetic fibers (accelerator nerves), with possible deleterious effects in this condition

Glaucoma can be considered a relative contraindication to stellate ganglion block, because provocation of glaucoma by repeated stellate ganglion blocks has been reported. Marked impairment of cardiac stimulus conduction (e.g., atrioventricular block) is also to be regarded as a relative contraindication, because blockade of the upper thoracic sympathetic ganglia aggravates bradycardia.

EQUIPMENT

- 25-gauge local infiltration needle
- 22-gauge, 1 inch of 1½-inch block needle
- 5- or 10-cm (2- or 5-mm tip) sharp Sluijter-Mehta or Racz-Finch Kit needle for radiofrequency (RF)
- RF machine

DRUGS

Local Anesthetic Block
- 0.2% to 0.5% bupivacaine or ropivacaine (5 to 8 mL)
- 1% to 2% lidocaine
- Steroids (optional)

Phenol
- 3% phenol in iohexol (Omnipaque 240)—total 6 mL
- 0.9% normal saline—2 mL

Radiofrequency Thermocoagulation
- Local anesthetics same as for block with steroids

PREPARATION OF THE PATIENT

PHYSICAL EXAMINATION

- Check neck extension mobility
- Check for prior radical neck surgery
- Examine for infection at injection site
- Examine for thyroid surgery
- Check for anatomic variations related to surgery

PREOPERATIVE MEDICATION

For preoperative medication, use the standard American Society of Anesthesiologists' recommendations for conscious sedation.

PROCEDURE

PATIENT PREPARATION

Ideally, proper patient preparation for the stellate ganglion block begins at the visit before the procedure. The patient is much more likely to remember discharge instructions and expected side effects if they are explained during a visit when the patient is not apprehensive about the imminent procedure, what side effects may be expected, and potential complications. Discussions of the realistic expectations of sympathetic blockade should be held before any procedure. The goals of blockade and the number of blocks in a given series differ with each pain syndrome, and these variables should be discussed, when possible, at visits before the actual blockade. Patients are much less likely to experience frustration or despair if they understand beforehand what can be expected. If the cause of pain is unclear and the intended block is considered diagnostic, a complete explanation allows the patient to record valuable information on the effectiveness of the procedure.

Informed consent must be obtained. Potential risks, complications, and possible side effects should be explained in detail. The patient should share responsibility for decision making and must understand the risks and the fact that complications do occur.

Placement of an intravenous (IV) line before the block is not mandatory at all pain clinics, but it facilitates use of IV sedation, when indicated, and provides access for administration of resuscitative drugs should a complication occur. In skilled hands, a stellate ganglion block can be performed quickly and relatively painlessly, so IV administration may not be necessary. All standard resuscitative drugs, suction apparatus, oxygen delivery system, cardiac defibrillators, and equipment for endotracheal intubation, however, need to be readily accessible. For anxious patients and in teaching institutions when the operator is inexperienced or when "hands-on" teaching is expected, preblock sedation through an IV line is beneficial.

PARATRACHEAL APPROACH

The patient is made to lie supine with the head resting flat on the table without a pillow. A folded sheet or thin pillow should be placed under the shoulders of most patients to facilitate extension of the neck and accentuate landmarks. The head should be kept straight with the mouth slightly open to relax the tension on the anterior cervical musculature. Hyperextension of the neck also causes the esophagus to move midline, away from the transverse processes on the left.

To ensure proper needle positioning, the operator must correctly identify the C6 tubercle. Identification is most easily performed using firm pressure with the index finger (Fig. 12–2). In either a left-handed or right-handed stellate ganglion block, the operator's nondominant hand should be used for palpating landmarks. Patients do not tolerate jabbing; rather, gentle but firm probing can easily define the borders of the tubercle. A single finger, the index finger, relays the most specific tactile information. An alternative approach traps the tubercle between the index and middle fingers.[8]

The skin is antiseptically prepared, and the needle is inserted posteriorly, penetrating the skin at the tip of the operator's index finger. Making a skin wheal with local anesthetic is rarely necessary, except in some teaching situations or in patients with obese necks. In both situations, a 5-cm needle (or a 22-gauge B-bevel needle) is used and should puncture the skin directly downward (posterior), perpendicular to the table in all planes. Although a smaller (e.g., 25-gauge) needle can be used, the added flexibility and smaller caliber make it more difficult to reliably ascertain when bone is encountered and then maintain the proper location for injection.

The needle passes through the underlying tissue until it contacts either the C6 tubercle or the junction between the C6 vertebral body and the tubercle. The depths of these structures differ, the tubercle itself being more anterior than the junction between body and tubercle. Regardless of the specific location encountered at C6, if the skin is being properly displaced posteriorly by the nondominant index finger, the depth is rarely more than 2.0 to 2.5 cm. The important difference between medial and lateral location of bone at C6 relates to the presence of the longus colli muscle, which is located over the lateral aspect of the vertebral body and the medial aspect of the transverse process. It does not cover the C6 tubercle; only the prevertebral fascia that invests the longus colli muscle also covers the C6 tubercle. Therefore, if the needle contacts the medial aspect of the transverse process at a depth somewhat greater than expected, the operator should be prepared to withdraw the needle 0.5 cm to avoid injecting into the longus colli muscle. Injection into the muscle belly can prevent caudad diffusion of local anesthetic to the stellate ganglion. Location of the needle on the superficial tip of the C6 anterior tubercle requires withdrawal of the needle from periosteum before injection.

The procedure is most easily performed if the syringe is attached before the needle is positioned. This prevents accidental dislodgment of the needle from the bone during syringe attachment after the needle is placed. Once bone is encountered, the palpating finger maintains its pressure, the needle is withdrawn 2 to 5 mm, and the medication is injected. Alternatively, once bone is met, the operator's palpating hand can release and fix the needle by grasping its hub, leaving the dominant hand free to aspirate and inject. Even though this technique can be performed blindly, more often fluoroscopy is used to confirm contrast spread

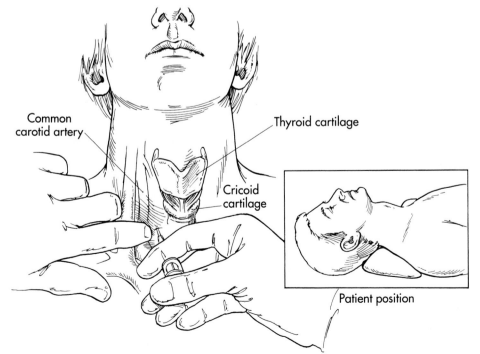

Common carotid artery

Thyroid cartilage

Cricoid cartilage

Patient position

FIGURE 12–2

Stellate ganglion block. C6 anterior tubercle is directly beneath the operator's index finger. The carotid artery is retracted laterally when necessary. The needle is perpendicular to all skin planes and is inserted directly posterior from the point of entry. *Inset,* The patient is positioned for stellate ganglion block. A pillow or roll should be placed between the shoulders to extend the neck, bring the esophagus to the midline, and facilitate palpation of Chassaignac's tubercle. (From Raj PP [ed]: Practical Management of Pain, 3rd ed. St Louis, Mosby, 2000, p 656.)

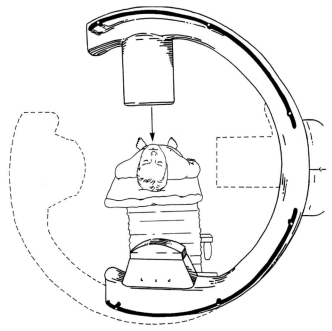

FIGURE 12–3

The patient lies supine. If the fluoroscope is used, the C-arm should visualize the C6–C7 vertebral region in the anteroposterior and lateral views.

(Fig. 12–3). With fluoroscopy correct placement of the needle should be demonstrated by anteroposterior and lateral views with spread of the contrast solution (Fig. 12–4*A* to *D*).

Final Injection

Once proper needle placement is confirmed, injection of medication must be performed in a routine and systematic fashion. A 50:50 mixture of 2% lidocaine with 0.5% ropivacaine and 1 mL of 40 mg/mL of triamcinolone may be used. An initial test dose must be injected in all cases. Less than 1 mL of solution injected IV has produced loss of consciousness and seizure activity. Before any injection, careful aspiration for blood and cerebrospinal fluid (CSF) must be performed. If the aspiration is negative, 0.5 to 1.0 mL of solution is administered, and the patient is asked to raise the thumb to indicate the absence of adverse symptoms. The patient should be informed beforehand and reminded during the blockade procedure that talking might cause movement of the neck musculature that could dislodge the needle from its proper location. To communicate during the block, the patient can be asked to point a thumb or finger upward in response to questions. After the initial test dose, the operator can inject the remainder of the solution, carefully aspirating after each 3 to 4 mL.

During injection or needle placement, paresthesia of the arm or hand may be elicited. It should always be interpreted to mean that the needle has been placed deeper to the anterior tubercle, adjacent to the C6 or C7 nerve root. Repositioning of the needle is necessary.

Aspiration of blood or CSF also demands repositioning of the needle. Even though the needle may be in the correct position, sometimes it is necessary to confirm that the injected solution is not flowing where it is not desired. The correct total volume of solution depends on what block is desired.[7] Properly placed, 5 mL of solution blocks the stellate ganglion.

C7 ANTERIOR APPROACH

The anterior approach to the stellate ganglion at C7 is similar to the approach described at C6. Unlike C6, C7 has only a vestigial tubercle, hence it is necessary to find Chassaignac's tubercle (C6). Then the palpating finger moves 1 fingerbreadth caudad from the inferior tip.

The advantage of blockade at C7 is manifested by the lower volume of local anesthetic needed to provide complete interruption of the upper extremity sympathetic innervation. Only 6 to 9 mL of solution suffices. The bothersome side effect of recurrent laryngeal nerve block is less common with this approach. The technique has two drawbacks: The less pronounced landmarks make needle positioning less reliable, and the risk of pneumothorax increases because the dome of the lung is close to the site of entry. The use of radiographic imaging during the approach helps avoid the complications possible with the blind technique.

CHEMICAL NEUROLYSIS OF STELLATE GANGLION

The approach for chemical neurolysis is similar to that for stellate ganglion block performed at C7. The patient must be positioned with the neck and head in a neutral position (see Fig. 12–6). Under direct anteroposterior fluoroscopy, the C7 vertebral body is identified. A skin wheal is raised over the ventrolateral aspect of the body of C7 with 1 mL of local anesthetic and a 25-gauge needle. A 22-gauge, B-bevel needle is inserted through the skin wheal to contact the body of C7 in the ventrolateral aspect. This is at the junction of the transverse process with the vertebral body. Depth and direction should be confirmed with both anteroposterior and lateral views. The needle tip is positioned deep to the anterior longitudinal ligament. The longus colli lies lateral to the needle tip. The needle should be stabilized with a long-handled Kelly clamp or hemostat. An IV extension should be attached to the needle and used for injection. Approximately 5 mL of water-soluble, nonirritating, nonionic, preservative-free, hypoallergenic contrast medium is injected after negative aspiration. Dye should spread around the vertebra, avoiding IV, epidural, intrathecal, thyroidal, or myoneural (longus colli) uptake. If good spread of the contrast medium is visualized, a mixture of local anesthetic, phenol, and steroid is injected. The total

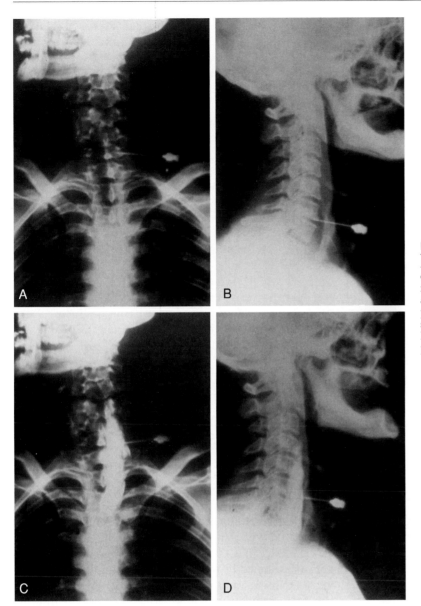

FIGURE 12–4

Anteroposterior and lateral views of correct placement of the needle and the contrast medium spread after injection for stellate ganglion block. Anteroposterior (A) and lateral (B) views of needle placement and anteroposterior (C) and lateral (D) views of contrast medium spread. (From Waldman SD [ed]: Interventional Pain Management, 2nd ed. Philadelphia, WB Saunders, 2001, p 367.)

volume of 5 mL should consist of 2.5 mL of 6% phenol in saline, 1 mL of 40-mg triamcinolone, and 1.5 mL of 0.5% ropivacaine. (The total 5-mL dose contains a final mixture of 3% phenol.) The previously injected contrast material serves as a marker for the spread of the phenol. In the anteroposterior view, the contrast should spread caudad to the first thoracic sympathetic ganglion, cephalad to the inferior cervical ganglion, and cephalad to the superior cervical ganglion. In the lateral view, spread should be observed in the retropharyngeal space and in front of the longus colli and anterior scalene muscles. After injection, the patient remains supine with the head elevated slightly for approximately 30 minutes to prevent spread of the phenol to other structures.[9]

RADIOFREQUENCY NEUROLYSIS

RF neurolysis of the stellate ganglion may be accomplished under fluoroscopic guidance. After the target area is identified as for chemical neurolysis, a 16-gauge angiocatheter is inserted through the skin wheal instead of the B-bevel needle. A 20-gauge, curved, blunt-tipped cannula with a 5-mm active tip is guided through the angiocatheter at the superolateral aspect. The tip should rest at the junction of the transverse process and the vertebral body. The depth and direction should be confirmed with anteroposterior and lateral views. Correct placement may be confirmed conclusively with the injection of contrast medium (Figs. 12–5 to 12–8). A sensory (50 Hz, 0.9 V) and a motor (2 Hz, 2 V)

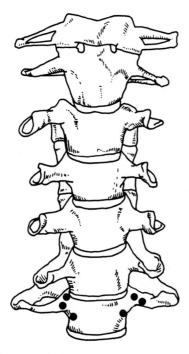

FIGURE 12–5

Drawing of a posteroanterior view of the cervical spine. *Dots* mark the target points for radiofrequency lesioning of the cervical sympathetic nerves. Note that these are at the junction of the medial aspect of the transverse process with the lateral aspect of its respective vertebral body.

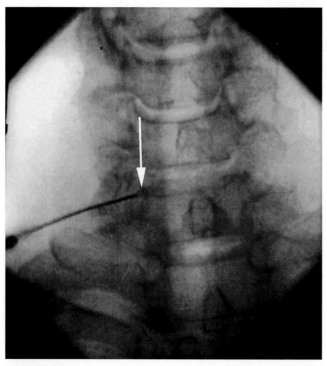

FIGURE 12–6

Posteroanterior radiograph of the cervical spine. Note that, at the C7 level, the radiofrequency cannula rests at the junction of the lateral aspect of the vertebral body and the medial aspect of the transverse process *(arrow)*. This represents the correct cannula position for lesioning of the C7 sympathetic fibers.

stimulation trial must be performed owing to the location of the phrenic nerve (lateral) and the recurrent laryngeal nerve (anterior and medial) relative to the proposed lesion. While motor stimulation is performed, the patient should say "ee" to ensure preservation of motor function. A small volume of local anesthetic (0.5 mL) should be injected before lesioning. The RF is applied for 60 seconds at 80°C. The cannula is then redirected to the most medial aspect of the transverse process in the same plane. Placement is in the ventral aspect of the transverse process in the same plane. Placement in the ventral aspect must be confirmed with a lateral view. Before lesioning, the patient must be retested for sensory and motor stimulation. A repeat dose of the local anesthetic should also be given through the cannula. A third (and final) lesion should be directed at the upper portion of the junction of the transverse process and the body of C7. Potential complications include injury to the phrenic or the recurrent laryngeal nerve, neuritis, and vertebral artery injury.[10, 11]

Side effects of a stellate ganglion block should be distinguished from complications. Most unpleasant side effects—ptosis, miosis, and nasal congestion—result from Horner's syndrome.

COMPLICATIONS

The two principal complications of stellate ganglion block are pneumothorax and intraspinal injection. A third risk when neurolysis is performed is the possibility of persistent Horner's syndrome. Pneumothorax can be avoided with careful placement of the needle, and, if care is taken that the needle angulation is never lateral and that the needle is advanced through the costotransverse ligaments (posterior and anterior) slowly and cautiously using the loss-of-resistance technique. Intraspinal injection most often occurs by diffusion through the intervertebral foramen and can be avoided by first injecting a water-soluble contrast dye and checking the needle position radiographically. The optimal method for checking needle position and solution spread is computed tomographic scan.

To check for possible subsequent Horner's syndrome, the clinician can first inject local anesthetic into the region and inspect the patient after 15 to 30 minutes. This practice does not always obviate Horner's syndrome with neurolytic injection, however, and prior local anesthetic injection may not be considered optimal in all situations.

Common complications of a stellate ganglion block result from diffusion of local anesthetic onto nearby nerve structures. These include the recurrent laryngeal nerve with complaints of hoarseness, feeling of a lump in the throat, and sometimes a subjective shortness of breath. Bilateral stellate blocks are rarely advised, because bilateral blocking of the recurrent laryngeal

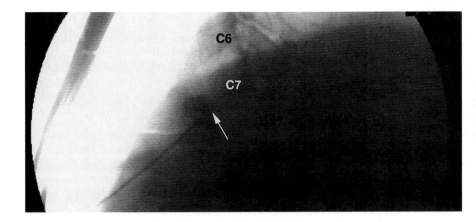

FIGURE 12–7

Lateral view of correct placement of the needle *(arrow)* and the contrast agent spread after injection for stellate ganglion block.

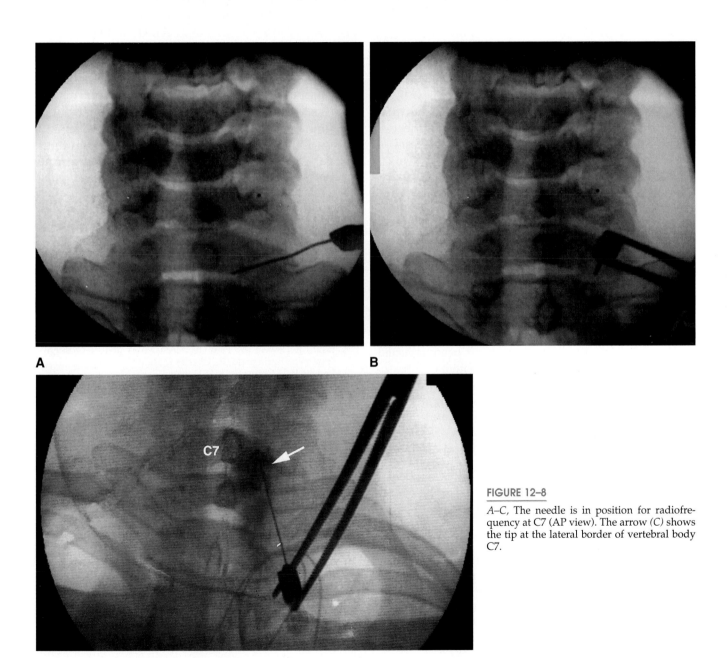

A

B

C

FIGURE 12–8

A–C, The needle is in position for radiofrequency at C7 (AP view). The arrow *(C)* shows the tip at the lateral border of vertebral body C7.

nerve can result in respiratory compromise and loss of laryngeal reflexes. Block of the phrenic nerve causes temporary paralysis of the diaphragm and can lead to respiratory embarrassment in patients whose respiratory reserve is already severely compromised. Partial brachial plexus block can also result secondary to spread along the prevertebral fascia[8] or positioning the needle too far posteriorly. The patient should be discharged with the arm in a sling and given careful instructions on how to care for a partially blocked arm, should this complication occur.

The two most feared complications of stellate ganglion block are intraspinal injection and seizures induced by intravascular injection. Respiratory embarrassment and the need for mechanical ventilation can result from injection into either the epidural space (if high concentrations of local anesthetic are used) or the intrathecal space. Should either occur, patients need continual reassurance that everything is being appropriately managed and that they will recover without sequelae. Some sedation is required while the local anesthetic wears off. No drugs are necessary for endotracheal cannulation, because profound anesthesia of the larynx can be expected.

IV injection most often involves the vertebral artery. Small amounts of local anesthetic cause unconsciousness, respiratory paralysis, seizures, and sometimes severe arterial hypotension. Increased IV fluids, vasopressors if indicated, oxygen, and endotracheal intubation may be necessary. If the amount of drug injected into the artery is less than 2 mL, the sequelae just listed are short-lived and self-limiting, with oxygen and increased fluid administration often being the only therapy needed. Care must be taken during a stellate ganglion block to ensure that no air is injected from the syringe. Cerebral air embolisms have been reported from this procedure, and they are preventable.[6, 12, 13]

The risk of pneumothorax also attends the anterior approach. If the C7 tubercle is used and the needle is inserted caudally, the dome of the lung can be penetrated. Unfortunately, some 10% to 15% of patients suffer postprocedure neuritis, which can last 3 to 6 weeks.[9, 14]

HELPFUL HINTS

Small amounts of local anesthetics (3 to 5 mL) do not reliably block all fibers to the upper extremities because contributions from T2 and T3 may be present. Injection of 10 mL of solution more reliably blocks all sympathetic innervation to the upper extremity, even in patients with the anomalous Kuntz's nerves. If blockade is being performed for sympathetic-mediated pain of the thoracic viscera, including the heart, 15 to 20 mL of solution should be administered.

Anomalous pathways, termed *Kuntz's nerves*, can be reliably blocked only by a posterior approach,[7] although the posterior approach is technically more difficult than the anterior approach taught traditionally.

EFFICACY

Sympathetic interruption to the head, supplied by the stellate ganglion, can easily be documented by evidence of Horner's syndrome: miosis (pinpoint pupil), ptosis (drooping of the upper eyelid), and enophthalmos (sinking of the eyeball). Associated findings include conjunctival injection, nasal congestion, and facial anhidrosis. These signs can be present without complete interruption of the sympathetic nerves to the upper extremity.

Evidence of sympathetic blockade to the upper extremity includes visible engorgement of the veins on the back of the hand and forearm, diminution of psychogalvanic reflex, and plethysmographic and thermographic changes. Skin temperature rises also, provided that the preblock temperature did not exceed 33°C to 34°C.

Stellate ganglion 64510; RFTC other nerve 64640.

REFERENCES

1. Kappis M: Weitere Erfahrungen mit der Sympathektomie. Klin Wehr 2:1441, 1923.
2. Brumm F, Mandl F: Die paravertebral Injektion zur Bekampfung visceraler Schmerzen. Wien Klin Aschsch 37:511, 1924.
3. White JC, Sweet W: Pain: Its Mechanisms and Neurosurgical Treatment. Springfield, IL, Charles C Thomas, 1955.
4. Leriche R: la Chirurgie de la Douleur. Paris, Masson et Cie, 1949.
5. Bonica JJ (ed): The Management of Pain. Philadelphia, Lea & Febiger, 1953.
6. Moore DC: Stellate Ganglion Block. Springfield, IL, Charles C Thomas, 1954.
7. Bonica JJ: Sympathetic Nerve Blocks for Pain Diagnosis and Therapy. New York, Breon Laboratories, 1984.
8. Cousins MJ, Bridenbaugh PO (eds): Neural Blockade in Clinical Anesthesia and Management of Pain, 2nd ed. Philadelphia, JB Lippincott, 1988.
9. Racz G: Techniques of Neurolysis. Boston, Kluwer Academic, 1989.
10. Wenger C, Christopher C: Radiofrequency lesions for the treatment of spinal pain. Pain Digest 8:1–16, 1998.
11. Sluijter ME: Radiofrequency Lesions in the Treatment of Cervical Pain Syndromes. Burlington, MA, Radionics, 1990, pp 1–19.
12. Moore DC: Regional Block, 4th ed. Springfield, IL, Charles C Thomas, 1975.
13. Adelman MH: Cerebral air embolism complicating stellate ganglion block. J Mt Sinai Hosp 15:28–30, 1948.
14. Skabelund C, Racz G: Indications and technique of thoracic neurolysis. Curr Rev Pain 3:400–405, 1999.

Atlanto-occipital Joint Block

13

HISTORY

A lateral approach to the atlanto-occipital joint block has been described by Dreyfuss and associates,[1, 2] who appear to use it with safety and facility.

ANATOMY

The atlas (C1) is unique in that it lacks a vertebral body and, instead, functions as a disc, or "relay center," between the occiput and C2. The cranial articular surfaces for the occiput are large and biconcave, complementing the occipital articular surfaces. The posterior arch lies deep under the skin, hence palpation is challenging. The anterior and posterior arches form the triangular spinal foramen that accommodates the brain stem. The transverse processes are long and perforated, accommodating the passage of the vertebral arteries through the transverse foramina. After exiting these transverse foramina, they course through grooves that can be observed posterior to the lateral masses. These grooves, or occasional tunnels, accommodate the vertebral arteries as they loop for a second time in the upper cervical region (Fig. 13–1). Bone changes can occur here that have the potential to compromise vertebral artery function and promote symptoms associated with vertebral basilar insufficiency.[3] The architecture at these grooves is different in men and in women; as a consequence, women may be more susceptible to arterial compromise.[4]

Noteworthy is the location of the accessory nerve nuclei, found in the spinal cord between C1 and C4.[5] Patients who suffer from chronic upper cervical conditions may experience increased tone in their upper trapezius muscles ("tight traps") secondary to sensitization and reorganization of interneurons at those same levels. This reorganization sensitizes the cranial

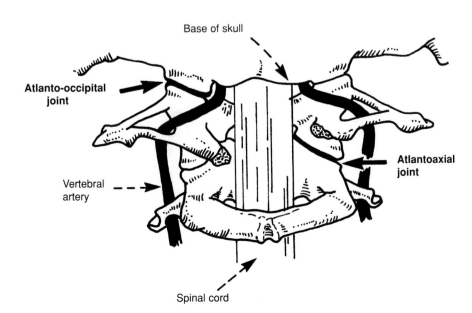

Base of skull

Atlanto-occipital joint

Atlantoaxial joint

Vertebral artery

Spinal cord

FIGURE 13–1

Anatomy of the atlanto-occipital joint. Note that (1) the anterior and posterior arches form the triangular spinal foramen, and (2) the transverse processes are long and perforated, with the vertebral arteries traversing through them.

nerve nuclei, increasing the efferent signals to the trapezius. A similar condition can arise from the trigeminal nuclei in the spinal cord between C1 and C4.[5] Chronic afferents from the cervical spine can also sensitize these cranial nerve nuclei, resulting in chronic headache in the cutaneous trigeminal distribution.[6] Note that the vertebral artery at this level lies lateral to the atlantoaxial articulation as it courses through the C1 and C2 foramina.

INDICATIONS

Deep suboccipital pain that is movement related can be one of the most elusive pains to diagnose and to treat. Busch and Wilson[7] used intracapsular injection of local anesthetic and steroid for suboccipital pain instead of putting the patient's head in a neurosurgical frame to immobilize it entirely.[8] Theoretically, once the motion ceases, the pain responds favorably to the stabilization of the fusion. Most patients, however, prefer repeat injections in the hope that the anti-inflammatory effect of injections will "settle the disease down" and limit pain from the swollen joint.[9]

Another indication is for headaches and pain caused by isolated injury to the atlanto-occipital and atlantoaxial joints. This is especially true when the pain is occipital or suboccipital and is exacerbated by the neck movements typically associated with these joints.[9]

CONTRAINDICATIONS

- Local infection
- Coagulopathy
- Cervical vertebrae/spine instability

EQUIPMENT

- 25-gauge, ¾-inch infiltration needle
- 22-gauge, 3½-inch spinal needle
- 3-mL syringe
- 1-mL syringe
- IV T-piece extension

DRUGS

- 1.5% lidocaine for infiltration
- 2% lidocaine preservative free
- 0.5% levobupivacaine/ropivacaine
- Iohexol (Omnipaque 240) radiographic contrast medium

PREPARATION OF THE PATIENT

PHYSICAL EXAMINATION

When rotation is performed at the end of the range of protraction or retraction, the segment most likely to be painful is C1–C2. On the other hand, when side bending is performed at the end of the range of protraction or retraction, the joint most likely affected is C0–C1.

A limitation of motion at the C0–C1 or C1–C2 segments renders the upper cervical spine incapable of compensating for coupling at cervical disc segments. This can manifest itself in a number of "deviated" patterns during active cervical motions.[10]

Nodding the head from a position of end-range cervical axial rotation allows assessment of the range of upper cervical spine flexion. It is primarily the C0–C1 segments that perform this movement; thus, a lesion at this level could cause pain or limitations of motion during this test.

LABORATORY

No special laboratory tests are required.

PREOPERATIVE MEDICATION

For preoperative medication, use the standard American Society of Anesthesiologists' (ASA) recommendations for conscious sedation.

MONITORING

Since this procedure is performed in the prone position, standard ASA monitoring is recommended.

PROCEDURE

POSITION OF THE PATIENT

The patient is placed in prone position with the neck slightly flexed; the fluoroscope is rotated in a caudal-cephalad direction to open up the atlanto-occipital joint (Fig. 13–2). The posterior approach to the atlanto-occipital and atlantoaxial joints is commonly used because of the safety it affords. Place several blankets under the chest to allow the head to be slightly flexed.

The fluoroscope C-arm approaches the table from the head in an anteroposterior direction. It is then rotated in the sagittal plane so that the beam passes from the anterosuperior aspect to the posteroinferior aspect (see Fig. 13–2).[11] This rotation is done under fluoroscopic visualization until the atlanto-occipital joint is visualized.

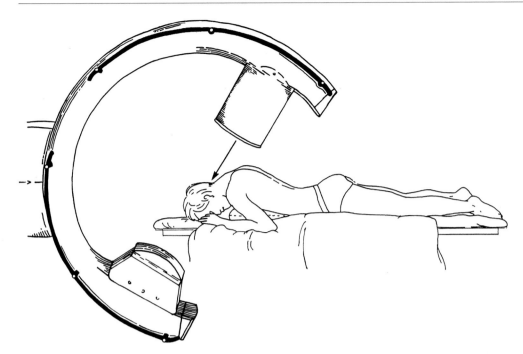

FIGURE 13–2
The drawing shows the position of the patient (prone) with neck flexed and support under the upper chest. The C-arm of the fluoroscope is turned from posteroanterior view to posteroinferior aspect.

TECHNIQUE OF NEEDLE ENTRY

The skin is prepared and draped in the usual sterile fashion, and a skin wheal is raised with local anesthetic at the insertion site. One can use a 22-gauge spinal needle to perform this procedure. For reasons of safety, an introducer needle is preferred to break the skin and direct the thinner block needle. A "through-the-eye-of-the-needle" or "gun barrel" technique is used, allowing the x-ray beam to define the course of the needle. The introducer needle, appearing as a small point on the screen (Fig. 13–3), is placed and directed toward the

posterolateral aspect of the atlanto-occipital joint. The vertebral artery lies medial to this facet, having passed from lateral to medial below it.

Generally speaking, the introducer needle's limited length prevents its entering the foramen magnum. If the atlanto-occipital joint is entered, a distinctive "pop" almost always is felt.

The C-arm can then be rotated to the horizontal plane, and the needle can be seen to have entered the joint (Fig. 13–4). The atlanto-occipital joint is anterior to the posterolateral columns of the spinal cord.[9] At this point the C-arm is turned lateral (Fig. 13–5). The

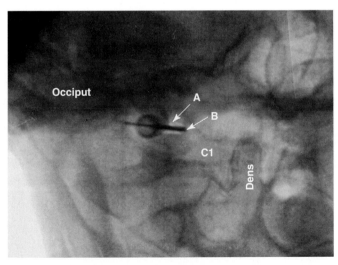

A

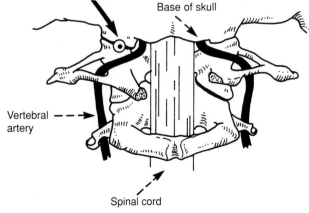

Needle in tunnel view position (atlanto-occipital joint)

Base of skull

Vertebral artery

Spinal cord

B

FIGURE 13–3

A, In a radiographic slightly oblique view, one can see the needle tip entering the atlanto-occipital joint. The following is a key to the letters shown on the figure: A, atlanto-occipital joint; B, needle tip in the atlanto-occipital joint. *B,* A drawing of posteroanterior (oblique) view of the atlanto-occipital joint showing the needle insertion in a tunneled view.

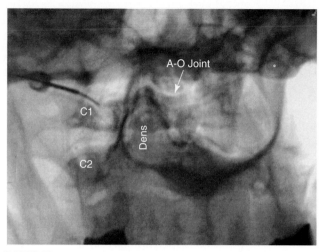

FIGURE 13–4

In the radiographic posteroanterior view, the needle is seen entering the atlanto-occipital (A-O) joint. Note the identification of atlanto-occipital joint on the opposite side.

fluoroscopic image then further confirms the needle in the atlanto-occipital joint (Fig. 13–6).

After removal of the stylet, and aspiration results prove negative, 1 mL of iohexol is injected under fluoroscopy using a flexible T-piece connected to the spinal needle (Fig. 13–7).

INJECTION OF CONTRAST AGENT AND ITS INTERPRETATION

With good placement, the classic bilateral concave dye pattern is seen on lateral fluoroscopic view, representing the dye's lining of the joint capsule (see Fig. 13–7). It is not uncommon, in the presence of trauma, for the dye to penetrate the torn capsule and enter the cervical epidural space.

Venous runoff of dye almost always heralds placement of the needle outside the joint, which is surrounded by a rich venous plexus. In the presence of

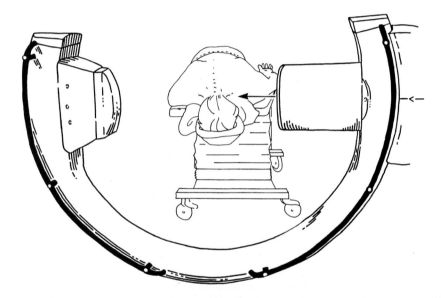

FIGURE 13–5

A drawing of the C-arm in the lateral position.

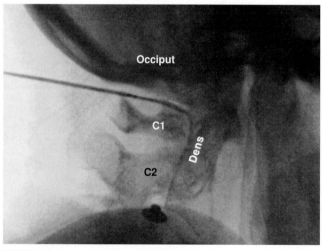

FIGURE 13–6

The lateral fluoroscopic image of the needle in correct position in the atlanto-occipital joint.

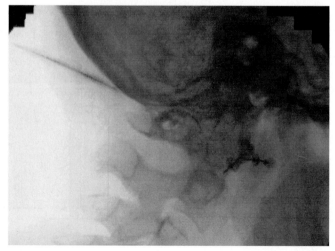

FIGURE 13–7

The lateral fluoroscopic image shows contrast agent spread after injection in the atlanto-occipital joint.

venous runoff or spread of dye into the epidural space, the injection is stopped, and either the needle is redirected (in the case of venous runoff) or the block is abandoned. Biplanar views are again checked before injection of local anesthetic to ensure safe and appropriate placement of the needle. If the dye spread remains circumscribed and the joint is outlined as described earlier, 1 to 1.5 mL of 0.2% ropivacaine with 20 mg of triamcinolone is slowly injected.[9]

HYALGAN INJECTION

Usually 1 mL of local anesthetic with steroid injected after negative aspiration for diagnostic and therapeutic block. Recently, hyaluronate sodium (Hyalgan), 1 mL, a lubricant used for knee injection, has also been employed. If helpful, this injection is repeated three to five times.

POSTPROCEDURE MONITORING

Brief periods of ataxia in the immediate postblock period have been noted by us and others.[7, 9] This ataxia may be secondary to the reproduction of pain by joint distention or by the absorption of local anesthetic into either the vertebral arteries or the valveless venous plexus that is posterior to the facets. Patients are therefore observed for approximately 30 minutes before discharge.[9]

COMPLICATIONS

Complications of atlanto-occipital blocks include epidural and intrathecal injections and intravascular injections into the adjacent venous plexus, vertebral artery, and possibly the carotid artery. Although only a small amount of local anesthetic is injected, its proximity to the brain ensures a higher intracranial concentration than would be anticipated, and it is possible for symptoms common to local anesthetic central nervous system toxicity to result.[9]

HELPFUL HINTS

The physician doing the procedure must avoid placing a needle into the brain stem or the vertebral artery and injecting either air or particulate matter such as precipitated steroids.

EFFICACY

No randomized, controlled, double-blind studies can be found. Efficacy can be based on individual anecdotal patient pain relief.

REFERENCES

1. Dreyfuss P, Michaelsen M, Fletcher D: Atlanto-occipital and lateral atlanto-axial joint pain patterns. Spine 19:1125–1131, 1994.
2. Dreyfuss P, Rogers J, Dreyer S, Fletcher D: Atlanto-occipital joint pain: A report of three cases and description of an intra-articular joint block technique [abstract]. Reg Anesth 19:344–351, 1994.
3. Aboumadwi A, Solanki G, Casey ATH, Crockard HA: Variation of the groove in the axis vertebra for the vertebral artery: Implications for instrumentation. J Bone Joint Surg Br 79:820–823, 1997.
4. Ebraheim NA, Xu RM, Ahmad M, Heck B: The quantitative anatomy of the vertebral artery groove of the atlas and its relation to the posterior atlantoaxial approach. Spine 23:320–323, 1998.
5. Oostendorp R: [Functional Vertebrobasilar Insufficiency] [thesis]. University of Nijmegen, Netherlands, 1988.
6. Gawel MJ, Rothbart PJ: Occipital nerve block in the management of headache and cervical pain. Cephalalgia 12:9–13, 1992.
7. Busch E, Wilson P: Atlanto-occipital and altantoaxial injections in the treatment of headache and neck pain. Reg Anesth 14:45, 1989.
8. Taylor JR, Finch P: Acute injury of the neck: Anatomical and pathological basis of pain. Ann Acad Med Singapore 22:187–192, 1993.
9. Racz GB, Sanel H, Diede JH: Atlanto-occipital and atlantoaxial injections in the treatment of headache and neck pain. In Waldman S, Winnie A (eds): Interventional Pain Management. Philadelphia, WB Saunders, 1996, pp 220–222.
10. Jirout J: Funktionelle Pathologie und Klinik der Wirbelsaule. Stuttgart, Gustav Fischer, 1990.
11. Ballinger P (ed): Merrill's Atlas of Radiographic Positions and Radiographic Procedures, 6th ed. St. Louis, CV Mosby, 1986, pp 238–243.

14 Atlantoaxial Joint Block

HISTORY

A lateral approach to the atlantoaxial joint block has been described by Dreyfuss and associates,[1, 2] who appear to use it with safety and facility.

ANATOMY

The axis, or C2, is most characterized by the dens, which looks like an asparagus spear projecting craniad from the front of the bony segment. With the dens, or odontoid process, C2 forms a pivot around which C1 and the head turn (Fig. 14–1).[3]

The anterior atlantoaxial (or atlantodental) joint is interposed between the dens and the anterior arch of

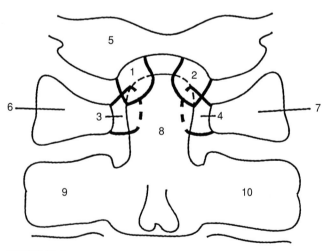

FIGURE 14–1

This posterior view of the atlanto-occipital and atlantoaxial joints shows the attachments of the alar ligaments. The following is a key to the numbers shown on the figure: 1, left occipital alar ligament; 2, right occipital alar ligament; 3, left atlantoalar ligament; 4, right atlantoalar ligament; 5, occiput; 6, left C1; 7, right C1; 8, dens; 9, left C2; 10, right C2. (Courtesy of the International Academy of Orthopedic Medicine—US.)

the atlas. Posterior to the dens is the joint between the dens and the transverse ligament of the atlas (TLA), the lower component of the cruciform ligament, which can also be interpreted as the bursa atlantodentalis.[3] From a sagittal view, the lateral atlantoaxial joint is biconvex on both the left and the right side, and its convexities are accentuated by increased thickness in articular cartilage (1.4 to 3.2 mm). These incongruences are accommodated by large, intra-articular menisci that emerge from flaccid, roomy joint capsules. The menisci are subject to degradation, producing interposition with rotation between C1 and C2 and resulting in sharp, local, catching pain. These four systems allow for flexion, extension, and rotation but afford very little lateral bending. Virtually no axial separation is allowed between C1 and C2, owing to the strong stabilizing influence of the TLA on a normally configured dens.

The TLA courses between lateral masses of C2 behind the dens, precluding any separation between C1 and C2 (Fig. 14–2). Additionally, this ligament prevents posterior tipping of the dens into the brain stem and spinal cord during forward flexion of the head, which could cause the patient to have a "drop attack." Compromise to this ligament, for example, after a whiplash injury, puts the brain stem and cord at risk for compression by the dens during normal flexion.

The vertebral artery at this level lies lateral to the atlantoaxial articulation as it courses through the C1 and C2 foramina membrane (Fig. 14–3).

The atlantoaxial joint has the widest range of motion of all articulations in the neck. Motion at C1–C2 is limited to anterior and posterior rocking (20 degrees[4]) and rotation, without allowing any side bending. Rotation around an axis coursing through the dens is limited to 40 to 45 degrees to each side.[5–9] The odontoid process permits stable rotation and allows 5 to 10 degrees of flexion and 10 degrees of extension.[5, 10] With rightward rotation, the right facet of C1 translates posterior to the right facet of C2 and the left C1 facet anterior

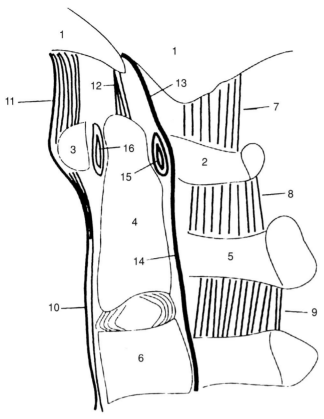

FIGURE 14–2

The relationship between the AA and AO joint is illustrated in this sagittal view. The following is a key to the numbers shown on the figure: 1, occiput; 2, posterior arch of atlas; 3, anterior arch of atlas; 4, dens; 5, posterior arch of C2; 6, vertebral body of C3; 7, posterior atlanto-occipital membrane; 8, ligamentum flavum C1–C2; 9, ligamentum flavum C2–C3; 10, anterior longitudinal ligament; 11, anterior atlanto-occipital membrane; 12, apical ligament of atlas; 13, tectorial membrane; 14, posterior longitudinal ligament; 15, transverse ligament of atlas; 16, synovial space between the dens and anterior arch of atlas. (Courtesy of the International Academy of Orthopedic Medicine—US.)

to left C2. Additionally, C1 demonstrates slight caudal translation on C1, owing to the convex-convex relationships of the C1–C2 zygapophyseal joints.

INDICATIONS

OCCIPITAL HEADACHE

Although we have rarely seen pain caused by isolated injury to the atlanto-occipital and atlantoaxial joints, injecting them may have a place in the treatment of some patients' headaches. This is especially true when the pain is occipital or suboccipital and is exacerbated by the neck movements typically associated with these joints.[10]

PAIN OF C1–C2 ROTATION

A patient with C1–C2 hypomobility is often unable to perform a pure lateral bending motion, in one or both directions. For instance, if leftward rotation is limited at the C1–C2 segment, the patient cannot bend the cervical spine to the right side while keeping the eyes in the frontal plane. Instead, rightward bending is coupled with rightward rotation.

When rotation is performed at the end of the range of protraction or retraction and it is painful, the segment most likely affected is C1–C2.

Although loss of motion can be subtle in patients with severe atlantoaxial osteoarthritis, Star and colleagues[11] reported severe limitations (>50%) of axial rotation and lateral bending of the cervical spine. Radiography demonstrated lateral mass degeneration in all of their patients.

Dreyfuss and coworkers reported that the C1–C2 joint pain referral pattern is small and rather localized in the suboccipital region.[1]

CONTRAINDICATIONS

Absolute
- Local infections
- Previous surgical fusion
- Previous cervical surgery

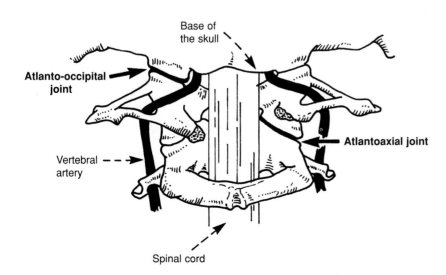

FIGURE 14–3

Anatomy of the atlantoaxial joint. Note that the vertebral artery lies lateral to the atlantoaxial joint.

Relative

- Arnold-Chiari syndrome
- Metastasis of cervical vertebral body
- Fracture of the dens
- Abnormal bleeding disorders

EQUIPMENT

- 25-gauge, ¾-inch infiltration needle
- 22-gauge, 3½-inch spinal needle
- 18-gauge introducer needle
- Flexible IV T-piece extension

DRUGS

- 1.5% lidocaine for skin infiltration
- 1 mL of iohexol (Omnipaque 240) radiographic contrast solution
- 20 mg of triamcinolone diacetate
- 1 to 1.5 mL of 0.2% ropivacaine or 0.25% bupivacaine
- Hyaluronate sodium (Hyalgan) (optional)

PREPARATION OF THE PATIENT

PHYSICAL EXAMINATION

Active range of motion of the cervical spine is generally performed to provoke the patient's symptoms and to assess limitation of motion. Pain provocation can be isolated to, or emphasized in, the upper cervical spine by means of testing rotation or lateral bending from a position of protraction and retraction. The flexion and exten-

sion of the C0–C2 segment are greatest during retraction and protraction, respectively.[4] Thus, an affliction of these segments is more accurately elicited by protraction or retraction rather than by general extension or flexion of the entire cervical spine.

LABORATORY

No laboratory studies are required in a typical patient.

PREOPERATIVE MEDICATION

For preoperative medication, use the standard American Society of Anesthesiologists' (ASA) recommendations for conscious sedation.

MONITORING

For monitoring, use the standard ASA monitoring recommendations.

PROCEDURE

POSITION OF THE PATIENT

The patient is placed in a prone position with several blankets positioned under the chest to allow the head to be slightly flexed. The fluoroscopy C-arm is positioned at the table from the head in an anteroposterior direction. It is then rotated in the sagittal plane so that the beam passes from the anterosuperior aspect to the posteroinferior aspect (Fig. 14–4).[5] This rotation is done under fluoroscopic visualization until the atlantoaxial joint is visualized.

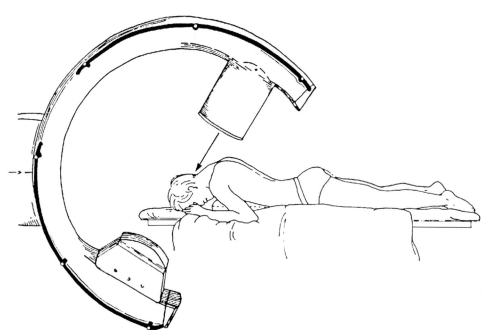

FIGURE 14–4

The drawing shows the positions of the patient and the C-arm to view the atlantoaxial joint optimally.

The skin is prepared and draped in the usual sterile fashion, and a skin wheal is raised with local anesthetic at the insertion site. The beam is placed for an antero-posterior view to identify the foramen magnum and the atlas. The introducer needle is directed at the postero-lateral aspect of the atlantoaxial joint, because the C2 ganglion lies at the middle point of the space. The needle is advanced in the anterior and medial direction until it enters the joint cavity, when a distinctive "pop" is felt (Fig. 14–5). The lateral view demonstrates the tip of the needle in the middle of the joint (Figs. 14–6 and 14–7).[9, 13] One milliliter of nonionic, water-soluble contrast agent (iohexol) is injected after negative aspiration for blood or cerebrospinal fluid (Fig. 14–8). The image should demonstrate the bilateral concavity of the joint, and the dye should remain confined to the joint space. If the dye remains circumscribed, 1 to 1.5 mL of 0.2% ropivacaine with 20 mg of triamcinolone is slowly injected.

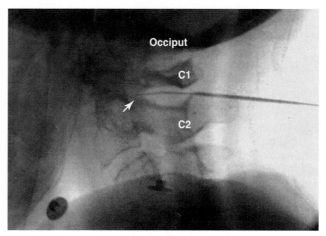

FIGURE 14–7

The radiographic lateral view of the needle placement (*arrow*) in the atlantoaxial joint.

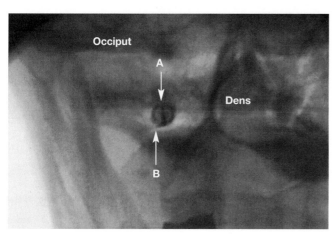

FIGURE 14–5

The radiographic posteroanterior view of the atlantoaxial joint with the needle placed in the right atlantoaxial joint (tunnel view). The following is a key to the letters shown on the figure: A, hub of the needle; B, atlantoaxial joint.

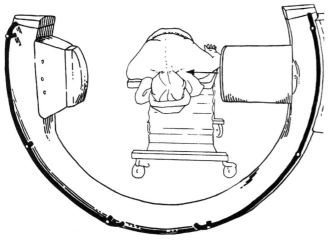

FIGURE 14–6

The drawing shows the C-arm in a lateral position for viewing of the atlantoaxial joint.

It is not uncommon for the patient to experience an exacerbation of the occipital headache during the injection.[1, 10]

INJECTION OF CONTRAST AGENT AND ITS INTERPRETATION

When injecting the contrast agent, it is not uncommon for the solution to penetrate the torn capsule and enter the cervical epidural space. Venous run-off of the contrast agent almost always heralds placement of the needle outside the joint, which is surrounded by a rich venous plexus. In the presence of venous run-off or spread of contrast agent into the epidural space, the injection is stopped, and either the needle is redirected (in the case of venous run-off) or the block is abandoned.

INJECTION OF DRUGS

After needle position is confirmed in the atlantoaxial joint, 1 mL of 0.2% ropivacaine or 1 mL of 1% lidocaine is injected after negative aspiration. In addition, 40 mg of triamcinolone diacetate in 1 mL can be added if the initial test dose is negative for vascular or spinal/intracranial injection. Another alternative is to inject 1 mL of hyaluronate sodium instead of steroids for prolongation of benefits. No neurolytic solutions are recommended.

COMPLICATIONS

Brief periods of ataxia in the immediate postblock period have been noted.[9, 10] This ataxia may be secondary to the reproduction of pain by joint distention or by absorption of local anesthetic into either the

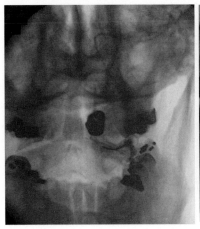

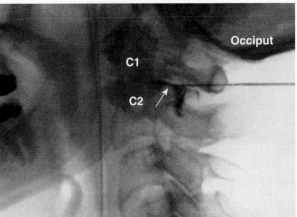

A **B**

FIGURE 14–8

A, The radiographic image shows the spread of the contrast agent from the atlantoaxial joint injection. *B,* The radiographic image shows the spillover of the contrast agent after injection in the atlantoaxial joint.

vertebral arteries or the valveless venous plexus that is posterior to the facets.

Complications of atlanto-occipital and atlantoaxial blocks include epidural and intrathecal injections and intravascular injections into the adjacent venous plexus, vertebral artery, and possibly the carotid artery. Although only a small amount of local anesthetic is injected, its proximity to the brain ensures a higher intracranial concentration than would be anticipated, and it is possible that symptoms common to local anesthetic central nervous system toxicity may occur.

HELPFUL HINTS

The physician doing the procedure must avoid placing a needle into the brain stem or the vertebral artery and injecting either air or particulate matter such as precipitated steroids. Therefore, it is strongly urged that the procedure be carried out by clinicians who are experienced in working under fluoroscopic guidance and who recognize the three-dimensional hazards of placing a needle so close to the foramen magnum and the brain stem.

EFFICACY

Only anecdotal reports of benefits from this procedure have been noted. No patient-controlled, double-blind studies are available.

REFERENCES

1. Dreyfuss P, Michaelsen M, Fletcher D: Atlanto-occipital and lateral atlantoaxial joint pain patterns. Spine 19:1125–1131, 1994.
2. Dreyfuss P, Rogers J, Dreyer S, Fletcher D: Atlanto-occipital joint pain: A report of three cases and description of an intra-articular joint block technique [abstract]. Reg Anesth 19:344–351, 1994.
3. Winkel D, Aufdemkampe G, Matthijs O, et al: Cervical spine: Functional anatomy. In Diagnosis and Treatment of the Spine: Nonoperative Orthopaedic Medicine and Manual Therapy. Gaithersburg, MD, Aspen, 1996, pp 546–558.
4. Ordway NP, Seymour RJ, Donelson RG, et al: Cervical flexion, extension, protrusion, and retraction: A radiographic segmental analysis. Spine 24:240–247, 1999.
5. Bogduk N: The clinical anatomy of the cervical dorsal rami. Spine 7:319–330, 1982.
6. Jofe M, White A, Panjabi M: Clinically relevant kinematics of the cervical spine. In Sherk H, Dunn E, Eismont F, et al (eds): The Cervical Spine, 2nd ed. Philadelphia, JB Lippincott, 1989, pp 57–69.
7. Worth DR, Selvik G: Movements of the craniovertebral joints. In Grieve GP (ed): Modern Manual Therapy of the Vertebral Column. London, Churchill Livingstone, 1987, pp 53–63.
8. Panjabi MM: Three-dimensional movements of the upper cervix spine. Spine 13:726–728, 1988.
9. Penning L: Normal movements of the cervical spine. AJR Am J Roentgenol 130:317–326, 1979.
10. Racz GB, Sanel H, Diede JH: Atlanto-occipital and atlantoaxial injections in the treatment of headache and neck pain. In Waldman S, Winnie A (eds): Interventional Pain Management. Philadelphia, WB Saunders, 1996, pp 220–222.
11. Star MJ, Curd JG, Thorne RP: Atlantoaxial lateral mass osteoarthritis: A frequently overlooked cause of severe occipitocervical pain. Spine 17(Suppl):71–76, 1992.

C H A P T E R

15

Cervical Facets Median Branch Block and Radiofrequency Thermocoagulation

HISTORY

Cervical facet joints have gained the attention of clinicians owing to the implications of a cervical origin for headache. Explanation of the cervical facet joints in headache can, in part, be attributed to Pawl in 1971.[1] Similar publications can be found dating as far back as 1940 with Hadden,[2] 1948 with Raney and Raney,[3] 1962 with Tarem and Kahn,[4] and finally 1967 with Brain and Wilkinson[5] and 1973 with McNab[6] and Mehta.[7]

ANATOMY

The apophyseal articulations are formed by the superior articular facet of one vertebra and the inferior articular facet of the adjacent vertebra above (Fig. 15–1). The articular surfaces of the facets are covered by hyaline cartilage. The joints are lined by synovium and, where the surfaces of the facets are not in contact, tabs of synovial tissue project into the joint from the joint margins.[8] The fibrous joint capsule forms superior and inferior joint recesses that may contain small synovial villi.[9] The inferior and posterior portions of the recesses are larger, allowing a wide range of motion. Medially and anteriorly, the capsule blends with the ligamentum flavum and is adjacent to the neural foramen and the nerve root.

The joint capsule is richly innervated.[8, 10–13] Each dorsal ramus sends branches to the facet joint at its own level and to the level below (Fig. 15–2). Consequently, each posterior ramus innervates two facet joints, and each facet joint has innervation from two levels.

The articular facets in the cervical spine extend laterally from the junction of the lamina and pedicles and are oriented in the coronal plane to permit flexion, extension, and lateral bending.

The C2–C3 through C5–C6 facet joints are angled 35 degrees from the coronal plane. The C6–C7 joint is in

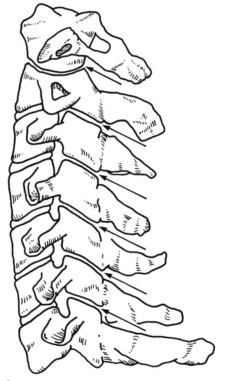

FIGURE 15–1

Cervical facets, lateral view (*arrows* indicate facets).

transition between the orientation of the C5–C6 facet joint and that of C7–T1, which is tipped 22 degrees from the coronal plane.[13, 14] All of the cervical facet joints from C2–C3 caudad to C7–T1 are angled 110 degrees from the midline posterior sagittal plane. This makes their orientation very much like that of the thoracic facet joints, only not quite as close to the vertical plane. The cervical facet joints play a physically larger role in the spinal articular tripod structure and are actually best described as the superior and inferior ends of articular pillars. Also unique to the cervical spine is the vertebral artery,

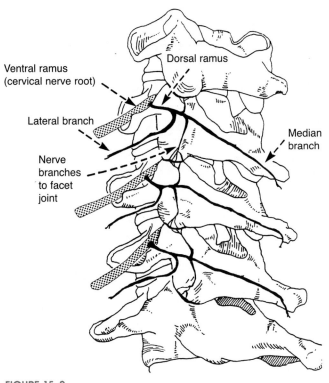

Ventral ramus
(cervical nerve root)

Dorsal ramus

Lateral branch

Nerve
branches
to facet
joint

Median
branch

FIGURE 15–2
Oblique view of cervical spine (C3–C7).

which passes through the transverse foramen of the transverse processes of the C6–C1 vertebrae.[15]

Given this description, the facet joints appear anatomically designed to limit excessive mobility and distribute axial loading over a broad area. They help resist the shearing motion produced by forward bending and the compression produced by rotation.[16]

The C2–C3 facet joint is innervated mainly by the large third occipital nerve, which is one of the two median branches of the C3 dorsal ramus, and to some degree also by the C2 dorsal rami.[16–18] The C2 dorsal ramus has five branches. The median branch is commonly known as the greater occipital nerve. There are several communicating branches between the dorsal branches of C1, C2, and C3, which may play a role in the anatomic basis for cervicogenic headaches. Unfortunately, there are no reliable radiologic coordinates for the C2 dorsal ramus, since it runs in the soft tissue dorsal to the C2 lamina. Because there are eight cervical nerves but only seven cervical vertebrae, the first seven cervical nerve roots exit the spine above the vertebral body whose "number" they share. Therefore, the C3 nerve root exits via the intervertebral foramen between the C2 and C3 vertebral bodies. The C3 dorsal ramus curves dorsally through the intertransverse space.

Two median branches usually arise separately from the C3 dorsal ramus. The superior and larger branch is the third occipital nerve (also known as the *superficial*

median branch), and the inferior branch is the deep median branch. The third occipital nerve curves dorsally and medially around the superior articular process of the C3 vertebra. It crosses the C2–C3 facet joint either just below or across the joint margin. The innervation of the C2–C3 facet joint may come from the third occipital nerve and an articular nerve that branches off the dorsal ramus itself. Because the C2–C3 facet innervation is complex, the practical implication is that blocking the third occipital nerve on the C3 articular process will denervate this joint (see Fig. 15–2).[19] The deep median branch of the C3 dorsal ramus is parallel but caudad to the third occipital nerve in the C3 articular pillar. The location of this nerve on the articular pillar is essentially the same as those of nerve C4–C8.

The C3–C4 to C7–T1 facet joints are supplied by the median branches of the cervical posterior rami at the same level and from the segmental level above.[15, 17] Therefore, the C3–C4 facet is innervated by the C3 and C4 median branch nerves. These nerves arise from the posterior primary rami in the cervical intertransverse spaces and then curve dorsally and medially to wrap around the waist of their respective articular pillars. As they start to wrap around the articular pillars, the nerves are 2.2 mm (C3) to 1.2 mm (C7) in vertical extent.[20] They are also 7.3 mm (C3) to 5.5 mm (C7) caudad to the tip of the superior articular pillar at this location. The median branches are bound to the periosteum by an investing fascia and are held against the articular pillars by tendons of the semispinalis capitis.[16, 17, 19] The median branches are seen on a lateral view of the cervical spine to pass through the "waist" of the articular pillar (see Fig. 15–2). Rostral and caudal branches from each nerve then pass into the joints immediately above and below. The C7 median branch crosses the root of the C7 transverse process and therefore lies higher on the lateral projection of the C7 articular pillar.[21]

INDICATIONS

Patients with cervical pain may have progressive facet joint arthritis and may develop vertical, lateral, and rotatory subluxation of the odontoid process with lateral mass collapse. This often causes neurologic deterioration as well as pain.[17] Whiplash injuries of the cervical spine causing muscle ligamentous sprains of the cervical facet joints with periosteal tearing have also been suggested as the most common cause of neck pain and nerve root irritation. In fact, recent research strongly suggests that for 50% to 60% of patients with neck pain after whiplash injury, the cervical facet joints are the primary source of pain. There is also growing evidence that the upper cervical spine (C1–C3), including the facet joints, contributes significantly to neck and head pain of cervicogenic headaches.

CONTRAINDICATIONS

- Local infection
- Coagulopathy

EQUIPMENT

- 22-gauge, 2-inch B-bevel needle
- 25-gauge, ¾-inch infiltration needle
- 3-mL syringe
- 10-mL syringe
- IV T-piece
- 19-gauge needle

Radiofrequency

- 5- or 10-cm curved Racz-Finch radiofrequency thermocoagulation (RFTC) needle with 10-mm active tip
- 20-gauge IV catheter

DRUGS

- 1% lidocaine for infiltration
- 2% lidocaine
- 0.25% bupivacaine or 0.2% ropivacaine
- Steroids (dexamethasone or triamcinolone diacetate)

PREPARATION OF THE PATIENT

PHYSICAL EXAMINATION

The clinical criteria for facet syndrome are nonspecific and still unreliable. Intra-articular facet injections or median branch blocks should be reserved for patients with no neurologic deficit, when no other cause for their chronic pain can be identified. Also, the pain should be unresponsive to simpler therapies such as rest during acute exacerbations and oral medications, including nonsteroidal anti-inflammatory drugs. The facets to be blocked can be identified by physical examination and analysis of the patient's symptoms. If the patient has marked tenderness to palpation over a particular facet joint or if pain increases with motion or loading of the joint, trial blockade of the joint should be considered.

For cervical facet joints, distinctive upper, lower, and pancervical neck pain syndromes have been described.[15] The pain is described as deep and aching.[22] It extends beyond the immediate vicinity of the joint and, therefore, is to some degree referred pain. Pain from the atlanto-occipital joint (C0–C1) is referred unilaterally to the suboccipital area.[23] Pain from the atlantoaxial joint (C1–C2) is described as unilateral, focused at the occipitocervical junction, and radiating to the postauricular region. There may be associated physical signs, such as limited head rotation, tender trigger points confined to the occipital area, palpable cervical crepitus, and abnormal head position. Pain from the C2–C3 facet joint pattern is located in the upper cervical region and extends at least to the occiput and sometimes into the head, toward the ear, vertex, forehead, or eye.[22, 25, 26] The C3–C4 facet joint produces pain over the posterolateral cervical region, following the course of the levator scapulae muscle. It extends craniad as far as the suboccipital region and then caudad over the posterolateral aspect of the neck without entering the region of the shoulder girdle. The C4–C5 facet joint pain involves a triangular area, its two sides consisting of the posterior midline and posterolateral border of the neck and its base running parallel to the spine of the scapula muscle. It extends craniad as far as the suboccipital region and then caudad over the posterolateral aspect of the neck without entering the region of the shoulder girdle. The C5–C6 facet joint produces pain in a triangular distribution with the apex directed toward the midcervical region posteriorly, the main area draped over the top of the shoulder girdle, both front and back, and the base coinciding with the spine of the scapula. The C6–C7 facet joint produces pain described as covering the supraspinous and infraspinous fossae.[25, 27]

PREOPERATIVE MEDICATION

For preoperative medication, use the standard American Society of Anesthesiologists' recommendations for conscious sedation.

PROCEDURE

POSITION OF THE PATIENT AND PHYSICIAN

Prone Technique

The purpose of this technique is to perform a block with local anesthetic and/or steroid of the median branches that innervates the facet joints. These can be performed in the prone position (Fig. 15–3). The patient's posterior aspect of the neck is prepared under sterile conditions and draped. As with any other surgical technique, a generous enough area should be allowed to perform these blocks properly. Under fluoroscopy a posteroanterior view is obtained to identify the posterior aspect of the waists of the articular pillars from C3 to C7. In some patients the articular pillars of the superior cervical spine (C3 and C4) may be hard to identify with the patient's head in neutral position. Two maneuvers that help in this situation are slightly hyperextending the patient's head or asking the patient to open their mouth to remove the mandible from the radiologic field. Once the waists of the articular pillars of the levels wanted to be blocked are identified, the needle (10-cm, 22-gauge

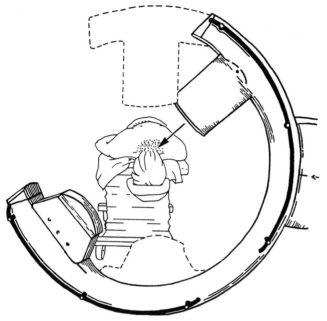

FIGURE 15–3

The drawing shows the optimal targets in the cervical spine for median branch localization and block with the correct position of the C-arm.

spinal needle or short-bevel needle) is advanced in a gun barrel fashion with the needle aligned with the fluoroscopic beam (Fig. 15–4). Once bone has been contacted, the fluoroscopic ray is rotated to the lateral view. In this view the needle should be seen in the posterior aspect of the waist of the articular pillar. Extreme caution must be taken with this projection, and one must ensure that the target is addressed in a direct fashion, because a deviation toward the midline in this view will direct the needle into the epidural and subarachnoid space. At this point, the needle is incrementally advanced under this view until the tip is seen in the center of the pedicle where the median branch lies. To advance the needle under this projection, a slight deviation toward lateral should be applied carefully and slowly to position the needle tip in the most lateral aspect of the articular pillar in the posteroanterior view. A confirmation of the needle tip should be done in both posteroanterior and lateral views before injecting any local anesthetic or steroid. As one approaches the lower articular pillars (C5, C6, and C7), the lateral view may be obscured or blocked by the bone and soft tissues of the shoulder.

To obtain a satisfactory image, the patient can be asked to reach for his or her feet or an assistant can pull on the patient's hands to help shift these tissues out of the way. Careful aspiration should be done prior to injection. To be safe, a very small amount of water-soluble contrast material can be injected to check the kind of spread the local anesthetic agent will have and to ensure that there will be no intravascular spread. It is important to emphasize that very little contrast material

should be used (maximum of 1 mL) to not obscure the views of the lower articular pillars. The maximum amount of local anesthetic agent to be injected per level is 2 mL.

Supine Technique

In the supine position the landmarks to be identified are the posterior border of the sternocleidomastoid muscle as well as the facet joints.[28] Once these are identified the area is prepared and draped in a sterile fashion. With the patient's neck in a neutral position the fluoroscopic ray is first brought in an anteroposterior view to identify the vertebral level, then shifted into an oblique view. Under active fluoroscopy the ray is rotated laterally approximately 30 degrees (Fig. 15–5). At this point, the neural foramen should come into view. To appreciate the neural foramen more clearly, some caudal-cephalad tilt of the fluoroscope C-arm may be necessary. Immediately posterior to the neural foramen, the articular pillars appear as elliptical-shaped structures, or "beads" (Fig. 15–6). The beads at each level form a string of pearls. These structures are the targets for the needles. A point between the most superior third of the elliptical structure and the middle third should be the ideal point of contact. One of the disadvantages of this approach is that a "tunnel" technique cannot be used. The insertion point of the needle is slightly posterior to the sternocleidomastoid muscle or a point slightly posterior to the facet joint. The needle is slowly advanced toward the target until bone contact is made. Confirmation of the needle position should be done under the anteroposterior view and the tip of the needle should be seen in the waist of the articular pillar (Fig. 15–7). Caution should be used during needle advancement, because there is no notion of how median or lateral the needle is in relation to the spinal cord, the nerve root, or the vertebral artery. If bone contact is not made at the bead, then the needle should be withdrawn and redirected. Following confirmation in the oblique view, the C-arm is directed in the anteroposterior view (Fig. 15–8). The needle is confirmed also in that position (Fig. 15–9).

CERVICAL FACET RADIOFREQUENCY

When denervating a facet joint, we use RFTC. It is performed in the same manner as described earlier, with some crucial differences. The needle used for radiofrequency is blunt and has a curved tip, it is 10 cm long with a 10-mm active uninsulated tip. To facilitate placement of the RFTC needle and minimize exposure to infection, an intravenous catheter is used to penetrate the skin and to guide the RFTC needle into the target. Proper placement of the RFTC needle is the same technique as used for the nerve block. Caution should be taken in ensuring that the active tip is outside the neural

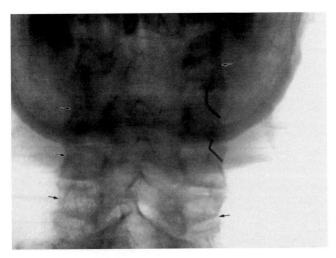

A

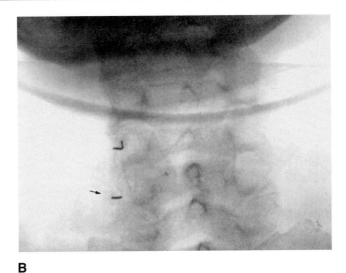

B

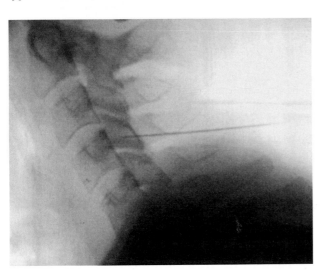

C

FIGURE 15–4

The radiographic images show the patient in prone position for cervical facet median branch block. *A,* Arrows at the waist of the vertebral body in AP view. *B,* The needle in position *(arrow)* in the AP view. *C,* Position of the needle in lateral view. (From Raj PP [ed]: Textbook of Regional Anesthesia. Philadelphia, WB Saunders, 2002.)

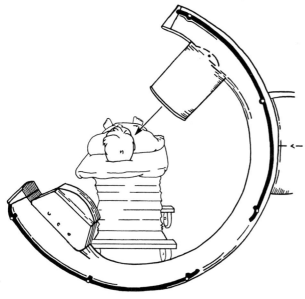

FIGURE 15–5

Patient in supine position with the C-arm directed toward the cervical facet with the oblique view.

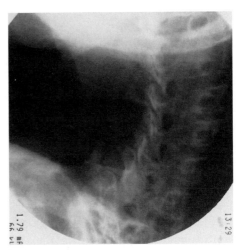

FIGURE 15–6

Oblique view of the cervical spine.

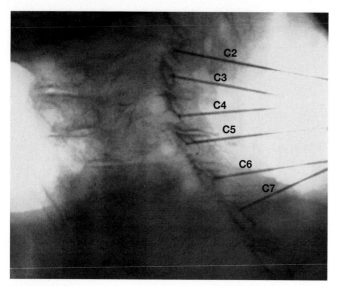

FIGURE 15–7

Oblique view. The needle is at C2–C7 median branches of the facets.

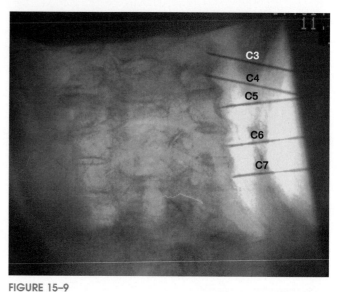

FIGURE 15–9

Cervical facet median branch, anteroposterior view. Needles at the waist show correct position for median branch block.

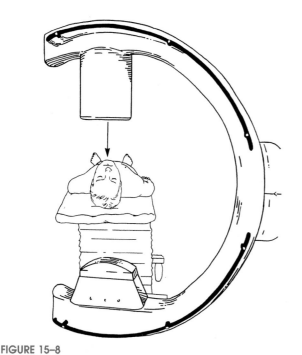

FIGURE 15–8

Anteroposterior drawing of fluoroscope with patient in supine position.

foramen to avoid lesioning of the spinal root. Confirmation of optimal needle positioning should again be done with posteroanterior and lateral views. Before lesioning, careful sensory and motor stimulation should be performed. During sensory stimulation, the generator should be set at 50 Hz, the output slowly increased from 0 to 1.0 V. This should elicit stimulation in the cervical area corresponding to the level being stimulated, and no stimulation should be felt by the patient in a radicular manner from nerve root stimula-

tion. Motor stimulation should be performed with the generator set at 2 Hz and maximum output of 2 V. Motor contraction may be seen in the paraspinous muscles in the neck, but no stimulation should be felt by the patient down the upper extremity or in the shoulder. A sensory stimulation should be greater than 0.3 V to avoid nerve root lesioning. Once these two modes of stimulation are adequate, the radiofrequency lesioning can be started after anesthetizing the median branch with a volume of maximum of 2 mL of local anesthetic. Lesioning is at 80°C. Once the first cycle is complete, the radiofrequency needle is then rotated 90 degrees from its first position and second cycle of lesioning is performed. This has the objective of performing two lesions with a higher likelihood of lesioning the median branch completely. It is important to mention some of the characteristics of the lesion created by the radiofrequency probe. Essentially, the lesion created is elliptical surrounding the active uninsulated tip as well as does not extend beyond the tip of the probe. It is also important to position the probe parallel to the structure or nerve to lesion to obtain a higher likelihood of success. For this reason, two lesions are performed.

COMPLICATIONS OF FACET BLOCK AND RADIOFREQUENCY

In general, the most common complication of cervical facet blocks and radiofrequency is a transient increase in pain immediately following the procedure. The overall incidence is 2%, with a variable period lasting between weeks to a maximum of 8 months.[29] Reports of spinal anesthesia following intra-articular lumbar facet joint injections have occurred.[30] This is one of the reasons why median branch blocks and radiofrequency are encouraged instead of intra-articular injections. With the popularity of fluoroscopy, these complications should decrease. Chemical meningism has also been reported after a median branch block.[31, 32] This could also be explained by inadvertent dural puncture. It has also been emphasized that it is important to confirm needle placement in more than one projection, particularly in the lateral view, to ensure that the needle tip is posterior to the neural foramen. An inadvertent injection into the dural sleeve with resultant deposit of local anesthetic or steroid into the subarachnoid space could result in the complications mentioned earlier. Other less severe complications include paraspinous tissue infections in the form of an abscess.[33–35] This places crucial importance in the preservation of a sterile technique throughout the entire procedure. The same complication described for the lumbar facet injections and blocks can occur for their cervical counterparts. Inadvertent injection of local anesthetic or non–water-soluble steroid into the vertebral artery is more likely to occur during intra-articular injections rather than median branch blocks. However, if the needle tip during a supine approach median branch block is too far anterior, this could definitely result in vertebral artery puncture. This is one of the reasons why we should emphasize the use of water-soluble steroids in the cervical region such as dexamethasone because the injection of a depot steroid into the central nervous system circulation via the vertebral artery could have catastrophic consequences, such as cerebrovascular accidents with resultant deficits. One particular complication in the cervical region relates specifically to the denervation of the C2–C3 facet joint by targeting the third occipital nerve. This could result in anesthesia of the suboccipital region as well as dizziness and vertigo most likely due to the blockade of the upper cervical proprioceptive afferents.[35] This, however, appears to be a transient complication, and no long-term effects have been reported.

In radiofrequency lesioning of the median branches, one of the not so common complications is that of neuritis. Fortunately, it is not common, but when it occurs it is uncomfortable and worrisome to the patient. It is manifested by a new-onset radicular-type burning pain. This is neuritis caused by the closeness of the radiofrequency needle to a large nerve root. It is a self-limited process that will most likely respond to conservative therapy and systemic steroids and is not expected to last more than 2 to 3 weeks.

It is crucial to check the needle insulation along the shaft before insertion. If there is a break in the insulation, a lesion could be done inadvertently on nontargeted tissue. Another precaution that should be taken is if during the lesioning cycle the patient experiences a sudden onset of burning sensation or pain down the extremity, then the cycle should be stopped immediately and the needle position checked or the procedure

aborted. It cannot be emphasized enough in this chapter that the use of fluoroscopy not only guarantees accuracy but also safety. In the cervical region the hazards of a needle misdirected and displaced medially could result in spinal cord injury in the cervical region.

HELPFUL HINTS

When the patient has significant degenerative disease of the spine or has had spine surgery (particularly fusion), the difficulty of the procedure increases and the success rate decreases. In the case of previous surgery, it is possible that pain may result from scar or bony entrapment of the nerves. Sometimes it simply takes longer to do the procedure, and sometimes it is simply wiser to abandon the procedure.

Some practitioners advocate use of larger volumes (2 to 5 mL) for pericapsular, rather than intra-articular, injection. This type of injection bathes the ligaments, paraspinal muscles, and supporting structures with local anesthetic and steroid in a nonspecific manner and has been beneficial to some patients with chronic low back pain, probably because the pain has multiple causes and the volume used provides analgesic and anti-inflammatory effects over a larger area of affected tissue.

Because of the anatomy of the cervical facets, median branch block is the superior procedure. Although the median branches of the dorsal rami innervate both joints and neck muscles, pain that is relieved by median branch block is most likely coming from the facet joint and not from the overlying muscles and ligaments. The small-volume diagnostic injections for median branch nerves, although fairly specific for assessing facet pain, produced false-negative results 8% of the time in the lumbar spine. This complication occurs when the injectate is inadvertently delivered to the vessels accompanying the median branch nerves (an event confirmed with radiocontrast dye). The result is that the injectate is either carried away or diluted by a small hematoma, and the pain is not relieved. It is then often falsely assumed that facet joint pain is not the problem. A similar problem may happen in the cervical spine, but this is not proven at this time.

Until the role of the facet as a cause of low back and neck pain is better defined, it is likely that, in clinical practice, facet joint denervation will continue to be considered for patients with intractable back and neck pain not responsive to conservative therapies and epidural steroid injections.

EFFICACY

As mentioned earlier, one cannot find any conclusive evidence in the literature showing superiority of median branch blocks over intra-articular injections. One of the most complete revisions of the literature regarding the efficacy of cervical median branch radiofrequency has been done by Lord and associates in 1995.[21] Seven series were included in this revision. The results demonstrated that all studies reported a percentage of patients between 37% and 89%, which experienced more than 40% relief for more than 2 months. Even though these studies were flawed due to technical and anatomic errors, these results show encouraging evidence that median branch radiofrequency could be beneficial in well-selected patients. In another study by the same authors in 1996,[36] they compared a group of control patients to a radiofrequency group. In conclusion, the radiofrequency patients had significantly longer pain relief (median time 263 days) compared with the control group. It has also been concluded that 71% of patients undergoing denervation by radiofrequency had a good response when they were chosen by double diagnostic blocks.

Cervical/thoracic facet-single level 64470; cervical/thoracic facet-additional levels 64472; RFTC cervical/thoracic facet-single level 64626; RFTC cervical/thoracic facet-additional levels 64627.

REFERENCES

1. Pawl RP: Headache, cervical spondylosis, and anterior cervical fusion. Surg Annu 9:391, 1971.
2. Hadden SB: Neurologic headache and facial pain. Arch Neurol 43:405, 1940.
3. Raney A, Raney RB: Headache: A common symptom of cervical disc lesions. Arch Neurol 59:603, 1948.
4. Taren JA, Kahn EA: Anatomic pathways related to pain in face and neck. J Neurosurg 19:116, 1962.
5. Brain L, Wilkinson M (eds): Cervical Spondylosis and Other Disorders of the Cervical Spine. London, Heinemann Medical, 1967.
6. McNab I: The whiplash syndrome. Clin Neurosurg 20:232, 1973.
7. Mehta M: Intractable Pain. Philadelphia, WB Saunders, 1973.
8. Hadley LA: Anatomico-roentgenographic studies of the posterior spinal articulations. AJR Am J Roentgenol 86:270–276, 1961.
9. Lewin T, Moffett B, Viidik A: The morphology of the lumbar synovial intervertebral joints. Acta Morphol Neurol Scand 4:299–319, 1961.
10. Mooney V, Robertson J: The facet syndrome. Clin Orthop 115:149–156, 1976.
11. Pederson HE, Blunck CFJ, Gardiner E: The anatomy of lumbosacral posterior rami and meningeal branches of spinal nerves (sinu-vertebral nerves). J Bone Joint Surg Am 38:377–391, 1956.
12. Nade S, Bell E, Wyke BD: The innervation of the lumbar spinal joints and its significance. J Bone Joint Surg 62:255, 1980.
13. Panjabi MM, Oxland T, Takata K, et al: Articular facets of the human spine: Quantitative three-dimensional anatomy. Spine 18:1298–1310, 1993.
14. Milne N: The role of zygapophyseal joint orientation and uncinate processes in controlling motion in the cervical spine. J Anat 178:189–201, 1991.
15. Bogduk N, Marsland A: The cervical zygapophyseal joints as a source of neck pain. Spine 13:610–617, 1988.
16. Selby DK, Paris SV: Anatomy of facet joints and its clinical correlation with low back pain. Contemp Orthop 3:1097–1103, 1981.
17. Santavirta S, Hopfner-Hallikainen D, Paukku P, et al: Atlantoaxial facet joint arthritis in the rheumatoid cervical spine: A panoramic zonography study. J Rheumatol 15:217–223, 1988.
18. Bovim G, Berg R, Gunnar Dale L: Cervicogenic headache: Anesthetic blockades of cervical nerves and facet joint (C2/C3). Pain 49:315–320, 1992.
19. Barnsley L, Bogduk N: Median branch blocks are specific for the diagnosis of cervical zygapophyseal joint pain. Reg Anesth 18:343–350, 1993.
20. Ebraheim NA, Haman ST, Xu R, et al: The anatomical location of the dorsal ramus of the cervical nerve and its relation to the superior articular process of the lateral mass. Spine 23:1968–1971, 1998.
21. Lord SM, Barnsley L, Bogduk N: Percutaneous radiofrequency neurotomy in the treatment of cervical zygapophyseal joint pain: A caution. Neurosurgery 36:732–739, 1995.
22. Dwyer A, Aprill C, Bogduk N: Cervical zygapophyseal joint pain patterns: I. A study in normal volunteers. Spine 15:453–457, 1990.
23. Dreyfuss P, Michaelsen M, Fletcher D: Atlanto-occipital and lateral atlanto-axial joint pain patterns. Spine 19:1125–1131, 1994.
24. Halla JT, Hardin JG: Atlantoaxial (C1–C2) facet joint osteoarthritis: A distinctive clinical syndrome. Arthritis Rheum 30:577–582, 1987.
25. Aprill C, Dwyer A, Bogduk N: Cervical zygapophyseal joint pain patterns: II. A clinical evaluation. Spine 15:458–461, 1990.
26. Santavirta S, Konttinen Y, Lindqvist C, Sandelin J: Occipital headache in rheumatoid cervical facet joint arthritis. Lancet 2:695, 1986.
27. Fukui S, Ohseto K, Shiotani M, et al: Referred pain distribution of the cervical zygapophyseal joints and cervical dorsal rami. Pain 68:79–83, 1996.
28. Wenger C: Radiofrequency lesions for the treatment of spinal pain. Pain Dig 8:1–16, 1998.
29. Bous RA: Facet joint injections. In Stanton-Hicks M, Bous R (eds): Chronic Low Back Pain. New York, Raven, 1982, pp 199–211.
30. Goldstone JC, Pennant JH: Spinal anesthesia following facet joint injection: A report of two cases. Anaesthesia 42:754–756, 1987.
31. Thomson SJ, Lomas DM, Collett BJ: Chemical meningism after lumbar facet joint block with local anesthetic and steroids. Anaesthesia 46:563–564, 1991.
32. Berrigan T: Chemical meningism after lumbar facet joint block. Anaesthesia 47:905–906, 1992.
33. Magee M, Kannangara S, Dennieen B: Paraspinal abscess complicating facet joint injection. Clin Nucl Med 25:71–73, 2000.
34. Cook NJ, Hanrahan P, Song S: Paraspinal abscess following facet joint injection. Clin Rheumatol 8:52–53, 1999.
35. Bogduk N, Marsland A: The cervical zygapophyseal joints as a source of neck pain. Spine 13:610–617, 1988.
36. Lord SM, Barnsley L, Wallis BJ, et al: Percutaneous radiofrequency neurotomy for chronic cervical zygapophyseal joint pain. N Engl J Med 335:1721–1726, 1996.

Cervical Epidural Nerve Block

HISTORY

Although Pages' description[1] of the paramidline approach to the lumbar epidural space in 1921 is considered the first clinically relevant report of the technique of lumbar epidural nerve block, it appears that Dogliotti[2] was the first to describe the technique of epidural block in the cervical region.[3]

Owing to the problem inherent in complete sensory blockade of the cervical nerve roots when cervical epidural nerve block is performed for surgical anesthesia, many anesthesiologists believed that cervical epidural nerve block was too risky, given the general anesthetic techniques available at the time. This fact led to two persistent beliefs that, unfortunately, have colored contemporary thinking about the use of cervical epidural nerve block for pain management. The first belief is that cervical epidural nerve block is too risky for routine clinical use. The second belief is that it has a limited number of applications. Cervical epidural steroid administration for management of cervical radiculopathy, tension-type headache, and other painful conditions is clinically common.

ANATOMY

The superior boundary of the cervical epidural space is the point at which the periosteal and spinal layers of dura fuse at the foramen magnum.[4] It should be recognized that these structures allow drugs injected into the cervical epidural space to travel beyond their confines if the volume of injectate is large enough. This fact probably explains many of the early problems associated with the use of cervical epidural nerve block for surgical anesthesia, when large volumes of local anesthetics were injected.

The epidural space continues inferiorly to the sacrococcygeal membrane.[5] The cervical epidural space is bounded anteriorly by the posterior longitudinal ligament and posteriorly by the vertebral laminae and the ligamentum flavum (Fig. 16–1). The ligamentum flavum is relatively thin in the cervical region and becomes thicker farther caudad, closer to the lumbar spine.[4] This fact has direct clinical implications, in that the loss of resistance felt during cervical epidural nerve block is more subtle than it is in the lumbar or lower thoracic region.

The vertebral pedicles and intervertebral foramina form the lateral limits of the epidural space. The degenerative changes and narrowing of the intervertebral foramina associated with aging may be marked in the cervical region. The distance between the ligamentum flavum and dura is greatest at the L2 interspace, measuring 5.0 to 6.0 mm in adults.[4] Because of the enlargement of the cervical spinal cord, the distance from the ligamentum flavum and dura is only 1.5 to 2.0 mm at C7.[4] It should be noted that flexion of the neck moves this cervical enlargement more cephalad, resulting in widening of the epidural space to 3.0 to 4.0 mm at the C7–T1 interspace.[5] This fact has important clinical implications if cervical epidural block is performed with the patient in the lateral or prone position.

CONTENTS OF THE EPIDURAL SPACE

Fat

The epidural space is filled with fatty areolar tissue. The amount of epidural fat varies in direct proportion to the amount of fat stored elsewhere in the body.[4] The epidural fat is relatively vascular and appears to change to a denser consistency with aging. The epidural fat appears to perform the following two functions:

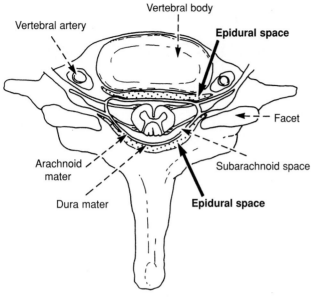

FIGURE 16–1

A drawing that shows the relationship of the cervical epidural contents.

1. It serves as a shock absorber for the other contents of the epidural space and for the dura and the contents of the dural sac.
2. It serves as a depot for drugs injected into the cervical epidural space.

The second function has direct clinical implications for the choice of opioids for cervical epidural administration.

Epidural Veins

The epidural veins are concentrated principally in the anterolateral portion of the epidural space.[4] These veins are valveless and so transmit both intrathoracic and intra-abdominal pressures. As pressure in either of these body cavities increases, owing to Valsalva's maneuver or compression of the inferior vena cava by a gravid uterus or a tumor mass, the epidural veins distend and reduce the volume of the epidural space. This decrease in volume can directly affect how much drug is needed to obtain a given level of neural blockade. Because this venous plexus serves the entire spinal column, it becomes a ready conduit for hematogenous infection.

Epidural Arteries

The arteries that supply the bony and ligamentous confines of the cervical epidural space as well as the cervical spinal cord enter the cervical epidural space via two routes: through the intervertebral foramina and via direct anastomoses from the intracranial portions of the vertebral arteries.[4,6] There are significant anastomoses between the epidural arteries, most of which lie in the lateral portions of the epidural arteries. Trauma to the epidural

arteries can result in epidural hematoma formation and compromise the blood supply to the spinal cord itself.

Lymphatics

The lymphatics of the epidural space are concentrated in the region of the dural roots, where they remove foreign material from the subarachnoid and epidural spaces (Table 16–1).

CONTRAINDICATIONS

Absolute
- Local infection
- Sepsis
- Anticoagulant medication or coagulopathy

Relative
- Hypovolemia

EQUIPMENT

- Tuohy epidural needle or similar needle
- 25-gauge, ¾-inch infiltration needle
- 3-mL syringe
- 10-mL syringe
- Loss-of-resistance (LOR) syringe

DRUGS

- Steroids (e.g., triamcinolone diacetate)
- 0.25% to 0.5% bupivacaine/ropivacaine
- Normal saline (0.9%), preservative free

PREPARATION OF THE PATIENT

PHYSICAL EXAMINATION

Examine the area for local infection and the ability to flex the cervical spine at C6, C7, and C8. The ability to sit upright is important.

LABORATORY

- Complete blood count with platelets
- Prothrombin time, partial thromboplastin time, platelet function studies, or bleeding times

PREOPERATIVE MEDICATION

For preoperative medication, use the standard American Society of Anesthesiologists' recommendations for conscious sedation.

▽ TABLE 16–1 Indications for Cervical Approach to the
              Epidural Space

Category	Type of Pain
Surgical, diagnostic, prognostic	Surgical anesthesia
	Differential neural blockade to evaluate head, neck, face, shoulder, and upper extremity pain
	Prognostic indicator before destruction of the cervical nerves
Pain	
Acute	Palliation in acute pain emergencies
	Postoperative pain
	Head, face, neck, shoulder, and upper extremity pain secondary to trauma
	Pain of acute herpes zoster
	Acute vascular insufficiency of the upper extremities
Prophylactic and preemptive	Pain of tension-type headache
	Prior to amputation of ischemic limbs
Chronic benign	Cervical radiculopathy
	Cervical spondylosis
	Cervicalgia
	Vertebral compression fractures
	Diabetic polyneuropathy
	Postherpetic neuralgia
	Reflex sympathetic dystrophy
	Shoulder pain syndromes
	Upper extremity pain syndromes
	Phantom limb syndrome
	Peripheral neuropathy
	Postlaminectomy syndrome
	Pain of tension-type headache
Cancer related	Pain secondary to head, face, neck shoulder, and upper extremity malignancies
	Bony metastases to head, face, cervical spine, shoulder girdle, and upper extremity
	Chemotherapy-related peripheral neuropathy

PROCEDURE

POSITION OF THE PATIENT AND PHYSICIAN

Sitting Position

The sitting position is easiest for the patient and pain management specialist. It also ensures that the cervical spine is flexed, which widens the lower cervical epidural space. The sitting position avoids the rotation of the spine inherent in the lateral position, which makes identification of the midline epidural space difficult (Fig. 16–2). A history of vasovagal syncope with previous needle punctures precludes the use of this position. In such situations, the lateral position is preferred.

Lateral Position

The lateral position is preferred for patients who cannot assume the sitting position or who are prone to vasovagal attacks. For the patient's comfort, the lateral position is more suitable for placement of tunneled epidural catheters or other implantable devices. If the lateral position is chosen, care must be taken to ensure that there is no rotation of the patient's spine, which would make epidural nerve block exceedingly difficult, if not impossible. Furthermore, flexion of the cervical spine is mandatory to maximize the width of the epidural space (Fig. 16–3).

Prone Position

The prone position is used principally for placement of tunneled epidural catheters and spinal stimulator

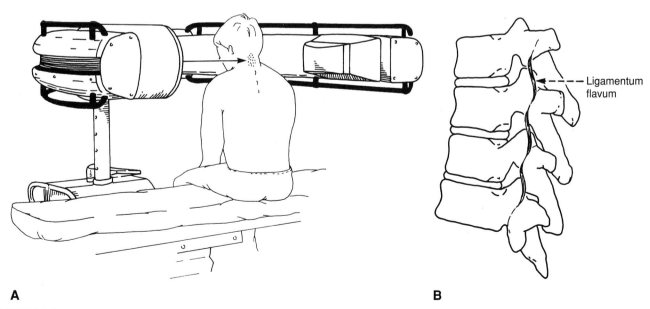

A

B

Ligamentum flavum

FIGURE 16–2

A, The fluoroscope is positioned to obtain a lateral image of the cervical spine in the sitting position. *B*, In a drawing of the lateral view, the "straight line" of the posterior bony canal can be seen radiographically. This straight line provides a guide for the physician to avoid damaging the dura and dural contents.

electrodes. As with the other positions, care must be taken to flex the cervical spine to widen the epidural space (Fig. 16–4). The prone position should be avoided if access to the airway is necessary for maintenance of the patient's respiratory function.

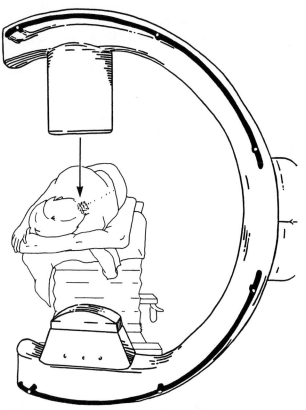

FIGURE 16–3

The patient is seen in a lateral decubitus position. The fluoroscopic C-arm is positioned for obtaining a lateral radiographic image. If it is difficult to keep the patient in a "true" lateral decubitus position, the fluoroscopic C-arm or the fluoroscopic table may be rotated obliquely to create an ideal lateral radiographic image.

LOSS-OF-RESISTANCE TECHNIQUE

After careful identification of the midline at the chosen interspace, 1 mL of local anesthetic is used to infiltrate the skin, the subcutaneous tissues, and the supraspinous and interspinous ligaments. Large amounts of local anesthetic should be avoided, because they disrupt the ligamentous fibers and contribute to postprocedure pain.

The styleted needle is inserted exactly in the midline in the previously anesthetized area through the supraspinous ligament into the interspinous ligament.[7] The needle stylet is removed, and a well-lubricated 5-mL LOR syringe filled with 2 mL of preservative-free sterile saline is attached. Because saline is not compressible, it provides better tactile feedback than air. Additionally, saline avoids the risk of air embolism via the cervical epidural veins.[7]

The operator holds the epidural needle firmly at the hub with the left thumb and index finger. The left hand is placed firmly against the patient's neck to ensure against uncontrolled needle movements should the patient move unexpectedly. The right hand holds the syringe with the thumb exerting continuous firm pressure on the plunger.[8] Bromage[4] admonished, "Never advance the needle without simultaneous pressure on the plunger to tell you where you are." Ballottement of the plunger, advocated by some clinicians, should not be used because it would increase the risk of inadvertent dural puncture.

As constant pressure is applied to the plunger of the syringe with the thumb of the physician's right hand, the needle and syringe are continuously advanced in a slow and deliberate manner with the left hand. As the needle bevel passes through the ligamentum flavum and enters the epidural space, there is a sudden LOR and the plunger slides effortlessly forward. This LOR

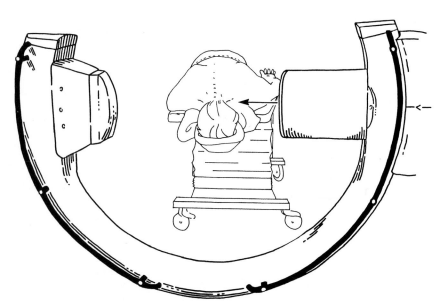

FIGURE 16–4

The typical position of the patient and of the fluoroscopic C-arm for the prone position is shown. Note the flexion of the cervical spine for enhanced epidural needle placement.

provides the operator visual and tactile confirmation that the needle bevel has entered the epidural space. The syringe is gently removed from the needle.

An air or saline acceptance test is carried out by injecting 0.5 to 1.0 mL of air or sterile, preservative-free saline with a well-lubricated sterile glass syringe to help confirm that the needle lies within the epidural space. The force required for injection should not exceed that necessary to overcome the resistance of the needle. Any significant pain or sudden increase in resistance during injection suggests incorrect needle placement. The injection should be stopped immediately and the position of the needle reassessed.

HANGING DROP TECHNIQUE

The "hanging drop," or Gutierrez, technique[9] relies on the presence of apparent negative pressure in the epidural space.[10] A drop of saline or local anesthetic solution is placed in the hub of the epidural needle, once the tip of the needle is located in the interspinous ligament (Fig. 16–5). The needle is then carefully advanced through the ligamentum flavum until the drop of fluid is drawn into the needle by the negative pressure in the epidural space. The negative pressure in the thoracic epidural space is thought to be related to transmitted negative pleural pressure.[10] Optimal conditions for the hanging drop test are found in the thoracic region, with the patient sitting. Most investigators attribute the existence of negative pressure in the lumbar epidural space to tenting of the dura by the epidural needle.[11] In the lumbar epidural space, pressure is not reliably below atmospheric pressure, particularly if the patient is sitting, if intra-abdominal pressure is increased, or if uterine contractions are in progress. Bromage[11] recommended that this test not be used in the lumbar region. One must be careful deciding when to use this technique, particularly when the technique is performed at a level where spinal cord is underlying the dura.

To add safety and efficacy to the blind cervical epidural steroid injection, lateral fluoroscopic images are most critically used. The epidural needle can be safely advanced short of the "straight line" formed by the anterior aspect of the spine process (Fig. 16–6A). After stopping short of the epidural space, the LOR or the hanging drop techniques are used to confirm correct placement of the needle if water-soluble contrast agent is injected (Fig. 16–6B)

The spread of drugs injected into the cervical epidural space depends on the volume and speed of injection; the anatomic variations of the epidural space; the extent of dilation of the epidural veins; and the position, age, and height of the patient.[12] Pregnant patients require a significantly smaller amount of drug to achieve a given level of blockade than do nongravid control subjects.[13]

For diagnostic and prognostic blocks, 1.0% preservative-free lidocaine is a suitable local anesthetic.[8] For therapeutic blocks, 0.25% preservative-free bupivacaine in combination with triamcinolone diacetate (Aristocort) 40 mg is injected.[7, 8] Subsequent nerve blocks are carried out in a similar manner, with 40 mg of steroids instead of the initial 80-mg dose.

COMPLICATIONS

- Inadvertent dural puncture
- Inadvertent subdural puncture
- Inadvertent IV needle and catheter placement
- Hematoma and ecchymosis
- Infection
- Neurologic complications
- Urinary retention and incontinence

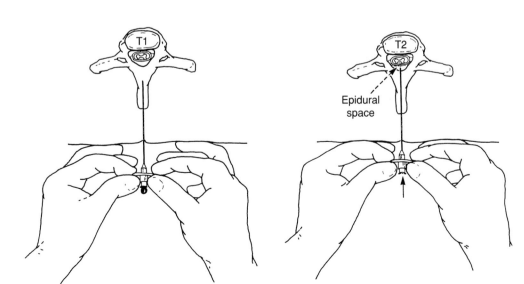

Epidural space

FIGURE 16–5

The "hanging drop or Gutierrez" technique for identifying needle entry into the epidural space. The presence of negative pressure is reliable only in the thoracic epidural space.

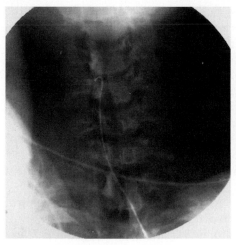
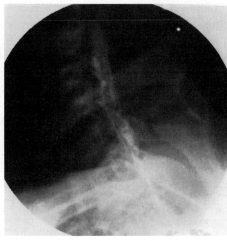

FIGURE 16–6
Radiographic images in the anteroposterior *(A)* and lateral *(B)* views. The image shows the epidural needle safely posterior and the contrast agent in the epidural space.

A   B

HELPFUL HINTS

In the cervical region, after traversing the skin and subcutaneous tissues, the styleted epidural needle impinges on the ligamentum nuchae, which runs vertically between the apices of the cervical spinous processes.[14] The ligamentum nuchae offers some resistance to the advancing needle. This ligament is dense enough to hold a needle in position even when the needle is released.

The interspinous ligament, which runs obliquely between the spinous processes, is encountered next and offers additional resistance to needle advancement. Because the interspinous ligament is contiguous with the ligamentum flavum, the operator may perceive a "false" LOR when the needle tip enters the space between the interspinous ligament and the ligamentum flavum. This phenomenon is more pronounced in the cervical region than in the lumbar region because the ligaments are less well defined.

A significant increase in resistance to needle advancement signals that the needle tip is impinging on the dense ligamentum flavum. Because the ligament is made up almost entirely of elastin fibers, resistance increases as the needle traverses the ligamentum flavum because of the drag of the ligament on the needle. A sudden LOR occurs as the needle tip enters the epidural space. There should be essentially no resistance to injection of drug into the normal epidural space.

CHOICE OF NEEDLE

For most adult patients, the 18-gauge, 3.5-inch Hustead or Tuohy needle is suitable for cervical epidural block; however, with the sharper Tuohy needle, the incidence of dural punctures may be higher.[15] Some centers are now using smaller epidural needles with equally good results. These smaller needles decrease the amount of procedure-related and postprocedure pain.

INJECTION OF DRUGS

When satisfactory needle position is confirmed, a syringe containing the drugs to be injected is carefully attached to the needle. Gentle aspiration is carried out to identify cerebrospinal fluid or blood.[8] Inadvertent dural puncture can occur in the best of hands, and careful observation for spinal fluid is mandatory.[16] If cerebrospinal fluid is aspirated, the epidural block may by attempted at a different interspace. In this situation, drug doses should be adjusted accordingly because subarachnoid migration of drugs through the dural rent can occur. Aspiration of blood can result from either damage to veins during insertion of the needle into the cervical epidural space or, less commonly, IV placement of the needle.[8] If blood is aspirated, the needle should be rotated slightly and the aspiration test repeated. If no blood is present, incremental doses of local anesthetic and other drugs may be administered while the patient is monitored closely for signs of local anesthetic toxicity or untoward reactions to the other drugs.

EFFICACY

No clear efficacy studies for cervical epidural steroid blocks could be found. However, the results of lumbar epidural steroid blocks have been positive.

Injection, catheter placement, continuous, cervical or thoracic 62318.

REFERENCES

1. Pages E: Anesthesia metameric. Rev Sanid Mil Madr 11:351–385, 1921.

2. Dogliotti AM: Segmental peridural anesthesia. Am J Surg 20:107, 1933.

3. Waldman SD: Epidural nerve block. In Weiner RS (ed): Innovations in Pain Management. Orlando, FL, PMD Press, 1990, pp 4–5.

4. Bromage PR: Anatomy. In Bromage PR (ed): Epidural Analgesia. Philadelphia, WB Saunders, 1978, pp 8–20.

5. Reynolds AF, Roberts PA, Pollay M, et al: Quantitative anatomy of the thoracolumbar epidural space. Neurosurgery 17:905, 1985.

6. Woollam DHM, Millen JW: An anatomical background to vascular disease of the spinal cord. Proc R Soc Med 51:540, 1958.

7. Cousins MJ, Bromage PR: Epidural neural blockade. In Cousins MJ, Bridenbaugh DO (eds): Neural Blockade in Clinical Anesthesia and Management of Pain, 2nd ed. Philadelphia, JB Lippincott, 1988, pp 340–341.

8. Cousins MJ, Bromage PR: Epidural neural blockade. In Cousins MJ, Bridenbaugh DO (eds): Neural Blockade in Clinical Anesthesia and Management of Pain, 2nd ed. Philadelphia, JB Lippincott, 1988, pp 333–334.

9. Gutierrez A: Valor de la aspiracion liquida en el espacio peridural en la anesthesia peridural. Rev Cir Buenos Aires 12:225–227, 1933.

10. Bromage PR: Epidural Analgesia. Philadelphia, WB Saunders, 1978, pp 160–175.

11. Bromage PR: Epidural Analgesia. Philadelphia, WB Saunders, 1978, pp 176–214.

12. Burn JM, Guyer PB, Langdon L: The spread of solutions injected into the epidural space: A study using epidurograms in patients with the lumbosciatic syndrome. Br J Anesth 45:338, 1973.

13. Bromage PR: Mechanism of action. In Bromage PR (ed): Epidural Analgesia. Philadelphia, WB Saunders, 1978, pp 141–142.

14. Katz J: Cervical approach: Single-injection technique. In Katz J (ed): Atlas of Regional Anesthesia, 2nd ed. Norwalk, CT, Appleton & Lange, 1994, pp 204–205.

15. Bromage PR: Epidural needles. Anesthesiology 22:1018, 1961.

16. Waldman SD, Feldstein GS, Allen ML: Cervical epidural blood patch for treatment of cervical dural puncture headache. Anesth Rev 14:1, 23–25, 1987.

17 Cervical Discogram

HISTORY

Knut Lindblom, a radiologist in Stockholm, Sweden, first described diagnostic disc puncture and coined the term *discography*.[1] It was Carl Hirsch who employed the procedure to identify painful discs in patients with lumbago and sciatica. The diagnostic parameter of the procedure was the pain response, thus, the concept of provocative discography. Lindblom continued to modify the technique to use the injection of contrast material to visualize the radial ruptures of the discs, and the diagnostic criteria were expanded to include the radiographic appearance of the disc and the patient's response to the injection (i.e., to provocation).

Wise and Weiford were the first in the United States to visualize and study internal disc morphology.[2] Cloward and Busade continued the work and described the technique of and indications for discography and the evaluation of normal and abnormal discs.[3]

ANATOMY

Cervical discs are distinct from lumbar discs. Radicular symptoms attributable solely to disc herniation are much less common in the cervical region than in the lumbar region. The reasons for this are that for the cervical disc to impinge on the cervical nerve roots, it must herniate posteriorly and laterally. Cervical nerve roots are protected from impingement from cervical disc herniation in part by the facet joints, which interpose a bony wall between the disc and the nerve root. Second, the disc is completely enclosed posteriorly by the dense, double-layered posterior longitudinal ligament. This ligament is much denser than its lumbar counterpart (Fig. 17–1).

In the cervical disc, the nuclear material lies farther anterior than it does in its lumbar counterpart (Fig. 17–2). The anterior portion of the cervical disc space is larger than the posterior portion, which makes it difficult for the nuclear material to move posteriorly unless great forces are applied to the disc. The tough outer annulus is also thicker in the posterior portion of the cervical disc, so posterior bulging is less likely. It is this annular layer that receives sensory innervation from a variety of sources. Posteriorly, the annulus receives fibers from the sinuvertebral nerves, which also provide sensory innervation to the posterior elements, including portions of the facet joints. Laterally, fibers from the exiting spinal nerve roots provide sensory innervation and the anterior portion of the disc receives fibers from the sympathetic chain. Whether some or all of these fibers play a role in discogenic pain is a subject of controversy among pain specialists.

The cervical nerve roots leave the spinal cord and travel laterally through the intervertebral foramina. If the posterior cervical disc herniates laterally, it can impinge on the cervical root as it travels through the intervertebral foramen, producing radicular symptoms. If the cervical disc herniates posteromedially, it may impinge on the spinal cord itself, producing myelopathy that may cause upper and lower extremity neurologic signs and symptoms and bowel and bladder dysfunction. Severe compression of the cervical spinal cord may result in quadriparesis or, rarely, quadriplegia.

INDICATIONS

Cervical discography is indicated as a diagnostic maneuver for a carefully selected subset of patients suffering from neck and cervical radicular pain. Patients who may benefit from discography include the following:

- Patients with persistent neck and/or cervical radicular pain when traditional diagnostic modalities, such as magnetic resonance imaging,

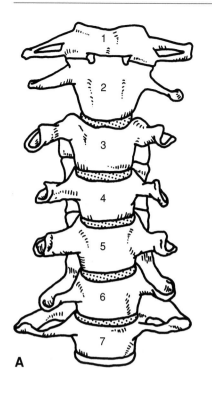

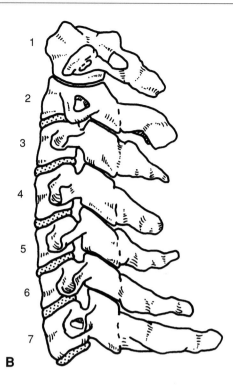

FIGURE 17-1

A drawing of the anatomy of the cervical region with particular reference to the disc and its relations: anterior (A) and lateral (B) views.

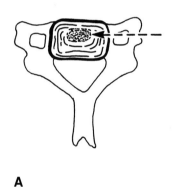

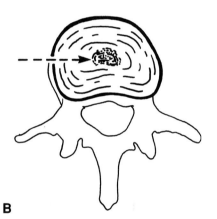

Disc nuclear material

A   B

FIGURE 17-2

This drawing shows the transverse section of the disc at the cervical (A) and lumbar (B) regions. Note that the nuclear material lies farther anterior in the cervical region than does its lumbar counterpart.

computed tomograpy, and electromyography, have failed to identify the cause of the pain.

- Patients in whom findings, such as bulging cervical disc identified on traditional diagnostic modalities, are equivocal (to determine whether such abnormalities are, in fact, responsible for the pain).
- Patients who are to undergo cervical fusion (to help to identify which levels need to be fused).
- Patients who have previously undergone fusion of the cervical spine (to help to identify whether levels above and below the fusion are causing persistent pain).
- Patients in whom traditional imaging techniques cannot distinguish recurrent disc herniation from scar tissue.

EQUIPMENT

- 25-gauge, ¾-inch infiltration needle
- 22-gauge, 3½-inch spinal needle
- 3-mL syringe
- 5-mL syringe
- IV T-piece extension

DRUGS

- 1.5% lidocaine
- Normal saline, preservative free
- Iohexol (Omnipaque 240) radiographic contrast medium

- Cefazolin (Kefzol) 5 mg/mL for intradiscal injections
- Ceftriaxone (Rocephin) 1 g for systemic injection

PREPARATION OF THE PATIENT

PHYSICAL EXAMINATION

The patient should be able to lie in a supine position and should be free of local infection. The cervical anatomy should be normal, and conditions such as collapsed vertebrae should be avoided.

LABORATORY

- Complete blood count with platelets
- Prothrombin time, partial thromboplastin time
- Platelet function studies, including bleeding time

PREOPERATIVE MEDICATION

For preoperative medication, use the standard American Society of Anesthesiologists' recommendations for conscious sedation.

PROCEDURE

TECHNIQUE OF CERVICAL DISCOGRAPHY

The patient is placed supine with the neck in neutral position, as if for a stellate ganglion block (Fig. 17–3). The anterior right side of the neck is usually chosen for the needle entry, because the esophagus tracks to the left as it descends through the neck (Fig. 17–4). The skin of the anterior neck is then prepared with antiseptic solution. When fluoroscopy is used, a skin wheal of local anesthetic is placed at the medial border of the sternocleidomastoid muscle at the level to be evaluated. A 22-gauge, 13-cm styleted needle is advanced toward the superior margin of the vertebral body just below the disc of interest, carefully to avoid the carotid artery, jugular vein, trachea, and esophagus.

After the needle impinges on bone, the depth at which bone contact is made is noted and the needle is withdrawn into the subcutaneous tissues and then advanced in a more superior trajectory into the anterior disc annulus (Fig. 17–5). The needle is advanced in increments into the nucleus (Fig. 17–6). Sequential scanning or fluoroscopy is indicated to avoid advancing the needle completely through the disc and into the cervical spinal cord. Water-soluble contrast medium suitable for intrathecal use is then slowly injected through the needle into the disc in a volume of 0.2 to 0.6 mL (Fig. 17–7). The resistance to injection

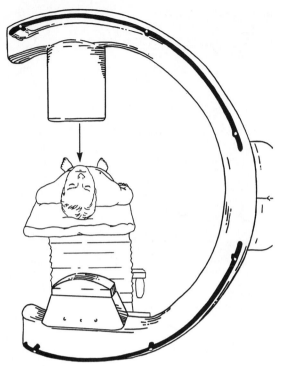

FIGURE 17–3

The patient lies supine with the C-arm in position for a posteroanterior view of the cervical spine.

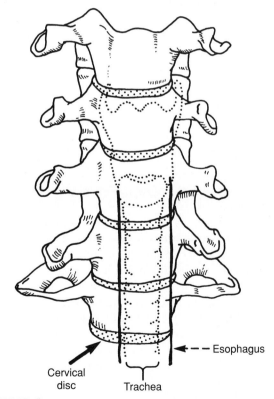

Esophagus

Cervical disc

Trachea

FIGURE 17–4

This drawing shows the relationship of the esophagus to the cervical spine on the left side. Because of this relationship, the needle is usually put on the right side of the disc.

should be noted—intact discs offer firm resistance to these volumes. Simultaneously, the patient's pain response during injection is noted. The site of the pain and its quality and similarity to the patient's ongoing clinical complaint are evaluated. A verbal analogue scale may be useful to help the patient quantify the degree of pain as compared with that from injection of adjacent discs.

INJECTION OF CONTRAST MEDIUM AND ITS INTERPRETATION

The nucleogram of a normal cervical disc shows a lobulated mass with posterolateral clefts, which develop as part of the normal aging process of the disc. In a damaged disc, the contrast material may flow into tears in the inter annulus, producing a characteristic transverse pattern. If the tears in the annulus extend to the outer layer, a radial pattern is produced. Contrast

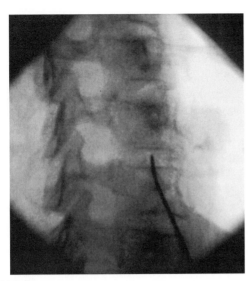

FIGURE 17–5

A radiographic image in the oblique view that shows the needle entry anterior to the facet joint.

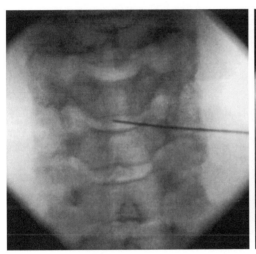

A

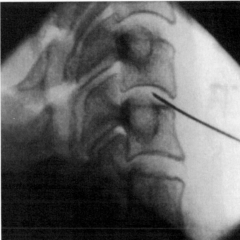

B

FIGURE 17–6

Anteroposterior (A) and lateral (B) views of the needle in the cervical disc in its final position.

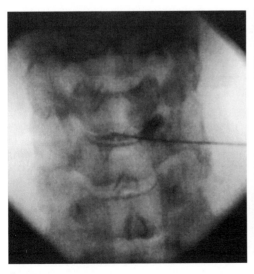

A

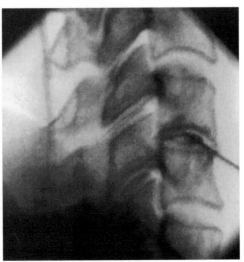

B

FIGURE 17–7

The spread of the contrast material in the cervical disc in anteroposterior (A) and lateral (B) views. This is a normal spread of contrast agent in a disc.

material may also flow between the layers of annulus, producing a circumferential pattern. Complete disruption of the annulus allows the contrast medium to flow into the epidural space or into the cartilaginous end plate of the vertebra itself. Although the likelihood that the disc being evaluated is the source of the patient's pain is directly proportional to the damage to the annulus, the pain management specialist must evaluate all information obtained during the discography procedure in the context of the pain symptoms. After evaluation of the nucleogram, a decision must be made to proceed with discography of adjacent discs or to inject local anesthetic into the disc currently being imaged. Analgesic discography is useful when the clinical pain pattern is reproduced or provoked during injection of contrast material and is relieved by a subsequent injection of local anesthetic into the disc. The inference can be drawn that the disc is the likely source of the patient's pain. It must be remembered that, if the annulus is disrupted, the injected local anesthetic may spread into the epidural space and anesthetize somatic and sympathetic nerves that may subserve discs at adjacent levels. Should that occur, findings obtained from subsequent discography on adjacent discs might be misleading.

POSTPROCEDURE MONITORING

After the procedure is completed, the patient should be observed for 30 minutes before discharge. The patient should be warned to expect minor postprocedure discomfort, including some difficulty in swallowing. Ice packs placed on the injection site for 20-minute periods help decrease these untoward effects. The patient should be instructed to call immediately if any fever or other systemic symptoms develop that might suggest infection.

EFFICACY

Cervical discogram is a diagnostic procedure. There are no data available to evaluate its efficacy.

REFERENCES

1. Bernard T: Lumbar discography followed by computed tomography: Refining the diagnosis of low back pain. Spine 15:690–707, 1990.
2. Wise RE, Weiford EC: X-ray visualization of the intervertebral disc. Cleve Clin Q 18:127–130, 1951.
3. Cloward RB, Busade LL: Discography: Technique, indications, and evaluation of the normal and abnormal intervertebral disc. AJR Am J Roentgenol 68:552–564, 1952.

CHAPTER 18

Brachial Plexus Block

HISTORY

Brachial plexus block was first performed in 1885 by William Steward Halsted, who used cocaine and direct exposure of the roots in the neck to accomplish the block. In 1911, Hirschel and Kulenkampff described the first percutaneous brachial plexus block by the axillary and supraclavicular routes, respectively. Since these historic reports, the efficacy of brachial plexus block has been confirmed, and the block is now commonly used to provide upper extremity anesthesia.

SUPRACLAVICULAR APPROACH

Kulenkampff described the first percutaneous supraclavicular approach in 1911.[3] Perthes attempted to improve the success rate of the technique by using an electric stimulator. The first significant modification of the technique was achieved by Labat in 1922, when he advocated injection of the local anesthetic agent at three separate points. In 1929, Livingston described a technique similar to what is now called the *subclavian perivascular approach*. In 1940, Patrick described a new technique that made it possible to lay down a wall of anesthetic through which the plexus must pass. Over time, many others have described various modified techniques.

INFRACLAVICULAR APPROACH

Soon after Hirschel described the first axillary block, Bazy reported in 1917 the first infraclavicular approach to the brachial plexus. In this technique, the needle was inserted below the clavicle, just medial to the coracoid process and advanced toward Chassaignac's tubercle. Minor modifications of Bazy's technique were proposed by Babitzky 2 years later. In 1973, Raj reintroduced a modified infraclavicular approach to the brachial plexus.

This modified approach provides adequate anesthesia of the entire arm. Although the danger of penetrating blood vessels is the same as in other approaches, there is less risk of pneumothorax because the needle is directed laterally from the midpoint of the clavicle. The lung lies behind the medial one third of the clavicle and thus escapes potential damage from the needle tip.

For consistently good results with the infraclavicular approach, it is necessary to use a peripheral nerve stimulator. The neurostimulator technique simplifies the process of locating the brachial plexus, which is deeper in the infraclavicular region than at other sites and improves the success rate of the block.

AXILLARY APPROACH

Hirschel in 1911 described the first percutaneous axillary approach to the brachial plexus, followed by Capelle, who in 1917 described the forerunner of the axillary perivascular technique. Since then, Labat (1922), Pitkin (1927), Accardo and Adriani (1949), Burnham (1958), Eriksson and Skarby (1962), and De Jong (1961) all have modified the technique somewhat, resulting in the approach commonly used today. This technique is described in the following sections.

EQUIPMENT

Continuous Infusion
- 18- to 20-gauge BD Longdwel catheter, 6 to 8 inches *or*
- 16-gauge R-K epidural needle and Tun-L-XL epidural catheter

DRUGS

Although lidocaine and mepivacaine have been used for continuous infusion, the most commonly chosen local anesthetic is bupivacaine. In a typical case, after the catheter is placed on the brachial plexus, a bolus of 20 to 30 mL of 0.5% bupivacaine only or a 1:1 mixture of 2% lidocaine and 0.5% bupivacaine is administered. Monitoring is mandatory for at least 45 minutes, during which time the onset of the block is tested. If adequate block is present, then up to 10 mL/hr of either 0.25% or 0.0625% bupivacaine with 5 μg fentanyl solution is administered via an infusion pump. Steady state is reached in five half-lives (~18 hours). The infusion should be started within 2 hours, before the bolus effect wears off. Before 18 hours is reached, however, the bolus block is expected to wear off (usually after 6 hours). The infusion of 0.25% bupivacaine would not be effective to maintain analgesia for another 12 hours. If there is intolerable pain at 6 hours, it is imperative to provide another bolus of 20 mL of 0.5% bupivacaine. Monitoring is required for 45 minutes, as with the initial bolus.

Plasma concentration and pharmacokinetics of brachial plexus infusion in a steady state are similar to those seen with epidural infusion. Once the steady state is reached, the drugs infused do not accumulate if infused at the same rate. The metabolites also remain at insignificant levels without causing any deleterious effect. However, brachial plexus infusion should be used with caution in patients with liver and kidney disease. To minimize the amount of local anesthetics and to theoretically improve the efficacy of the block, adjuvant drugs such as opioids or clonidine can be used.

PREPARATION OF THE PATIENT

PHYSICAL EXAMINATION

Examine the area for local infection and distorted anatomy, and assess for the ability to properly position the arm. Neurologic examination should be performed to document any deficits.

PREOPERATIVE MEDICATION

For preoperative medication, use the standard American Society of Anesthesiologists' recommendations for conscious sedation.

PROCEDURE

SUPRACLAVICULAR APPROACH

Position of the Patient

The patient lies supine with a roll-shaped cushion between the scapulae. The arms are at the patient's side with the hands pointing toward the knee. The patient's head is turned contralateral to the affected side. For accentuation of the sternocleidomastoid and scalene muscles, the head may be lifted 30 degrees off the table.

Landmarks

The correct point of entry is determined by observing the following landmarks:

- The midpoint of the clavicle is located midway between the acromial end (the prominence at the top of the shoulder) and the sternal end of the clavicle.
- The point of entry is on the lateral border of the scalenus anterior muscle at the midpoint of the clavicle.

Technique

After sterile preparation of the region, the needle is inserted at the point of entry above the midpoint of the clavicle in a backward-inward-downward direction. The needle thus appears to be at right angles to all planes at this level of the neck. Even though the direction of the needle is toward the first rib, it is not necessary to touch the rib (Fig. 18–1). Paresthesia of the digits or wrist is sought. If obtained, after negative aspiration for air or blood, inject 1 to 3 mL of local anesthetic as a test dose. This is followed after 5 minutes by the total calculated volume of the local anesthetic if there are no systemic effects. If paresthesia is not obtained and the needle touches the first rib, it is usually at the subclavian groove. The needle should then be walked posteriorly to elicit paresthesia. If paresthesia is not obtained, contact with the rib will be lost. It is then necessary to regain contact with the rib and walk toward the vertebra. If no paresthesia is obtained at this point, repeat the

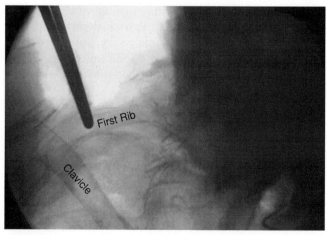

FIGURE 18–1

Radiographic supraclavicular view of the middle of the first rib as the site for skin entry toward the first rib.

procedure. A nerve stimulator can be used to aid in locating the brachial plexus.

Complications

Complications associated with this approach include hematomas of the neck and pneumothorax. In the event of the former, advise the patient, watch closely, and aspirate or evacuate the hematoma, if necessary; the hematoma will take 2 to 3 weeks to disappear by itself. For pneumothorax, conservative treatment is appropriate in fewer than 10% of cases, whereas chest tube insertion is advised for more than 20%.

INFRACLAVICULAR APPROACH

Position of the Patient and the Physician

The patient lies supine. The anesthesiologist should be standing opposite the arm to be blocked. Although the patient's arm is usually abducted to 90 degrees and the head turned away from the arm, the block can be performed with the patient's arm and head in any position (Fig. 18–2).

Landmarks

A line is drawn from the C6 tubercle to the brachial artery in the arm, which crosses the midpoint of the clavicle. This line provides the surface marking of the brachial plexus in the infraclavicular region.

- Before cleaning, the whole length of the clavicle and the subclavian artery where it dips under the clavicle should be identified by palpation and marked.
- If the artery cannot be felt, the midpoint of the clavicle should be identified.
- The point of needle entry is 2.5 cm below the midpoint of the clavicle (Fig. 18–3).

Technique

After the field has been sterilized and draped, the stimulator and the leads should be tested and the ground electrode attached to the patient's shoulder opposite the site of needle entry. The skin should be infiltrated with a small amount of local anesthetic 2.5 cm below the inferior border of the clavicle at its midpoint. A 22-gauge, unsheathed, standard 9-cm spinal needle should be introduced through the skin wheal with the needle point directed laterally toward the brachial artery (Fig. 18–4). After the needle has barely pierced the skin, the exploring electrode is attached either to the stem or to the metal hub of the needle with a sterile alligator clip. The voltage control of the peripheral nerve stimulator should be set to deliver 6 to 8 V or 3 to 5 mA at 1 or 2 impulses per second, and the needle should be advanced at a 45-degree angle to the skin. The pectoralis group of muscles will contract and adduct the shoulder. When that occurs, reduce the voltage until the patient is comfortable. When the needle tip is past the muscles, the contractions will stop. As the needle approaches the fibers of the brachial plexus, muscles supplied by the musculocutaneous, median, ulnar, and radial nerves will contract with each impulse (Fig. 18–5). Observe the forearm and hand carefully for these movements. When flexion or extension of the elbow, wrist, or

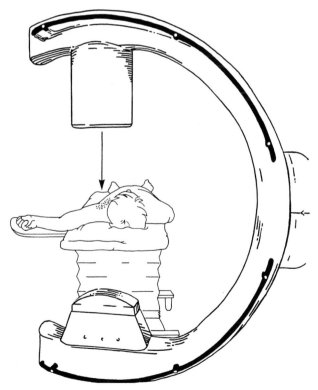

FIGURE 18–2

Drawing of the C-arm and the patient position for infraclavicular approach.

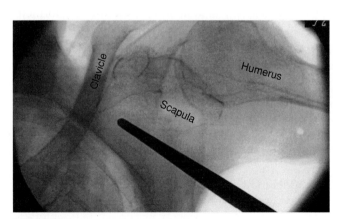

FIGURE 18–3

Radiographic anteroposterior view of the ipsilateral side for infraclavicular approaches, indicating the skin entry site in the middle of the scapula.

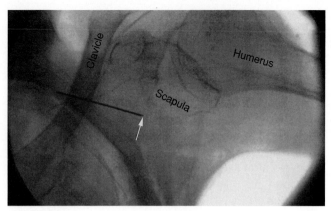

FIGURE 18–4

Radiographic anteroposterior view during insertion of the needle to the brachial plexus via the infraclavicular approach. The *arrow* shows the location of the needle tip conformed by a peripheral nerve stimulator.

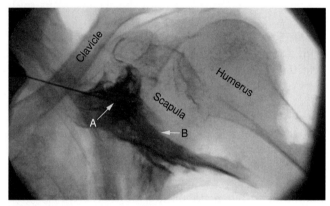

FIGURE 18–5

The contrast spread (20 mL) in the anteroposterior view during the performance of the infraclavicular block. The following is a key to the letters shown on the figure: A, width of the brachial plexus sheets; B, formation of the axillary sheath.

digits is observed, the needle point is close to nerve fibers of the brachial plexus (Fig. 18–6). When this occurs, decrease the voltage to the lowest level that still allows muscle movement to be observed. The needle should again be advanced until maximal muscle movements are seen and then begin to diminish. The diminution in muscle movement signals that the needle tip has passed the nerve.

Complications

The complications of continuous brachial plexus infusion are similar to those of a brachial plexus block: bleeding, infection, intravascular or intrathecal injection, pneumothorax, and phrenic nerve paralysis. The severity and length of phrenic nerve paralysis are related to the site of catheter placement (e.g., interscalene, supraclavicular) and what local anesthetic is used.[1–7] The plasma concentration and pharmacokinetics of the constant infusion in steady state are similar to

those observed in epidural infusion. Once steady state is reached, the drugs do not accumulate if infused at the same rate. The metabolites also remain at insignificant levels without causing any deleterious effects.[8]

AXILLARY APPROACH

Position of the Patient

The patient lies supine with the arm abducted 90 degrees at the shoulder joint and forearm placed in a supine position. Some anesthesiologists prefer to hyperabduct the arm at the shoulder joint with flexion at the elbow joint; this position should be avoided, because abduction beyond 90 degrees impedes the proximal spread of local anesthetic to the origin of the musculocutaneous nerve.

Technique

After the area is sterilized and draped, the anesthesiologist stands next to the arm to be blocked, palpating the axillary artery with the finger of one hand and with the palm of that hand resting comfortably on the upper arm. Next, the needle is inserted just proximal to the palpating finger. Since the width of the finger corresponds to the size of the brachial plexus sheath at that level, the needle insertion should be within the area delineated by the palpating finger. As the needle is inserted, any one of the following three different methods can be used to confirm the needle's position in the brachial plexus sheath (Fig. 18–7):

1. If the needle penetrates the axillary artery, withdraw the needle until the needle pulsates over the artery and blood can no longer be aspirated.
2. Paresthesia can be sought in the distribution of the ulnar, median, or radial nerves.

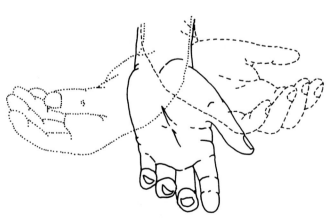

FIGURE 18–6

During the testing with peripheral nerve stimulation, one needs to identify the main nerves being stimulated. In this drawing, one can note palmar flexions of the wrist and flexion of all digits and ulnar deviation of the wrist. This suggests that median and ulnar nerves are being stimulated.

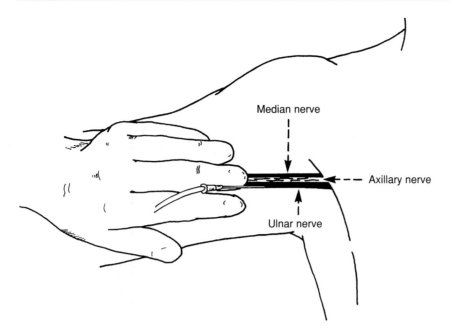

FIGURE 18-7
The drawing shows the axillary approaches with the middle finger on the brachial artery.

3. When a peripheral nerve stimulator is used, movements of the muscles in the hand are seen at the lowest current (0.5 mamp) voltage (2 V) and disappear after injection of 2 mL of local anesthetic solution.

Once the needle position has been confirmed, the axillary artery is compressed and an adequate volume and concentration of anesthetic solution is injected. Compression of the axillary artery during injection facilitates the proximal spread of the anesthetic solution to block the musculocutaneous nerves. A tourniquet is not needed.

After injection of the required volume of local anesthetic, the needle should be removed, the area massaged, and the patient's arm brought down the side while the anesthesiologist continues to compress the axilla for a few minutes. The block can be confirmed by clinical examination and, optionally, by neurostimulator. If signs of toxicity occur with injection, indicating that inadvertent intravascular injection has occurred, it is essential to stop the injection, withdraw the needle, and stabilize the patient.

Side Effects and Complications

The proximity of the nerves to the axillary artery and other large vessels carries the risk for inadvertent intravascular injection or local anesthetic toxicity from intravascular absorption. Given the large doses of local anesthetic required for axillary brachial plexus block, the pain specialist should carefully calculate the total milligram dose of local anesthetic that may safely be given. The dense vascularity also increases the risk of postblock ecchymosis and hematoma formation. In spite of the vascularity of this anatomic region, this technique can safely be attempted in a patient taking anticoagulant by using a 25- or 27-gauge needle, albeit at increased risk of hematoma, if the clinical situation dictates a favorable risk-to-benefit ratio. These complications can be reduced if manual pressure is applied to the area of the block immediately after injection. Applying cold packs for 20-minute periods after the block also reduces the amount of postprocedure pain and bleeding.

The distance of the nerves to be blocked from the neuraxis and phrenic nerve makes the complications associated with injection of drugs onto these structures highly unlikely, which is an advantage of the axial approach as compared with the intrascalene and supraclavicular approaches to brachial plexus block. Because paresthesias are elicited, the potential for postblock persistent paresthesia is a possibility and the patient should be so advised.

HELPFUL HINTS

SUPRACLAVICULAR APPROACHES

The key to performing safe and successful supraclavicular brachial plexus block is a clear understanding of the anatomy and careful identification of the necessary anatomic landmarks. Poking around for a paresthesia without first identifying the anatomic landmarks is a recipe for disaster. The pain specialist should remember that the brachial plexus is quite close to the surface at the level where this block is performed. The needle should rarely be inserted deeper than 1 inch in all but the most obese patients. If strict adherence to technique is observed and the needle is never advanced medially from the lateral border of the insertion of the sternocleidomastoid muscle on the clavicle, the incidence of pneumothorax should be less than 0.5%. Careful neurologic examination to identify preexisting neurologic deficits that might later be attributed to the nerve block should be performed before beginning the brachial plexus block.

INFRACLAVICULAR APPROACH

It is helpful to abduct the arm 90 degrees or more to open the axilla and allow the brachial plexus to traverse lateral to the first to fourth ribs by this measure. Because the brachial plexus is deeper than at other approaches, a stimulator to locate the plexus is important. The musculocutaneous nerve (C5–C6) should not be the target since it is too far lateral. The physician should aim for the median nerve for reliable success.

AXILLARY APPROACH

The axillary approach to brachial plexus block is a safe and simple way to anesthetize the distal upper extremity. For pain above the elbow, the interscalene or supraclavicular approach is probably a better choice. Careful neurologic examination for preexisting neurologic deficits that might later be attributed to the nerve block should be performed before any brachial plexus block.

EFFICACY

For periods up to 48 hours, continuous brachial plexus analgesia is reliably efficacious. After this period, the efficacy drops precipitously for A delta fiber blocking. Sympathetic blocking can still be maintained for as long as 2 to 3 weeks with 0.125% or 0.25% bupivacaine quite reliably if catheters are well anchored.

The best site for catheter insertion seems to be the infraclavicular region. The second best site is at the axilla. The interscalene site is too superficial for reliable anchoring over prolonged periods.

Brachial plexus 64415.

REFERENCES

1. Pere P, Pitkanen M, Rosenberg PH, et al: Effect of continuous interscalene brachial plexus block on diaphragm motion and on ventilatory function. Acta Anaesthesiol Scand 36:53–57, 1992.
2. Urmey WF, Talts KH, Sharrock NE: One hundred percent incidence of hemidiaphragmatic paresis associated with interscalene brachial plexus anesthesia as diagnosed by ultrasonography. Anesth Analg 52:897–004, 1973.
3. Urmey WF, McDonald M: Hemidiaphragmatic paresis during interscalene brachial plexus block: Effects on pulmonary function and chest wall mechanics. Anesth Analg 74:352–357, 1992.
4. Knoblanche GE: The incidence and etiology of phrenic nerve blockade associated with supraclavicular brachial plexus block. Anaesth Intensive Care 7:346–349, 1979.
5. Dhuner K-G, Moberg E, Onne L: Paresis of the phrenic nerve during brachial plexus block analgesia nd its importance. Acta Chir Scand 109:53–57, 1955.
6. Farrar MD, Scheybani M, Nolte H: Upper extremity block: Effectiveness and complications. Reg Anesth 6:133–134, 1981.
7. Kulenkampff D: Die Anasthesia des plexus brachialis. Zentralbl Chir 38:1337–1340, 1911.
8. Raj, PP, Montegomery SJ, Nettles D, et al: Infraclavicular brachial plexus block—a new approach. Anesth Analg 52:897–904, 1973.

CHAPTER

19

Intercostal Nerve Block

HISTORY

On reviewing the early writings of Schleich,[1] Braun,[2] Pauchet and associates,[3] and Labat,[4] one is struck with the idea that the technique of intercostal nerve blockade developed through a series of evolutionary steps. At the turn of the 20th century, surgeons were fascinated by infiltration anesthesia. Elaborate descriptions and recipes defined how surgery of the chest and abdomen could be accomplished using large volumes (100 to 150 mL) of dilute solutions of local anesthetic drugs, procaine being the mainstay after it was synthesized in 1904. Over time, many of the descriptions and illustrations began to define the reality of blocking the intercostal nerve trunk, in preference to the more elaborate process of infiltration or "field block" of the more peripheral twigs and branches. In addition, paravertebral injections began to be used as an alternative to spinal injections.[5] These lumbar and thoracic blocks became popular because of increasing doubt and concern about possible neurotoxicity from the injection of cocaine and its synthetic allies directly into the spinal canal. Techniques were defined whereby major nerve trunks could be blocked after they exited the vertebral canal. Thus, proximal and more distal sites for blocking intercostal nerves were gradually defined. By 1922, Labat's textbook contained an elaborate description of intercostal nerve block that is quite similar to our present-day conceptions.

ANATOMY

The intercostal nerves are composed of the ventral rami of the first through the twelfth thoracic nerves. The first, second, and twelfth nerves differ from the other nine in several respects. T1 gives off a small contribution to the brachial plexus. T2–T3 sends cutaneous branches to the arm as the intercostobrachial nerve. T12 is not strictly an intercostal nerve but, rather, is more appropriately called a *subcostal nerve*. It runs its course in the abdominal wall below the twelfth rib and sends fibers to join L1.

Evidence from cadaver studies indicates that the classic medical school teaching that the intercostal vein, artery, and nerve are located in precise order and comfortably tucked into the subcostal groove is unrealistic. The nerve may actually vary from a subcostal to midcostal to supracostal location. In his cadaver study, Hardy[6] found the frequencies of these variations: classic subcostal, 17%; mid-zone, 73%; and supracostal, 10%.

Another anatomic subtlety for the anesthesiologist's appreciation is intercostal nerve branching, of which there are two types. First, the nerve may split into separate bundles that have no common enclosing fascial sheath. These may rejoin or subdivide further as the nerve continues its lateral course; thus, there is not necessarily a single, well-defined nerve at every site in the intercostal space. Second, each intercostal nerve gives off four well-defined branches as it proceeds on its circuitous route anteriorly. The first is the gray rami communicantes, which goes to the appropriate sympathetic ganglion. The second branch arises as the posterior cutaneous branch and supplies skin and muscles in the paravertebral region and possibly as far lateral as the posterior axillary line. The third branch, the lateral cutaneous division, arises just anterior to the midaxillary line. The clinical importance of the takeoff of this branch historically has been emphasized, and perhaps exaggerated. This is a concern during blocking of intercostal nerves for pain relief, because the third branch sends subcutaneous fibers coursing both posteriorly and anteriorly, and a lateral injection could conceivably be directed too far anterior and miss the point of takeoff. The terminal or final branch is the anterior cutaneous branch, which provides cutaneous innervation to the midline of the chest and abdomen. Unlike the situation at the vertebral spines, there appears to be some slight overlap of sensory fibers across the anterior midline of the chest and abdomen.

The paravertebral space deserves separate discussion. The dura mater and the arachnoid membrane fuse with the epineurium as the nerve exits the vertebral foramen. This has two important implications. Local anesthetics or other drugs injected directly intraneurally to the peripheral nerve may spread centrally, to the nerve roots or spinal cord. It is also possible to produce epidural or spinal anesthesia if a large volume of local anesthetic is injected into the paravertebral region and then flows centrally around the nerve in the vertebral foramen. Conacher[7] has nicely demonstrated that even quick-setting resin can be thus propelled into the vertebral epidural space. He also showed that correctly placed paravertebral intercostal injections can spread over several intercostal spaces and can even dissect the pleura laterally from the vertebral bodies. In transverse section, the paravertebral space is wedge shaped. The posterior wall is the costotransverse ligament; anterolaterally is the parietal pleura; and medially lie the vertebral body and vertebral foramen. From the paravertebral space to the posterior angle of the rib, there is no structure between the intercostal nerve and the pleura. At the angle of the rib, the internal intercostal muscle arises and lies internal to the nerve, all the way around to the costosternal cartilages.

In the paravertebral region, the intercostal artery and vein are usually singular structures. Laterally, they show multiple branches. This has implications for intercostal block, because vessel puncture can lead to hematoma formation or rapid uptake of local anesthetic drug. Flank hematomas can become quite extensive in a patient taking anticoagulants.[8] Other high-risk scenarios involve patients with neurofibromatosis, Marfan's syndrome, and arterial dilatation or stretching, as, for example, in coarctation of the aorta or severe scoliosis.[9]

INDICATIONS

No method of pain relief is more specific and effective for fractured ribs than intercostal nerve block.[10] The pain from chest wall contusion, pleurisy, and flail chest is also quickly relieved.[11, 12] Often unappreciated is the fact that the pain from median sternotomy, pericardial window, or fractured sternum can be controlled successfully by blocks in the parasternal region (Fig. 19–1).[4] This point might well be applied to many cardiac and pulmonary surgery cases of today.[13, 14] Blockade of two or more nerves is a simple way to prepare for insertion of thoracostomy tubes and can also be used to provide analgesia for percutaneous biliary drainage or liver biopsy. Perhaps the most important but least exploited use of this block is for control of postoperative pain of the chest or abdomen.[15] A simple study by Bunting and McGeachie[16] vividly demonstrates this point. They performed lateral intercostal blocks of right T10, T11, and T12 at the conclusion of appendectomy. With this investment of a few milliliters of local anesthetic drug, the study patients required only a third as much postoperative narcotic as did the patients who did not receive intercostal blocks.

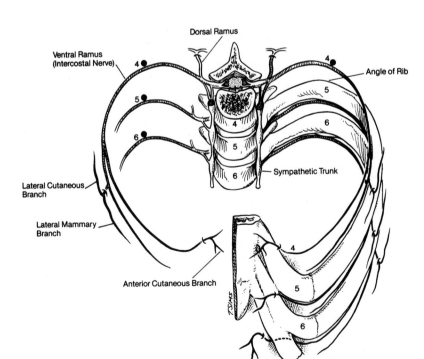

FIGURE 19–1

Anatomy of the intercostal nerve and its distribution with its branches along the ribs. (From Raj PP, Pai U, Rawal N: Techniques of regional anesthesia in adults. In Raj PP [ed]: Clinical Practice of Regional Anesthesia. New York, Churchill Livingstone, 1991, p 301.)

Intercostal blocks (Current Procedural Technology [CPT] Code 64420 [single], 64421 [multiple, regional]) are also useful in several chronic pain scenarios. For instance, when combined or alternated with celiac plexus blockade, they can help resolve a not uncommon diagnostic dilemma and distinguish abdominal wall pain from visceral pain. A unilateral paravertebral T12 and L1 nerve block (CPT Code 64440 [single], 64441 [multiple, regional]) can help unravel the question of nerve entrapment syndromes after inguinal hernia repair. Numerous references have been made to the diagnostic and therapeutic benefits of this block in patients with acute and chronic pain from herpes zoster.[17] There are also limited applications for a limited number of neurolytic intercostal blocks (CPT Code 64620) in some patients with terminal cancer.

CONTRAINDICATIONS

An intercostal nerve block is contraindicated if pneumothorax would be deleterious to the patient, if there is infection at the site of the injection, if the patient is on anticoagulant therapy, if the patient is allergic to local anesthetics, and if the patient is in shock.

EQUIPMENT

Local Block
- 25-gauge, ¾-inch needle
- 22-gauge, 1½-inch needle
- 3-mL syringe
- 5-mL syringe

Cryoneurolysis
- 12- or 14-gauge, 1½-inch angiocatheter
- Cryoprobe set

The intercostal nerve root block is performed with a 22-gauge, 1½-inch needle; a 23-gauge, ½-inch needle; 10-mL syringes; and the usual preparation tray.

DRUGS

- 1.5% lidocaine
- 0.5% bupivacaine/ropivicaine
- 2% lidocaine
- Steroids (optional)

The volume of injectate is 3 to 5 mL per intercostal nerve. For a short-duration block, 1% to 1.5% lidocaine is used; for a long-duration block, 0.5% bupivacaine or 1% etidocaine is used. For a neurolytic block, 6% to 8% phenol in diatrizoate is used.

PREPARATION OF THE PATIENT

PHYSICAL EXAMINATION

Physical examination should be performed to determine the level of patient pain and to rule out disease that may distort the anatomy.

PREOPERATIVE MEDICATION: USE OF SEDATIVE DRUGS

Intercostal nerve block may cause significant skin and periosteal stimulation that can be easily relieved by giving light sedation before the procedure. This is not to say that these nerve blocks cannot be performed without sedation. In fact, it may be mandatory to use little or no sedation when the blocks are performed on seriously ill patients or when a block is being used to help solve a diagnostic pain dilemma. Drugs commonly used to supplement these blocks include midazolam, fentanyl, ketamine, thiopental, and propofol.[18] The clinical situation should dictate which agent(s) should be used. Is there need for hypnosis, analgesia, tranquilization, or some combination of these effects? It is important to titrate all sedative drugs in small intravenous doses while observing closely for the desired action.

PROCEDURE

POSITION OF THE PATIENT AND PHYSICIAN

The blocks are easiest to learn and perform with the patient in a prone position with a pillow under the mid-abdomen. This position is optimal for rib identification by posterior palpation of the intercostal spaces. The patient's arms are kept hanging over the sides of the cart or operating table to rotate the scapula laterally and make it easier to block the nerves under the upper ribs.

SITE OF NEEDLE ENTRY

In the classic approach, intercostal nerve block is performed posteriorly at the angle of the ribs and just lateral to the sacrospinalis group of muscles (Fig. 19–2).[19] At this point, the thickness of the rib is about 8 mm.

After the patient is positioned, it is helpful to use a skin marking pen to identify the inferior edge of each rib. This constitutes a map to illustrate and review anatomic detail and ultimately makes the process of blocking smoother and quicker. First, a vertical line is drawn connecting the posterior thoracic vertebral spines. Then, by palpation, the lateral edge of the sacrospinalis group of muscles is identified and marked as another vertical line on each side. This lateral line is

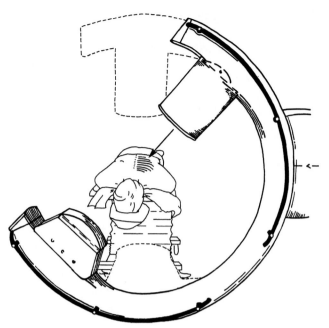

FIGURE 19–2

The patient is lying in the prone position beneath the fluoroscopic C-arm. After identifying the appropriate levels for blockade, the C-arm is rotated ipsilaterally to enhance the posterolateral ribs.

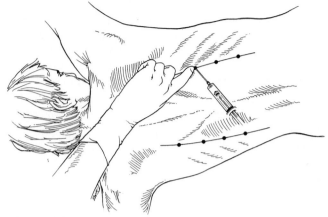

FIGURE 19–3

Intercostal block, showing the correct placement of anesthetist's finger on the inferior edge of patient's rib. Note that the needle with syringe touches rib before slipping under it to touch the intercostal nerve. The needle should be inserted obliquely under rib to prevent development of a pneumothorax. (From Raj PP, Pai U, Rawal N: Techniques of regional anesthesia in adults. In Raj PP [ed]: Clinical Practice of Regional Anesthesia. New York, Churchill Livingstone, 1991, p 302.)

usually 7 to 8 cm from the posterior midline and should angle medially at the upper levels to avoid the scapulae. The inferior border of each rib is then marked along these two lateral vertical lines.

Once these markings and local anesthetic mixing preparations have been completed, the initial step is to raise skin wheals (using a 30-gauge needle) at each of the previously marked intersections of vertical and horizontal lines. A 2- to 3-cm, 22- or 23-gauge needle is then used to inject each intercostal nerve. If a disposable long-beveled needle is used, the operator must remember that the tip may easily be bent with the repeated bone contacts necessary to do this block. The needle can thus become barbed and possibly cause bleeding or nerve damage (Fig. 19–3).

Beginning at the lowest rib, a right-handed operator uses the index finger of the left hand to pull the skin up and over at the lower edge of the rib. The needle is then introduced to the rib as the palpating left index finger defines it. Obviously, care should be taken to prevent the needle's penetrating beyond this palpated depth, because it could enter the interpleural or intra-alveolar space. The practitioner should think of the palpating finger as having sonar capabilities. Once the needle reaches the rib, the right hand pushes to maintain firm contact between needle and rib. The left hand is then shifted to gain control of the needle by holding the hub and shaft with thumb and the index and middle fingers. Firm placement of the left hand's hypothenar eminence against the patient's back is crucial. This allows precise and constant control of needle depth as the left hand

now "walks" the needle off the lower edge of the rib. While the needle is being advanced, a slight loss of resistance is often felt as the tip enters the correct space. From 3 to 5 mL of local anesthetic solution is injected at each interspace. The left hand then walks the needle back onto the rib and finally releases control to the right hand and to the left index finger for palpation of the next higher rib. Keeping the needle in firm contact with the previously injected rib until the next space is identified serves to avoid missing a rib or doing a second block of the same rib.

This process is repeated for each of the nerves to be blocked. An experienced operator can safely and successfully block 12 to 14 ribs in 3 to 5 minutes. Intercostal blocks may be repeated as needed (Fig. 19–4).

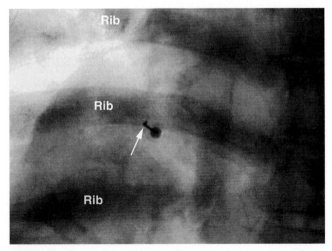

FIGURE 19–4

Intercostal nerve block, anteroposterior view. The *arrow* indicates where the needle touches and stops below the rib.

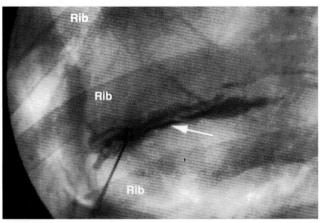

FIGURE 19–5

Intercostal nerve block with contrast medium, anteroposterior view. The *arrow* indicates the spread of contrast in the intercostal groove.

Cryoanalgesia has been advocated as a method of obtaining blocks of long duration by freezing the nerves. This technique, however, is unreliable, cumbersome, and declining in use (Fig. 19–5).[20, 21]

COMPLICATIONS

PNEUMOTHORAX

Careful performance of the block reduces the risk of development of pneumothorax. If it does develop, it should be recognized and treated as necessary. The patient must be reassured.

SUBARACHNOID BLOCK

An inadvertent subarachnoid block should be treated as a spinal block. This complication has been reported and proven with dye studies. Because the dura occasionally extends out along the intercostal nerve a variable distance before it adheres to the nerve as the neurilemma or nerve sheath, an anesthetic drug deposited in this potential space can dissect back into the subarachnoid space and result in spinal anesthesia. All the devices necessary to support the patient should be present (e.g., airway equipment, breathing bag, intravenous fluids, and vasopressors).

INTRAVASCULAR INJECTION LEADING TO SYSTEMIC TOXICITY

Treat the toxicity; intravascular absorption is much more problematic. Since the intercostal space is supplied by a rich network of vascular anastomoses because of the high metabolic activity of the intercostal muscles, there is a much greater absorption of the local anesthetic, leading to high plasma levels. Blood anesthetic levels are higher here and peak sooner than when the same amount of local anesthetic is injected elsewhere, such as axillary sheath or other nerve blocks. This may lead to toxic reactions. Pay careful attention to the maximum dosage allowed, and add a vasoconstrictor in small concentrations (i.e., a 1:200,000 to 1:400,000 concentration is useful).

HELPFUL HINTS

Large volumes of local anesthetics should not be used for intercostal blocks, since they are more readily absorbed at this site than at other sites. The risks associated with this block are intravascular injection and pneumothorax. Pneumothorax can be prevented if the operator is careful and slow and learns the anatomy of the areas before trying the technique. Resuscitative equipment and skilled personnel should be nearby.

EFFICACY

The success rate of intercostal nerve block should approach 100%.

Intercostal nerve, single 64420; intercostal nerve, multiple 64421.

REFERENCES

1. Schleich DS: Schmerzlose Operationen. Berlin, J Springer, 1894.
2. Braun H: Local Anesthesia: Its Scientific Basis and Practical Use. Philadelphia, Lea & Febiger, 1914.
3. Pauchet V, Sourdat P, Labat G: L'Anesthésie Régionale, 3rd ed. Paris, Librairie Octave Doin, 1921.
4. Labat G: Regional Anesthesia: Its Technic and Clinical Application. Philadelphia, WB Saunders, 1922.
5. Mandl F: Paravertebral Block. New York, Grune & Stratton, 1947.
6. Hardy PAJ: Anatomical variation in the position of the proximal intercostal nerve. Br J Anaesth 61:338, 1988.
7. Conacher ID: Resin injection of thoracic paravertebral spaces. Br J Anaesth 61:657, 1988.
8. Baxter AD, Flynn JF, Jennings FO: Continuous intercostal nerve blockade. Br J Anaesth 56:665, 1984.
9. Butchart EG, Grott GJ, Barnsley WC: Spontaneous rupture of an intercostal artery in a patient with neurofibromatosis and scoliosis. J Thorac Cardiovasc Surg 69:919, 1975.
10. Moore DC, Bridenbaugh LD: Intercostal nerve block in 4333 patients: Indications, technique, and complications. Anesth Analg 41:1, 1962.
11. Moore DC: Intercostal nerve block for postoperative somatic pain following surgery of thorax and upper abdomen. Br J Anaesth 47:284, 1975.
12. Mozell EJ, Sabanathan S, Mearns AJ, et al: Continuous extrapleural intercostal nerve block after pleurecotomy. Thorax 46:21, 1991.
13. Conacher I, Kokri M: Postoperative paravertebral blocks for thoracic surgery. Br J Anaesth 59:155, 1987.
14. Baxter AD, Jennings FO, Harris RS, et al: Continuous intercostal blockade after cardiac surgery. Br J Anaesth 59:162, 1987.
15. Nunn JF, Slavin C: Posterior intercostal nerve block for pain relief after cholecystectomy. Br J Anaesth 52:253, 1980.
16. Bunting P, McGeachie JF: Intercostal nerve blockade producing analgesia after appendicectomy. Br J Anaesth 61:169, 1988.

17. Sihota MK, Holmblad BR: Horner's syndrome after interpleural anesthesia with bupivacaine for postherpetic neuralgia. Acta Anesth Scand 32:593, 1988.
18. Thompson GE, Moore DC: Ketamine, diazepam, and Innovar: A computerized comparative study. Anesth Analg 50:458, 1971.
19. Thompson GE, Brown DL: The common nerve blocks. In Nunn FF, Utting JE, Brown BR (eds): General Anaesthesia, 5th ed. London, Butterworth, 1989, p 1070.
20. Lloyd JW, Barnard JDW, Glynn CJ: Cryoanalgesia: A new approach to pain relief. Lancet 2:932, 1976.
21. Maiwand O, Makey AR: Cryoanalgesia for relief of pain after thoracotomy. BMJ 282:1749, 1981.

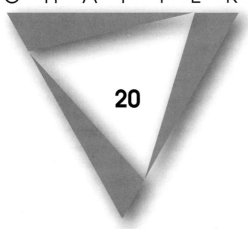

C H A P T E R

20

Thoracic Sleeve and Dorsal Root Ganglion Block and Neurolysis

HISTORY

The origin of selective nerve root blockade (SNRB) can be traced back to 1906 when Sellheim performed paravertebral blocks for urological surgery.[1] A few years later, in 1912, Kappis described the blockade of the brachial plexus via the cervical nerve roots. Over the ensuing century, selective root sleeve blocks have become commonplace in the diagnosis and treatment of many painful syndromes. For the purposes of this chapter, detailed knowledge of the nerve root and surrounding anatomic structures is of utmost importance to improve the efficacy of the block, and, more important, to decrease the incidence of complications. To complement the physician's knowledge base, the use of fluoroscopy is heavily stressed. It is even more important if the physician chooses to use a neurolytic agent.

ANATOMY

VERTEBRAL COLUMN

The spinal axis comprises 33 vertebral bodies: 7 cervical, 12 thoracic, 5 lumbar, 5 sacral, and 4 coccygeal. Each vertebra consists of two parts: the ventral vertebral body and the dorsal vertebral arch (Fig. 20–1).[2,3] In turn, the vertebral arch is composed of two pedicles anteriorly and two lamina posteriorly. Laterally, the pedicle and the laminae of each vertebra join to form the transverse process. In a similar fashion, the laminae join dorsally to form the spinous process that is often bifid in the cervical region. The junction of the ventral vertebral body with the dorsal vertebral arch creates the vertebral foramen, which in sequence form the vertebral canal. The vertebral canal is triangular in the cervical and lumbar regions but circular in the thoracic region.[4] The vertebral bodies are separated by the intervertebral discs, which are composed of an avascular gelatin-like

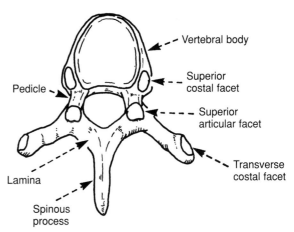

FIGURE 20–1

Thoracic vertebrae components.

core, the nucleus pulposus, surrounded by the annulus fibrosus, collagenous lamellae.

The intervertebral foramina are formed by the pedicles at the cephalad and caudal ends; posteriorly by the opposing articular surfaces and ligamentum flavum; and anteriorly by the vertebral body superiorly and intervertebral disc caudally (Fig. 20–2).

NERVE ROOTS

Exiting the neuroforamina are 31 pairs of spinal nerves: 8 cervical, 12 thoracic, 5 lumbar, 5 sacral, and 1 coccygeal. The eighth cervical nerve emerges between the C7 and T1 vertebral bodies, whereas the remaining seven cervical nerves emerge above their same-numbered vertebral bones. In the thoracic, lumbar, and sacral regions, the spinal nerves emerge below their same-numbered vertebral segments.

Each nerve is formed by the union of the anterior (ventral) motor root and the posterior (dorsal) sensory

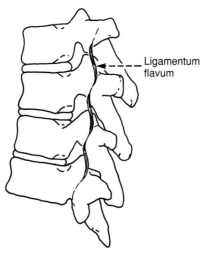

FIGURE 20–2

Lateral view of the thoracic vertebrae that shows the borders of the intervertebral foramina.

root, which remain separate within the subarachnoid space. The anterior root originates from the anterolateral columns of the cord and of four to eight filaments. It is generally smaller than its posterior counterpart. The posterior root originates from the posterolateral fissure of the cord and contains a ganglion that is not found in the anterior root. Likewise, the posterior root is composed of four to eight rootlets. The two roots form a mixed peripheral nerve only after becoming ensheathed by the dura-arachnoid distal to the dorsal root ganglion (DRG).[2] The nerve root is covered by a thin membranous structure (root sheath), which is permeable to cerebrospinal fluid.[5] The nerve root sheath is continuous with the pia mater at the junction with the spinal cord.[6] The epineurium of the peripheral nerve is continuous with the dura mater, and the endoneurium also continues from the peripheral nerve to the nerve root. The perineurium separates into two layers at the border of these

nervous tissues, and only part of it is included in the root sheath. Thus, the nerve root lacks both the perineurium and epineurium of the peripheral nerve.

Once the mixed nerve exits the intervertebral foramen, it divides into anterior and posterior rami, which innervate their respective parts of the body. The larger anterior rami form the major nerve plexus, whereas the smaller posterior rami divide almost immediately into lateral and medial branches and innervate the paraspinous musculature and the facet joints at their respective levels (Fig. 20–3A).[7] Branching almost immediately from the ventral roots from T1 to L2 are the white rami communicantes that carry preganglionic sympathetic information to the sympathetic ganglion. Some postganglionic sympathetic nerves exit the sympathetic ganglion and return to the ventral division via the gray rami communicantes, whereas others course through the sympathetic chain located along the vertebral column (Fig. 20–3B).

The nerve roots in the thoracic and lumbosacral regions also have a similar blood supply. The proximal radicular arteries also branch from the anterior and posterior spinal arteries. The posterior intercostal, lumbar segmental, and lateral sacral arteries give rise to the thoracic, lumbar, and sacral distal radicular arteries, respectively. At all levels, a branch of the posterior radicular artery supplies the DRG.

INDICATIONS

The SNRB, when combined with a careful history, physical examination, and quality radiographic studies, is an important tool in the diagnostic evaluation and treatment of patients with predominantly radicular symptoms.[8] It is helpful in patients with multiple level abnormalities, in complex postoperative patients, and in patients with clearly defined clinical symptoms

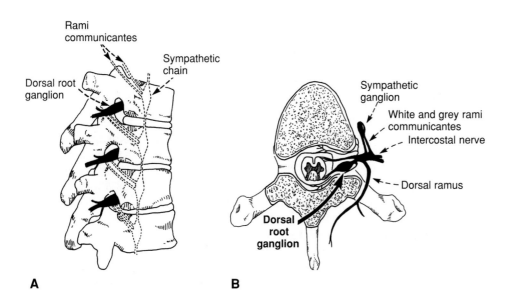

A   **B**

FIGURE 20–3

A, Lateral view of the thorax spine showing gray and white rami communicantes to the sympathetic chain. B, Coronal view. The course of the nerve roots and their connections are identified here.

without significant imaging findings.[9] More specifically, an SNRB is useful in helping to (1) ascertain the specific nociceptive pathway; (2) define the mechanisms of the chronic pain state; and (3) identify the differential diagnosis of the site of the pain.[10]

SNRBs are also performed for both prognostic and therapeutic purposes. Prognostically, the SNRB aids in predicting the efficacy of a neurolytic or neurosurgical treatment.[10–12] The prognostic block also affords the patient the opportunity to experience the numbness and other side effects that follow surgical resection or neurolytic block.[10] From this experience, the patient can decide whether or not to undergo the procedure. On a therapeutic basis, SNRBs are useful for treating pain not amenable to other methods of analgesia. This can be on a temporary or permanent basis, depending on the medication used.

Clinical indications include pain secondary to nerve root compression, pain from tumor invasion of a nerve root or in the distribution of a nerve root, vertebral fractures, acute herpetic neuralgia, postherpetic neuralgia, discogenic pain, segmental neuralgia, and postsurgical pain.[13, 14]

CONTRAINDICATIONS

- Local infection
- Coagulopathy

EQUIPMENT

Nerve Block
- 25-gauge, ¾-inch infiltration needle
- 20-gauge, 10-cm blunt-curved needle with 10-mm active tip
- 16-gauge, 1½-inch angiocatheter
- 3-mL syringe
- 5-mL syringe
- 10-mL syringe
- IV T-piece extension

Pulsed Electrode Magnetic Field and Radiofrequency Thermocoagulation
- Same as above, with the addition of a radiofrequency thermocoagulation electrode and connecting cables

PROCEDURE

The lower thoracic nerve roots are approached slightly differently. This is due to the changing orientation of the facet joints at the lower levels, which makes the neuroforamen more accessible. Obtain an anteroposterior view of the desired level. Mark the 4-cm line to

identify the most lateral margin. Oblique the C-arm 15 to 20 degrees to the ipsilateral side. The site of skin entry is the shadow of the tip of the superior pars articularis. Insert the angiocatheter and advance the needle until the tip of the superior pars articularis is touched. Rotate the needle and walk around the pars. Advance the needle a few millimeters and obtain a lateral view (Fig. 20–4).

On lateral view, advance the needle until it just enters the foramen below the inferior border of the pedicle (Fig. 20–5). Proper placement of the needle on the anteroposterior view is just below the pedicle with the tip touching an imaginary line drawn vertically through the center of each pedicle (Fig. 20–5B). Contrast medium and local anesthetic are then injected after negative aspirate.

DORSAL ROOT GANGLIONOTOMY (PARTIAL RHIZOTOMY)

Only after a successful diagnostic block should a partial rhizotomy of the DRG be attempted. This can be performed using conventional radiofrequency (RF), pulsed electrode magnetic field (pEMF), cryoanalgesia, and neurolytics. Epidural neurolytic blocks have been performed in the past, but with the advent of RF techniques, neurolytics are infrequently used. Therefore, only conventional and pulsed RF are discussed in this section.

The goal is to position the tip of the needle directly adjacent to the DRG of the desired nerve root. A sensory paresthesia should be felt in the desired dermatome at less than 1.0 V at 50-Hz stimulation. Ideal stimulation should be felt between 0.4 and 0.6 V. If stimulation is felt at less than 0.4 V, the tip of the needle is too close to the DRG, and if stimulation is felt at greater than 0.6 V, the tip is too far away from the DRG. Motor stimulation is then performed at 2 Hz. There should be a clear dissociation between motor and sensory stimulation; that is, the voltage required to see motor fasciculations at 2 Hz should be at least two times the voltage that produces sensory stimulation at 50 Hz.[13] Thus, if good sensory stimulation at 50 Hz was noted at 0.5 V, then motor fasciculations at 2 Hz should not be seen at voltages less than 1.0 V. The point of dissociation defines the position of the DRG. If dissociation between sensory and motor stimulation cannot be obtained, the tip of the needle is not in alignment with the DRG, and lesioning at this point is not recommended.

Once the proper stimulation parameters have been achieved, inject 2 mL of local anesthetic with 40 mg of triamcinolone diacetate. Wait 3 to 5 minutes and then lesion at 67°C for 90 seconds with conventional RF. With pEMF, local anesthetic is not required since the necessary temperature is just above body temperature.

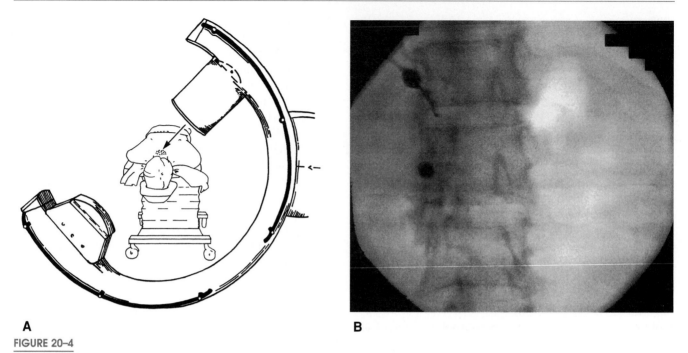

FIGURE 20-4

A, Drawing of the patient in the prone position and the fluoroscopic C-arm in the oblique "tunnel" position. *B*, Radiographic image of the oblique tunnel view with needles in place.

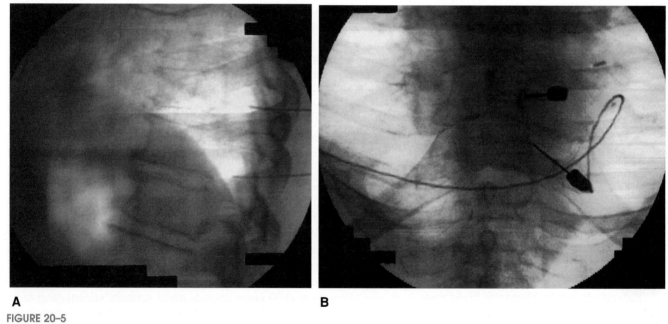

FIGURE 20-5

Radiographic images of the thoracic sleeve root needles in lateral *(A)* and anteroposterior *(B)* views.

Lesioning is carried out at 42°C for 120 seconds. There has been no reported neuritis with pEMF.

COMPLICATIONS

One of the biggest concerns is damage to the nerve root while the needle is being positioned. Using a blunt-tipped needle dramatically reduces this complication.

Neuritis after RF lesioning is the other big concern. This is the reason that sensory and motor testing is so important. If the proper parameters are not met, there is an increased incidence of postprocedure neuritis (30%). Injection of steroid prior to lesioning helps reduce, but not completely eliminate, the chance of neuritis.

Other complications include intravascular and intrathecal injection of medication, paralysis, bowel and bladder incontinence, pneumothorax, hemothorax, bruising, bleeding, increased pain, and infection.[14]

HELPFUL HINTS

Curved blunt-tipped needles have been useful in avoiding neural trauma and pneumothoraces in this procedure. In addition, by not inserting the needle beyond 4 cm laterally, the incidence of pneumothoraces is further decreased.

EFFICACY

Data cannot be found for thoracic DRG blockade. Individually, the blocks have been helpful in carefully selected patients.

Transforaminal epidural, cervical/thoracic single level 64479; transforaminal epidural, cervical/thoracic additional levels 64480.

REFERENCES

1. Fink B: History of neural blockade. In Cousins M, Bridenbaugh PO (eds): Neural Blockade in Clinical Anesthesia and Management of Pain, 2nd ed. Philadelphia, JB Lippincott, 1988, pp 13–21.
2. McQuillan P: Central nerve blocks: Subarachnoid. In Raj PP (ed): Practical Management of Pain, 3rd ed. St. Louis, Mosby, 2000, pp 631–636.
3. Raj P, Nolte H, Stanton-Hicks M: Central nerve blocks. In Raj PP (ed): Pain Medicine: A Comprehensive Review. St. Louis, Mosby, 1996, pp 185–199.
4. Hogan Q: Spinal anatomy. In Hahn M, McQuillan P, Sheplock G (eds): Regional Anesthesia: An Atlas of Anatomy and Technique. St. Louis, Mosby–Year Book, 1996, pp 205–220.
5. Hasue M: Pain and the nerve root. Spine 18:2053–2058, 1993.
6. Yoshizawa H, Kobayashi S, Hachiya Y: Blood supply of nerve roots and dorsal root ganglia. Orthop Clin North Am 22:195–211, 1991.
7. Bose K, Balasubramaniam P: Nerve root canals of the lumbar spine. Spine 9:16–18, 1984.
8. Slosar P, White A, Wetzel F: The use of selective nerve root blocks: Diagnostic, therapeutic, or placebo? 23:2253–2256, 1998.
9. Link S, El-Khoury G, Guilford WB: Percutaneous epidural and nerve root block and percutaneous lumbar sympatholysis. Radiol Clin North Am 36:509–521, 1998.
10. Levy B: Diagnostic, prognostic, and therapeutic nerve blocks. Arch Surg 112:870–879, 1977.
11. Lamacraft G, Cousins M: Neural blockade in chronic and cancer pain. Int Anesthesiol Clin 35:131–153, 1997.
12. Guarino A, Staats P: Diagnostic neural blockade in the management of pain. Pain Digest 7:194–199, 1997.
13. Kline M: Radiofrequency techniques in clinical practice. In Waldman S, Winnie A (eds): Interventional Pain Management. Philadelphia, WB Saunders, 1996, pp 185–218.
14. Botwin K, Gruber R, Bouchlas C, et al: Complications of fluoroscopically guided transforminal lumbar epidural injections. Arch Phys Med Rehabil 81:1045–1050, 2000.

Suprascapular Nerve Block

HISTORY

Historically, suprascapular nerve block was used as a primary treatment for conditions that limited the range of motion of the shoulder, including adhesive capsulitis and calcific tendinitis and bursitis.[1] The advent of corticosteroids allowed earlier treatment of these maladies. Subsequently, the use of a suprascapular nerve block as a primary treatment modality for shoulder lesions declined. Recently, there has been renewed interest in suprascapular nerve block to allow early range of motion and rehabilitation after shoulder reconstruction or joint replacement.

ANATOMY

The suprascapular nerve is formed from fibers originating from the C5 and C6 nerve roots of the brachial plexus and, in most patients, some fibers from the C4 root. The nerve passes inferiorly and posteriorly from the brachial plexus to pass underneath the coracoclavicular ligament through the suprascapular notch.[2] The suprascapular artery and vein accompany the nerve through the notch. The suprascapular nerve provides much of the sensory innervation to the shoulder joint and innervation to two of the muscles of the rotator cuff, the supraspinatus and infraspinatus (Fig. 21–1).

INDICATIONS

Suprascapular nerve block with local anesthetics can be used as a diagnostic tool when performing differential neural blockade on an anatomic basis to evaluate shoulder girdle and shoulder joint pain.[3] If destruction of the suprascapular nerve is being considered, this technique is useful as a prognostic indicator of the degree of motor

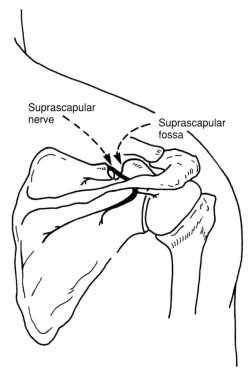

Suprascapular nerve

Suprascapular fossa

FIGURE 21–1

Drawing of the anatomy of the suprascapular nerve.

and sensory impairment that the patient might experience.[4] Suprascapular nerve block with local anesthetic may be used to palliate acute pain emergencies, including postoperative pain, pain secondary to trauma to the shoulder joint and girdle, and cancer pain while waiting for pharmacologic, surgical, or antiblastic treatment to become effective.[4] Suprascapular nerve block is also useful as adjunctive therapy for decreased range of motion of the shoulder secondary to reflex sympathetic dystrophy or adhesive capsulitis,[1,4] and it can be used to allow the patient to tolerate more aggressive physical therapy after shoulder reconstructive surgery.[4]

Destruction of the suprascapular nerve is indicated for palliation of cancer pain, including that of invasive tumors of the shoulder girdle.[4] It can be performed in patients who are taking anticoagulants, if the clinical situation dictates a favorable risk-to-benefit ratio.

CONTRAINDICATIONS

- Local infection
- Anatomic anomaly
- Coagulopathies

EQUIPMENT

- 3- or 5-mL syringe for local infiltration
- 5- or 10-mL syringe for local anesthetics/steroids
- 25-gauge needle for local infiltration
- 22-gauge spinal needle or 22-gauge, B-beveled needle for nerve block
- 10-cm curved-blunt radiofrequency (RF) needle with 10-mm active tip for pulsed RF

DRUGS

- 1% to 2% lidocaine
- 0.25% to 0.5% bupivacaine
- 0.2% to 0.5% ropivacaine
- 40- to 80-mg depot steroids

Neurolytic Solution
- 6% phenol

PREPARATION OF THE PATIENT

PHYSICAL EXAMINATION

Palpate the area for needle entry. In addition, examine the shoulder motion and document the range of motion for evaluation of success of the block.

PREOPERATIVE MEDICATION

For preoperative medication, use the standard American Society of Anesthesiologists' recommendations for conscious sedation.

PROCEDURE

POSITION OF THE PATIENT

The patient is placed in the prone position with the arms at the side (Fig. 21–2). A total of 10 mL of local

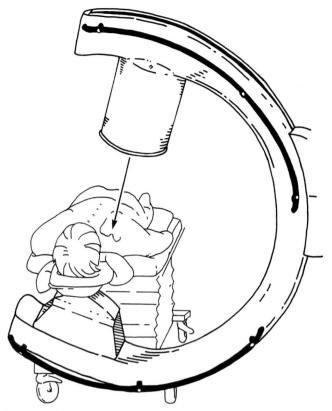

FIGURE 21–2

Drawing of the patient in the prone position with the fluoroscope slightly lateral to midline at the T2–T3 level with a slight cephalocaudad tilt.

anesthetic is drawn up in a 10-mL sterile syringe. When treating painful conditions that are mediated via the suprascapular nerve, a total of 80 mg of depot steroid is added to the local anesthetic with the first block and 40 mg of depot steroid with subsequent blocks.

TECHNIQUE

Suprascapular Nerve Block

The patient is placed in the prone position with the arms at the side (see Fig. 21–2). Local anesthetic is drawn up. When treating painful conditions that are mediated via the suprascapular nerve, a total of 80 mg of depot steroid is added to the local anesthetic with the first block and 40 mg of depot steroid with subsequent blocks.

The spine of the scapula is identified, and the pain specialist then palpates along the length of the scapular spine laterally to identify the acromion (Fig. 21–3). At the point where the thicker acromion fuses with the thinner scapular spine, the skin is prepared with antiseptic solution. At this point, the skin and subcutaneous tissues are anesthetized using a 1½-inch infiltration needle. After adequate anesthesia is obtained, a 25-gauge, 3½-inch needle or an RF needle with previously inserted catheter is inserted with an inferior trajectory

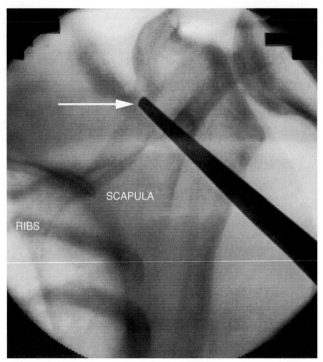

FIGURE 21–3

Radiographic image of the suprascapular notch *(arrow)* emphasized by the oblique angulation of the fluoroscope.

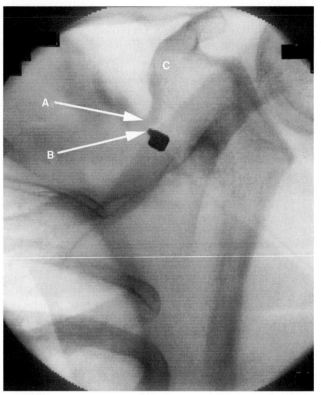

FIGURE 21–4

Suprascapular nerve block with needle in place contacting bone just below the suprascapular nerve. The following is a key to the letters shown on the figure: A, Suprascapular notch; B, Curved blunt needle tip at the notch.

toward the body of the scapula (Fig. 21–4). The needle should make contact with the body of the scapula at a depth of about 1 inch. The needle is then gently "walked" superiorly and medially until the tip walks off the scapular body into the suprascapular notch. If the notch is not identified, the same maneuver is repeated directing the needle superiorly and laterally until the needle tip is positioned in the suprascapular notch. A paresthesia is often encountered as the needle tip enters the notch, and the patient should be warned. If a paresthesia is not elicited after the needle has entered the suprascapular notch, it is advanced an additional ½ inch, to place the tip beyond the substance of the coracoclavicular ligament. The needle should never be advanced deeper, lest pneumothorax occurs.

After paresthesia is elicited or the needle has been advanced into the notch as described earlier, gentle aspiration is carried out to identify blood or air. If the aspiration test is negative, 10 mL of solution is slowly injected as the patient is monitored closely for signs of local anesthetic toxicity.

Neurolytic Block

After the needle is placed appropriately as described earlier, 3 to 4 mL of iohexol (Omnipaque) is injected. An anteroposterior radiographic image is taken. The contrast solution should fill the suprascapular notch and run toward the glenoid cavity (Fig. 21–5). When the physician is satisfied that the contrast solution is correctly placed, then 3 to 5 mL of local anesthetic is

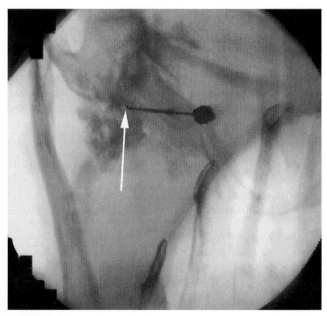

FIGURE 21–5

Suprascapular nerve block with contrast medium filling the suprascapular fossa *(arrow)*.

injected. If there are no side effects, then 3 to 5 mL of 6% phenol is injected.

Pulsed Electrode Magnetic Field of the Suprascapular Nerve

For pulsed electrode magnetic field (pEMF) of the suprascapular nerve, the landmarks and position are the same as described earlier. The needle chosen is a 10-cm curved-blunt Racz-Finch kit (RFK) needle with a 16-gauge introducer catheter. After the fluoroscopic view of the suprascapular notch is obtained, the catheter is inserted. This is done with a "tunnel view." Following the catheter insertion, the RFK needle is introduced until it reaches the suprascapular notch (see Fig. 21–4). Contrast solution is then injected to confirm the position of the needle on the suprascapular nerve (see Fig. 21–5).

Sensory stimulation is then done at 50 Hz ideally positive at 0.3 to 0.6 V to confirm proximity to the suprascapular nerve. Motor stimulation should not be more than two times the sensory stimulation voltage and at 2 Hz. Once proper placement is confirmed, the pEMF lesion is created at 42°C for 120 seconds for two cycles. The needle is then removed. No local anesthetic is injected.

COMPLICATIONS

The proximity of the suprascapular nerve to the suprascapular artery and vein suggests the potential for inadvertent intravascular injection or local anesthetic toxicity from intravascular absorption. The pain specialist should carefully calculate the total (milligram) dose of local anesthetic that may safely be given for suprascapular nerve block. Owing to the proximity of the lung, should the needle be advanced too deep through the suprascapular notch, pneumothorax is a possibility.

HELPFUL HINTS

Suprascapular nerve block is a safe and simple regional anesthesia technique that has many pain management applications. It is probably underutilized as an adjunct to rehabilitation after shoulder reconstruction and for the shoulder-hand variant of reflex sympathetic dystrophy. It is important that the pain specialist be sure that the physical and occupational therapists caring for the patient understand that suprascapular nerve block renders not only the shoulder girdle but also the shoulder joint insensate. This means that deep heat modalities and range-of-motion exercises must be carefully monitored to avoid burns and damage to the shoulder.

EFFICACY

No reliable data for efficacy are available. Block success is dependent on patient response and pain relief.

Suprascapular nerve 64418; RFTC other nerve 64640.

REFERENCES

1. Pitkin GP: Therapeutic nerve block. In Pitkin GP (ed): Conduction Anesthesia. Philadelphia, JB Lippincott, 1946, pp 884–886.
2. Waldman SD: Suprascapular nerve block. In Waldman SD (ed): Atlas of Interventional Pain Management. Philadelphia, WB Saunders, 1998, pp 144–147.
3. Bonica JJ: Musculoskeletal disorders of the upper limb. In Bonica JJ (ed): The Management of Pain, 2nd ed. Philadelphia, Lea & Febiger, 1990, pp 891–893.
4. Katz J: Suprascapular nerve block. In Katz J (ed): Atlas of Regional Anesthesia, 2nd ed. Norwalk, CT, Appleton & Lange, 1995, pp 72–73.

22

T2 and T3 Sympathetic Nerve Block and Neurolysis

HISTORY

Thoracic sympathectomies have been used for the past 80 years to manage painful conditions and vascular insufficiencies of the upper extremities. Indications for sympathectomies at the thoracic ganglia level are for treatment of complex regional pain syndrome (CRPS) type I (reflex sympathetic dystrophy), CRPS II (causalgia), arterial occlusions leading to ischemia, drug-resistant Raynaud's disease, Buerger's disease, and frost injuries of the upper extremities.[1]

In 1916, Jonnesco was the first surgeon to promote the stellate ganglion for the treatment of angina pectoris.[2] It soon was recognized that the ablation of the stellate ganglion function also provided pain relief in addition to vasodilation in patients with Raynaud's disease. Jonnesco further advocated stellate ganglionectomy for vascular diseases (Raynaud's) of the upper extremities, in 1921.[1] This was performed via the supraclavicular approach. In reality, it did not provide prolonged relief of vasospasticity and sympathetic tone would eventually return.[1] In 1927, Kuntz[3] observed that nerves from the T2 and T3 sympathetic ganglia would connect to the brachial plexus in 20% of people, bypassing the stellate ganglion. This contributed to the lack of success noted in stellate ganglionectomy alone. This new information led to multiple procedures to remove or block the T2 and T3 sympathetic ganglia.

The first operative procedure was the modification of the supraclavicular approach described above, which went through the neck down to T2 and T3 retropleurally.[4] Other approaches,[5] the transthoracic axillary approach,[6] and the anterior approach are discussed elsewhere.[7] In 1954, Kux[8] devised a transthoracic approach in which an endoscope was used for electrocoagulation. This approach was largely forgotten for 25 years and then rediscovered by a newer group of surgeons.[9, 10]

During the time when these surgical procedures were being developed, percutaneous blocks were also explored. In 1925, Leriche and Fontaine[11] first used a paravertebral approach for sympathetic blockade with procaine on patients with severe pain caused by angina pectoris, causalgia, and reflex sympathetic dystrophy. In 1926, Mandl[12] described paravertebral blocks for diagnosis and treatment of visceral pain and anginal pain. That same year, Swetlow[2] used 85% alcohol with this technique. The patient was placed in a lateral decubitus position with the side to be injected up. The knees were flexed to the abdomen and the head bowed down. The ribs were used as landmarks, and the intercostal space to be injected was carefully palpated. The skin was marked over the spinous processes. At a 4-cm mark from the spinous processes, the skin was anesthetized with procaine hydrochloride. This was used both as a marker and to numb the skin. The needle was introduced perpendicular to the rib, just above where the injection would be performed. The needle was advanced to touch the rib and then withdrawn in order to redirect the needle. The needle then was advanced caudal, medial, and anterior at a 45-degree angle. The needle was advanced 2 cm from the lateral border of the rib. The needle point was between the internal and external intercostal muscles. It was then attached to a water manometer to determine whether or not it was in the pleural cavity. The absence of extensive oscillation with respiratory movement indicated the needle was not in the pleural cavity. Then 2.5 cc of 85% alcohol was injected.[1, 2] White and White[13] noted that, in their experience, hyperesthesia occurred for 2 to 4 weeks' duration in all of the patients injected with 85% alcohol over the area of the injected nerve. Leriche and Fontaine,[11] in 1932, published a case of inadvertent tracing of alcohol through the root sleeve into subarachnoid space, causing paraplegia.

Mandl[12] noted that the sympathetic ganglia at the thoracic level lie so close to the intercostal nerves that alcohol infiltrated around the sympathetic chain bathed the intercostal nerve trunks. At first the patients became paralyzed, but anesthesia disappeared within 14 days, and at approximately 4 weeks, hyperesthesia to the chest wall increased and commonly persisted for a number of months. This procedure was thus rejected by many because of the frequency of neuritis that occurred in these patients. Many abandoned chemical interruption of sympathetic fibers and looked for surgical methods because of intercostal neuritis, as well as other side effects, caused by percutaneous alcohol infection.

In 1979, Wilkinson[14] devised a technique for radiofrequency thermocoagulation (RFTC) via percutaneous needle placement for ablation of the T2 and T3 blocks with minimal complications.

ANATOMY

Yarzebski and Wilkinson[15] noted the discrepancies in the description of the location of sympathetic chain ganglia in anatomy textbooks. They noted that the locations of T2 and T3 varied in 24 freshly embalmed cadavers. In the dorsoventral location, the T2 ganglia on the right side had a median location of 19 mm (range of 12 to 31 mm) dorsal to the ventral surface of the vertebral body, and the left side had a median location of 17 mm (range 6 to 27 mm) dorsal to the ventral surface. The right-sided T3 median location was 20 mm (range of 9 to 31 mm) dorsal to the ventral surface of the T3 vertebral body. The left-sided T3 median was 19.5 mm (range of 9 to 30 mm) to the ventral surface (Fig. 22–1A).

The relationship of the ganglia caudad and cephalad to the vertebral bodies was more constant. The median location of the T2 ganglia was 2 mm rostral to the midpoint of the T2 vertebral body on the right side (range of 1 to 7 mm), between the head of the ribs. The left median was 1.5 mm (range of 1 to 2 mm) rostral to the midpoint of the vertebral body. The T3 ganglia were located 2 mm (range of 2 to 3 mm) rostral to the midpoint of the T3 vertebral body bilaterally (Fig. 22–1B).[15]

Sympathetic ganglion cell bodies that supply the upper limbs are in the intermediolateral horn of the spinal cord from the T2 to T8 levels. Preganglionic fibers run to the sympathetic chain via white rami communicantes. Here, they ascend cephalad and synapse with postganglionic fibers, primarily in T2, but also in T3, in the stellate ganglia, and in the middle cervical ganglia. By blocking T2 and T3, which are the "key" synaptic stations, all the synaptic nerves destined for the upper limbs can be blocked.[16]

INDICATIONS

The T2 and T3 sympathetic block is considered for patients who have sympathetically maintained pain or upper extremity vascular disease.

CONTRAINDICATIONS

Absolute
- Local infection
- Systemic infection
- Coagulopathy

Relative
- Thoracic aortic aneurysm
- Respiratory insufficiency

EQUIPMENT

- 10-cm curved-blunt R-F RFTC needle
- 20-gauge, 1¼-inch IV introducer catheter

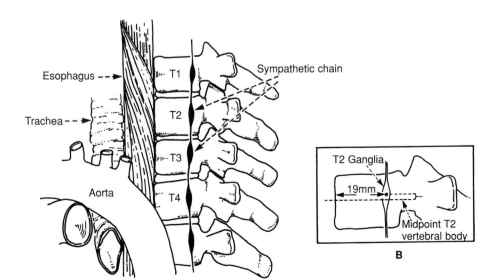

FIGURE 22–1

A, In this drawing, the thoracic sympathetic chain is approximately 20 mm dorsally from the anterior vertebral body. For practical purposes, this is equivalent to the posterior one third of the thoracic vertebrae in the lateral view. *B*, This close-up view shows the slightly (2-mm) rostral location of the thoracic sympathetic ganglion in relation to the midpoint of the vertebrae.

- IV T-piece
- Metal marking clamp
- 3-mL syringe
- 10-mL syringe
- 19-gauge, 1½-inch needle
- 25-gauge, ¾-inch needle

DRUGS

- Radiographic contrast: iohexol
- Local anesthetic (5 to 10 mL)
    Lidocaine
    Bupivacaine or ropivacaine
- Depot steroids: triamcinolone (40 mg)

PREPARATION OF THE PATIENT

Prior to the procedure, the patient should be cleared for any bleeding diathesis by obtaining prothrombin time, partial thromboplastin time, and bleeding time values. This reduces the risk of hematoma formation into the chest cavity. Any anticoagulants that the patient may be receiving should be discontinued 7 days prior to the procedure.

LABORATORY

- Complete blood count with platelets
- Prothrombin time, partial thromboplastin time, platelet function studies
- Anteroposterior chest plain film

PREOPERATIVE MEDICATION

For preoperative medication, use the standard American Society of Anesthesiologists' recommendations for conscious sedation.

PROCEDURE

POSITION OF THE PATIENT AND PHYSICIAN

The patient is put in a prone position on a fluoroscopic-compatible table. The back is prepared and draped in a sterile fashion. The fluoroscope is then used to identify the T2 vertebral body in an anteroposterior view. The fluoroscope is then obliqued approximately 20 degrees toward the ipsilateral side. The fluoroscope is then rotated in a cephalocaudad direction approximately 20 degrees. This helps open up the intervertebral space and "squares up" the T2 vertebral body (Fig. 22–2).

Kelly forceps are used to identify the point of skin entrance at the lateral edge of the T2 vertebral body just

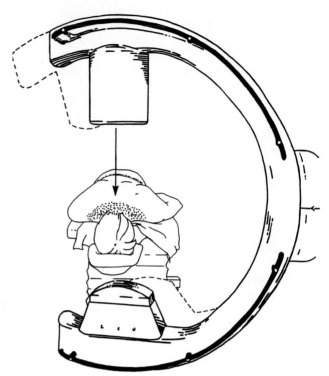

FIGURE 22–2

The drawing shows the arrangement of the patient and the fluoroscope in an anteroposterior view to first identify the appropriate vertebral level. The lateral stippling demonstrates the rotation of fluoroscope to create a tunneled view for radiographic needle placement.

cephalad to the third rib. The skin is anesthetized using a 25-gauge, short-beveled needle with 1.5% lidocaine. A 16-gauge, 2-inch angiocatheter is advanced toward the lateral border at T2 above the third rib, in a tunnel view, with the aid of fluoroscopy.

A tunnel view is maintained to keep straight orientation in deeper tissues. The stylet is removed from the angiocatheter at about 1 inch deep. A 20-gauge, 10-cm blunt-curved 10-mm active-tip RFTC needle is inserted. The needle is advanced using the "direction-depth-direction" technique with the fluoroscope to confirm placement of the needle (Fig. 22–3).

The needle is advanced, hugging the lateral edge of the T2 vertebral body. A lateral view confirms the posterior half of the T2 thoracic vertebral body (Fig. 22–4A) An anteroposterior view demonstrates the needle "hugging" the T2 vertebra at approximately the level of the pedicle (Fig. 22–4B). Iohexol 240 dye (approximately 2 mL) is then injected. The dye spread is up and down the thoracic vertebral column, and unilateral placement is confirmed if the spread follows the dome of the lung. If the needle is more lateral than the parietal pleura, the needle needs to be redirected medially.

If this is a diagnostic block, local anesthetic and steroid are injected. Approximately 6 to 8 mL of a 1:1 mixture 0.5% ropivacaine and 2% lidocaine with 40 mg/mL of triamcinolone are injected. This volume is

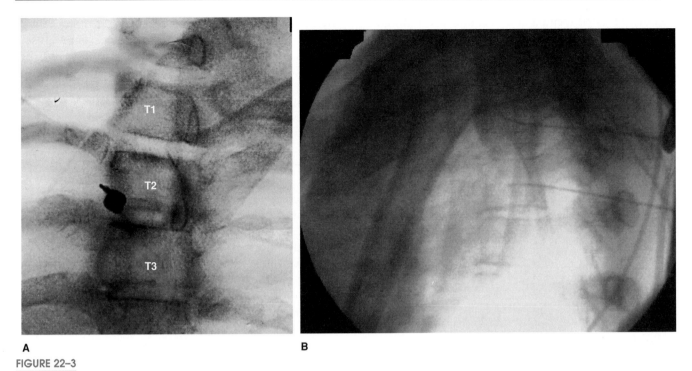

A   **B**

FIGURE 22–3

A, Oblique fluoroscopic view of T2 and T3 vertebrae. The curved, blunt needle is shown in a "tunnel" view at the T2 vertebral level. *B*, Lateral view. The needle tip is at the midpoint to the posterior one third of the thoracic vertebral body.

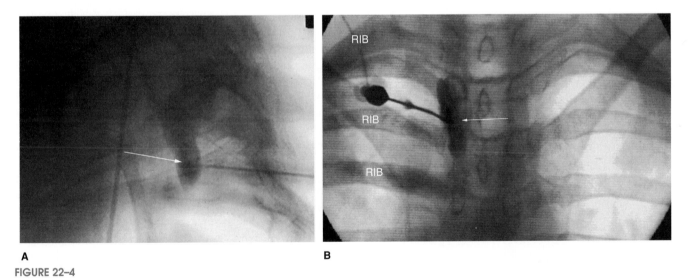

A   **B**

FIGURE 22–4

A, Lateral fluoroscopic view of T2 and T3 vertebrae. The contrast medium is seen over the vertebral body *(arrow)* without tracking of the contrast medium into the neuroforamina. *B*, Anteroposterior fluoroscopic view. The contrast medium is seen "hugging" the thoracic vertebral body *(arrow)*.

generally sufficient to block both the T2 and T3 sympathetic ganglia. This can be confirmed by watching the spread of dye before and after injection of local anesthetic.

Prior to the procedure, temperature probes are placed on each hand. A baseline temperature is noted and compared with postprocedural temperature. Fentanyl, midazolam, and lidocaine all produce vasodilation and affect sympathetic function for hours after the procedure. Bilateral temperature probes help avoid confusion. The patient is then followed for 1 month after the

diagnostic block. The duration of the block and the percentage of pain relief are noted.

RADIOFREQUENCY THERMOCOAGULATION OF T2 AND T3 SYMPATHETIC GANGLION

If the block was beneficial, the patient is then scheduled for an RFTC of the T2 and T3 sympathetic ganglia. The needle is placed as mentioned earlier at the T2 sympathetic ganglion. Iohexol dye is injected (Fig. 22–5), and stimulation is performed at 50 Hz and 2 V, noting any stimulation of intercostal nerves. Prior to lesioning and after stimulation, local anesthetic and steroids are injected. Thirty seconds is usually enough time to wait before lesioning occurs.

Lesioning occurs at 80°C for 90 seconds. When lesioning is complete, the needle hub is directed in a medial-caudad direction. The tip of the RFTC needle is curved approximately 15 degrees, and this gives a larger area of burn when rotated, increasing the chance of burning the ganglia. The process is repeated again for the T3 ganglia. At the end of lesioning, the needle and catheter are removed. The back is cleansed. A triple-antibiotic ointment and bandage are placed over the injection site.

COMPLICATIONS

The patient is transported to the recovery room. A chest radiograph is ordered to rule out a pneumothorax, and the pain level and temperature are re-evaluated. A quick examination is done to rule out any neurologic deficits. The patient is recovered in 45 minutes and sent home. The patients are advised of late-occurring pneumothorax and instructed that they should go to the emergency department for evaluation if they experience increased shortness of breath or chest pain.

Another side effect of this procedure is intercostal neuritis. Wilkinson[17] noted neuritis in approximately 40% of his procedures. This problem can be minimized

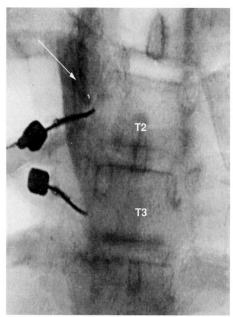

FIGURE 22–5

Anteroposterior fluoroscopic view. The two radiofrequency needles can be seen in place at the T2 and T3 vertebral levels. The arrow indicates the correct position of the needle tip on the T2-T3 sympathetic chain.

by meticulously performing sensory and motor stimulation prior to lesioning. If no dysesthesias or muscle contractions occur in the somatic nerve (intercostal) distribution, then one could deduce that the needle tip is at least 1 cm away from the nerve root. The data of the incidence of neuritis by this procedure are still scant and need to be further evaluated.

HELPFUL HINTS

The lack of significant side effects in our group can be attributed to the use of a blunt, curved-tip needle, which seems to push nerves and arteries out of its pathway rather than injuring them. Staying within 4 cm of the spinous process is another safety factor that contributes to the success of the technique and alleviates pneumothoraces. During radiofrequency lesioning, intercostal stimulation during motor testing can be resolved by advancing the needle 2 to 3 mm anteriorly.

EFFICACY

Retrospective data on T2 and T3 were reviewed, using the Current Procedural Technology coding for T2 and T3 sympathetic block or RFTC. Charts that were on microfilm were ignored, and charts that did not have a radiograph report or a dictated physician's note excluding a pneumothorax were also ignored. A total of 42 patients had 110 percutaneous thoracic sympathetic blocks or RFTC performed. Of these patients, 27 had complex regional pain syndrome type I of the upper extremities; 1 had a brachial plexus injury; 1 had postmedication neuritis of the brachial plexus; 2 had phantom limb pain; 1 had Arnold-Chiari syndrome and deafferentation pain following dorsal root entry zone lesioning; and 4 had chest wall pain due to multiple reasons (1 following breast removal, 1 had costochondritis, 1 had a chest tube, and 1 was unknown).

Of these 110 procedures, 36 were diagnostic blocks, 73 were T2 and T3 sympathetic RFTC blocks, and 1 was pulsed electrode magnetic field; T4 block was done in 8 blocks, T1 in 1 block, and T4 and T9 in another. A total of 193 needle punctures into the thoracic cavity were placed. From the 110 procedures, there were two pneumothoraces. One was in a 57-year-old woman with diffuse reflex sympathetic dystrophy. This was a diagnostic block, and it caused a 10% apical pneumothorax. It was not realized at the time the radiograph was read by the anesthesiologist but was confirmed by the radiologist at a later time. No treatment was necessary and the pneumothorax resolved on its own. The second pneumothorax occurred in a patient with deafferentation pain in the right upper extremity. This also was a diagnostic block at T2. The patient experienced a 20% pneumothorax on the right side. The patient's oxygen saturation levels were normal and no chest pain was noted. No chest tube was placed to treat the pneumothorax, and it resolved on its own. The incidence of pneumothoraces in this group was 1.82%. Wilkinson,[17] in his experience, had six pneumothoraces in 247 procedures, or an incidence of 2.4%. These were symptomatic pneumothoraces and required brief chest tube placement.

Lumbar/thoracic sympathetic 64520; RFTC other nerve 64640.

REFERENCES

1. Roos DB: Sympathectomy for the upper extremities: *Anatomy, indications and techniques In Rutherford R (ed): Vascular Surgery.* Philadelphia, WB Saunders, 1977, p 460.
2. Swetlow G: Paravertebral alcohol block in cardiac pain. Am Heart J 1:393–412, 1926.
3. Kuntz A: Distribution of the sympathetic nerve to the brachial plexus. Arch Surg 15:871–877, 1927.
4. Telford ED: The technique of sympathectomy. Br J Surg 23:448–450, 1935.
5. Adson AW, Brown GE: The treatment of Raynaud's disease by resection of the upper thoracic and lumbar sympathetic ganglia and trunks. Surg Gynecol Obstet 48:557–603, 1929.
6. Atkins HJB: Sympathectomy by the axillary approach. Lancet 1:536–539, 1954.
7. Palumbo LT: Anterior transthoracic approach for the upper extremity thoracic sympathectomy. Arch Surg 72:659–666, 1950.
8. Kux E: Thorakoskopische Eingriffe an Merran system. Stuttgart, Georg Thieme Verlag, 1954.
9. Weale FE, Felix E: Upper thoracic sympathectomy by transthoracic electrocoagulation. Br J Surg 67:71–72, 1980.
10. Malone PS, Duignan JP, Hederman WP: Thoracic electrocoagulation, a new and simple approach to upper limb sympathectomy. Ir Med J 75:20, 1982.
11. Leriche R, Fontaine R: L'aniskesie isolée du ganglion etile: Sa technique, ses indications, ses resultats. Presse Med 42:849–850, 1934.
12. Mandl F: Die Paravertebral Injection. Vienna, J Springer, 1926.
13. White JC, White RD: Angina retro treatment with paravertebral alcohol injection. JAMA 90:1099–1103, 1928.
14. Wilkinson H: Percutaneous radiofrequency upper thoracic sympathectomy: A new technique. Neurosurgery 15:811–814, 1984.
15. Yarzebski JL, Wilkinson H: T2 and T3 sympathetic ganglia in the adult human: A cadaver and clinical-radiographic study and its clinical application. Neurosurgery 21:339–342, 1987.
16. Kuntz A: Autonomic Nervous System, 4th ed. Philadelphia, Lea & Febiger, 1953.
17. Wilkinson HA: Percutaneous radiofrequency of upper thoracic sympathectomy. Neurosurgery 38:715–725, 1996.

C H A P T E R

23

Thoracic Facet Block and Radiofrequency Thermocoagulation

HISTORY

The facet joints of the spine may be otherwise known as the apophyseal joints. The Greek word apophysis means "offshoot," and the anatomic definition of the word is a natural outgrowth or process on a vertebra or other bone.[1] The degenerative changes and associated muscle spasm that develop when a facet joint is involved in a sprain from a forceful or violent twisting motion were termed the *facet syndrome* by Ghormley in 1933.[2] The intra-articular facet joints at all levels are subject to trauma.

ANATOMY

The T1–T2 facet joint is angled 66 degrees from a transverse plane, with the cephalad end more anterior than the caudad end.[3, 4] The angle steepens to 75 degrees by the T3–T4 facet joint and then remains constant to the T11–T12 facet joint. The T1–T2 to the T11–T12 facet joints are uniformly angled 110 degrees from the midline posterior sagittal plane. The thoracic facet joints are thus mostly vertically oriented and almost parallel to the coronal plane. The transition from the thoracic to the lumbar facet joints occurs primarily at the T11–T12 and T12–L1 joints.[5] There is some variability at the T11–T12 facet joint, but it is essentially oriented vertically (perpendicular to the sagittal plane) and faces directly anterior (parallel to the coronal plane). The T12–L1 facet joint assumes the more lumbar orientation and is approximately 25 degrees oblique to the sagittal plane from the midline posteriorly.

Medial branch nerves from two segmental levels innervate the joint at the same level plus the joint below. Below the T3 level this pattern is consistent, but it seems that the C7 and C8 nerves may travel caudad as far as the T2 and T3 levels (Fig. 23–1).[6]

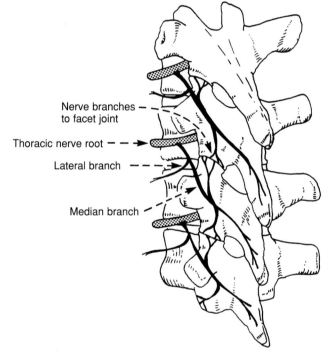

FIGURE 23–1

The drawing illustrates the distribution of the posterior primary rami on the thoracic vertebrae innervation of the facet joints by the median branches from and below the corresponding level.

INDICATIONS

The major indications for facet joint injection include (1) focal tenderness over a facet joint; (2) chronic back pain with or without radiation but with a normal radiographic evaluation; and (3) back pain with evidence of disc disease and facet arthritis.[7, 8]

The findings on conventional radiographs correlate poorly with the clinical symptoms.[7, 9] There may be better correlation between symptoms and findings on computed tomographic scans.[10, 11] Facet arthrography

138

with injection of local anesthetic and an anti-inflammatory agent is a diagnostic procedure that is often therapeutic, with relief of symptoms lasting much longer than expected from the pharmacologic effects of the injected agents.[7, 9, 12, 13]

The clinical picture of painful thoracic facet joints is thought to be analogous to that in the lumbar region, although there are little data at this time. No clearly delineated thoracic facet syndrome exists, and the research to date has been based on vague clinical features, continuous or nearly continuous unilateral or bilateral paravertebral pain and tenderness in a clearly identified thoracic area of the back, without objective neurologic signs.[14]

CONTRAINDICATIONS

Absolute
- Infection in the overlying soft tissue

Relative
- Allergy to injecting agents

As listed, the only absolute contraindication to facet joint block is infection in the overlying soft tissues. A relative contraindication is allergy to injecting agents. Facet joint block can be accomplished, however, without injection of contrast medium, and the newer non-ionic contrast agents also decrease the risk in allergic individuals.

EQUIPMENT

Injection and Nerve Block

- 22-gauge, 1½-inch B-bevel needle
- 25-gauge, ¾-inch skin infiltration needle
- 3-mL syringe
- 10-mL syringe
- IV T-piece extension
- Metal clamp for radiographic

Radiofrequency Thermocoagulation Lesioning

Same equipment used for the nerve block, plus

- 20-gauge, 3⁄4-inch angiocatheter
- 10 cm with 10-mm active-tip Racz-Finch radiofrequency thermocoagulation (RFTC) needle
- RFTC electrode and connecting cables

DRUGS

- Radiographic contrast: iohexol
- Local anesthetics: 1.5% lidocaine and 0.2% ropivacaine or 0.25% levobupivacaine
- Steroids: methylprednisolone or triamcinolone

PREPARATION OF THE PATIENT

PHYSICAL EXAMINATION

The thoracic facet joint syndrome is similar to that of the cervical facet syndrome, resulting from a sudden twisting motion, twisting while lifting overhead, or an unguarded rotating motion of the thoracic spine. The resultant pain may be mild, dull, and aching, with radiation encircling the chest, or it may be sharp, pleuritic-type pain that can affect functional vital capacity or become overwhelming to the patient. There is usually decreased motion in the portion of the spine involved. Examination of the patient may reveal a loss of the thoracic curve or muscle spasms, causing localized scoliosis.

Nonetheless, pain referral patterns from injection into normal joints have been described (Figs. 23–2 and 23–3).[6, 15] Distention of normal joints was not painful in 27.5% of volunteers, but, when it was painful, the referral patterns were always unilateral and reproducible for most of the thoracic spine. In all subjects for the T2–T3

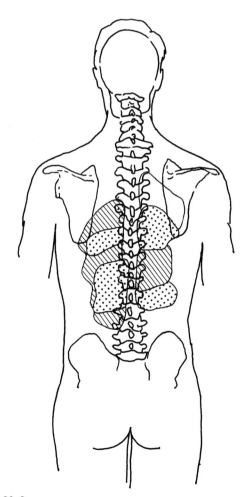

FIGURE 23–2

The drawing shows the skin referral patterns for the T3–T4 to T10–T12 facet joints. (Adapted from Dreyfuss P, Tibiletti C, Dreyer S: Thoracic zygapophyseal joint pain patterns. Spine 19:807–811, 1994.)

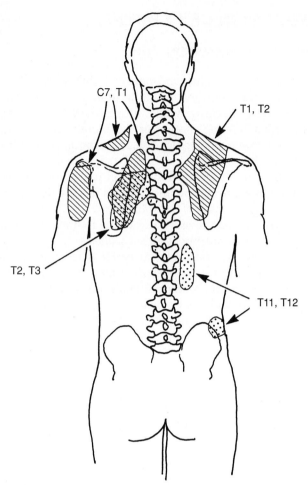

FIGURE 23–3

The drawing shows the skin referral patterns for the C7–T3 and T11–T12 facet joints. (Adapted from Fukui S, Ohseto K, Shiotani M: Patterns of pain induced by distending the thoracic zygapophyseal joints. Reg Anesth 22:332–336, 1997.)

to T11–T12 levels, the area of most intense pain was one segment inferior and slightly lateral to the involved joint and never crossed the midline. Although significant overlap occurred, pain was not referred more than 2½ segments inferior to the joint injected. At the C7–T1 joint, pain was felt in the paravertebral area over the injected point, which extended superiorly toward the superior angle of the scapula and inferiorly toward the inferior angle of the scapula. The pain was sometimes also referred toward the shoulder joint and suprascapular region. At the T1–T2 joint, pain was felt in the paravertebral region over the joint, below the inferior angle of the scapula, and sometimes into the suprascapular region. Because of the considerable overlap, the pain maps for the C7–T1 through T2–T3 joints were not thought to be reliable enough to identify the joint of origin.

LABORATORY

No laboratory studies are required.

PREOPERATIVE MEDICATION

For preoperative medication, use the standard American Society of Anesthesiologists' recommendations for conscious sedation.

PROCEDURE

MEDIAN BRANCH INJECTION

Position of the Patient

The patient is placed in the prone position for median branch block. In the anteroposterior view, the first level to be injected is identified by either counting cephalad from T12 or caudal from T1 under fluoroscopy with a radiographic marker. Once the desired level is identified, the fluoroscope is rotated laterally to create a "Scottie dog" image, via an ipsilateral oblique radiographic image (Fig. 23–4). Using fluoroscopy, the radiographic marker is positioned over the skin to mark the "eye of the Scottie dog" (Fig. 23–5). Local anesthetic (usually 0.5 to 1 mL) is injected for skin infiltration at the designated skin entry site. Then a 20- or 22-gauge B-beveled needle is inserted in a "tunnel" view at the eye of the Scottie dog (Fig. 23–6).

When bone is contacted, usually within 3.5 to 4.5 cm, the C-arm is rotated into a lateral view to confirm proper needle placement (Figs. 23–7 to 23–9). If final needle placement is satisfactory, the C-arm is rotated

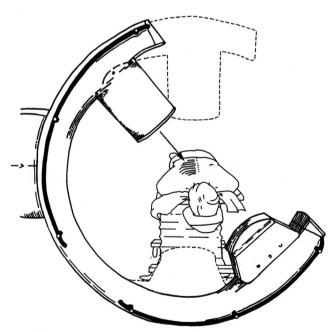

FIGURE 23–4

The fluoroscope is rotated into an oblique position to create a "Scottie dog" image of the posterior thoracic vertebrae components. The "eye of the Scottie dog" will be on the same side as the lateral rotation of the C-arm.

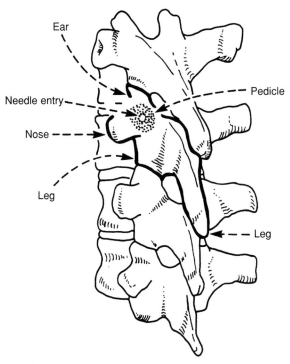

FIGURE 23–5

A drawing of the oblique view of thoracic vertebra showing a "Scottie dog" image.

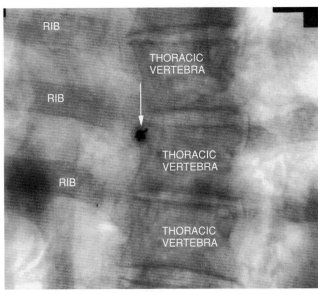

FIGURE 23–6

The *arrow* points to the needle on the left thoracic facet median nerve. The fluoroscopic image is an oblique view rotated laterally to the left.

into an anteroposterior view prior to the injection of radiographic contrast medium.

Technique

An intravenous (IV) T-piece extension set is connected to the 10-mL syringe containing the radiographic contrast medium. The T-piece is primed with contrast medium prior to connection with the needle to minimize the dead space air in the tubing. After the T-piece is attached to the needle the syringe should be aspirated for blood or air. If either blood or air is continuously obtained, the needle will need to be repositioned.

After negative aspiration is accomplished, 0.5 to 1 mL of contrast medium is injected and monitored under fluoroscopy for vascular run-off. If there is run-off present, the needle must be repositioned. With a negative aspiration test, 1 to 1.5 mL of local anesthetic/steroid mixture is injected. The needle is thereafter removed for the next level or left in place as a marker.

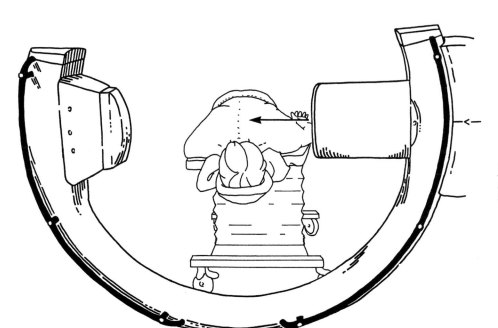

FIGURE 23–7

A drawing of the fluoroscope is shown in a lateral position.

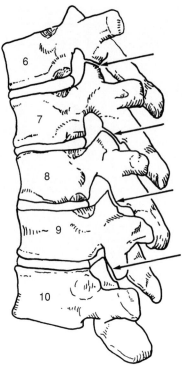

FIGURE 23–8

Thoracic facets—lateral view (*arrows* indicate facets).

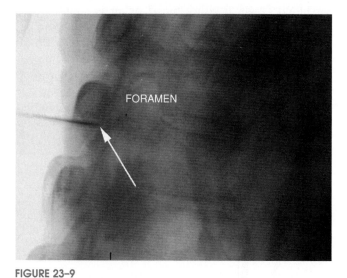

FORAMEN

FIGURE 23–9

Lateral fluoroscopic view shows the needle just below the rib and posterior to the facet joint and foramen.

INTRA-ARTICULAR INJECTION

Position of the Patient

For the articular injection technique the patient is positioned prone. The joint to be blocked is identified by counting the ribs from T1 caudad and from T12 cephalad. Once the joint is identified, a radiopaque marker on the skin over the joint may help in needle localization.

Technique

Because of the steep angle of the thoracic facet joints, the skin entry point may need to overlie the pedicle one or two segments caudad. After sterile preparation and draping, local anesthetic is injected into the skin and tissues along the needle path. A 20- or 22-gauge, 10-cm spinal needle is then directed steeply cephalad toward the joint. Using the skin marker and a combination of anteroposterior and lateral fluoroscopic images, the needle is then advanced into the joint. As in the lumbar spine, a combination of dye injection and needle "feel" confirms proper needle placement. The thoracic facet joints are small and can hold only 0.4 to 0.6 mL of injectate. The mixture of dye, local anesthetic, and steroid should not exceed this total joint volume. Additional solutions may be injected periarticularly for therapeutic purposes.

RADIOFREQUENCY THERMOCOAGULATION LESIONING

The approach and views for RFTC are the same as described for the median branch injection. An angiocatheter is inserted through the skin in a tunnel view instead of a block needle. The RFTC needle is passed through the angiocatheter until bone is contacted. Frequent monitoring of the needle's passage with fluoroscopy ensures proper placement.

Once satisfactory needle placement is confirmed via fluoroscopic imaging and contrast injection, the RF electrode is placed through the needle. Sensory testing at 50 Hz and up to 1 V and motor testing at 2 Hz and up to 2 V should be negative for anterior nerve root stimulation. If testing is positive, the needle must be repositioned posteriorly until testing is negative. After proper placement and satisfactory testing, 1 to 1.5 mL of local anesthetic and steroids is injected. The RF electrode is replaced into the needle. Lesioning is then performed twice for 20 seconds at 80°C.

COMPLICATIONS

Complications following facet blocks are rare but include infection, allergic reaction, transient radicular pain, and pneumothorax. Theoretically, the subarachnoid space can be entered during a facet block. It is important to aspirate before any injection to ensure that there is no return of cerebrospinal fluid. Placement of the needle under fluoroscopic visualization and proper technique are safeguards to prevent this possibility.

HELPFUL HINTS

Neuritis, subarachnoid injection, and pneumothorax risks are minimal if the needle is kept posterior and on the eye of the Scottie dog. To ensure accuracy of needle placement, incremental corrections and measured advancement of the needle minimize imprecise placement.

EFFICACY

Only three studies of thoracic facet denervation have been conducted, and, unfortunately, the results are unreliable because the anatomic location of the medial branch nerves in the thoracic spine has since been shown to be 12 mm away from the site of denervation.[14, 16] Therefore, until a reliable technique is developed, the only injection for thoracic facets is either intra-articular or periarticular. These may be useful therapeutically and perhaps also diagnostically.

Most patients experience little or no pain during injection of the facet joints. If the injected facet is the cause of the pain, frequently dramatic relief of pain immediately follows the injection. The patient is questioned concerning any immediate change in symptoms and is instructed to keep track of any change in pain over the next 24 hours as well as during the following weeks.

Cervical/thoracic facet single level 64470; cervical/thoracic facet additional levels 64472; RFTC cervical/thoracic facet-single level 64626; RFTC cervical/thoracic facet additional levels 64627.

REFERENCES

1. Webster's New Collegiate Dictionary, 9th ed. Springfield, MA, Merriam-Webster, 1985.
2. Ghormley RK: Low back pain: With special reference to the articular facets, with presentation of an operative procedure. JAMA 101:1773–1777, 1933.
3. Panjabi MM, Oxland T, Takata K, et al: Articular facets of the human spine: Quantitative three-dimensional anatomy. Spine 18:1311–1317, 1993.
4. Ebraheim NA, Su R, Ahmad M, et al: The quantitative anatomy of the thoracic facet and the posterior projection of its inferior facet. Spine 22:1811, 1997.
5. Malmivaara A, Videman T, Kuosma E, et al: Facet joint orientation, facet and costovertebral joint osteoarthrosis, disc degeneration, vertebral body osteophytosis, and Schmorl's nodes in the thoracolumbar junctional region of cadaveric spines. Spine 12:458–463, 1987.
6. Fukui S, Ohseto K, Shiotani M: Patterns of pain induced by distending the thoracic zygapophyseal joints. Reg Anesth 22:332–336, 1997.
7. Jackson RP: The facet syndrome: Myth or reality? Clin Orthop 279:110–121, 1992.
8. Helbig T, Lee C: The lumbar facet syndrome. Spine 12:61–64, 1988.
9. Mixter WJ, Barr JS: Rupture of the intervertebral disk with involvement of the spinal canal. N Engl J Med 211:210–215, 1934.
10. Bland JH, Boushey DR: Anatomy and physiology of the cervical spine. Semin Arthritis Rheum 20:1–20, 1990.
11. Revel ME, Listrat VM, Chevalier XJ, et al: Facet joint block for low back pain: Identifying predictors of a good response. Arch Phys Med Rehabil 73:824–828, 1992.
12. Manchikanti L: Facet joint pain and the role of neural blockade in its management. Curr Rev Pain 3:348–358, 1999.
13. Lord SM, Barnsley L, Wallis BJ, et al: Chronic cervical zygapophysial joint pain after whiplash. Spine 21:1737–1745, 1996.
14. Stolkre RJ, Vervest ACM, Groen GJ: Percutaneous facet denervation in chronic thoracic spinal pain. Acta Neurochir 122:82–90, 1993.
15. Dreyfuss P, Tibiletti C, Dreyer S: Thoracic zygapophyseal joint pain patterns. Spine 19:807–811, 1994.
16. Chua WH, Bogduk N: The surgical anatomy of thoracic facet denervation. Acta Neurochir 136:140–144, 1995.

24

Thoracic Epidural Block

HISTORY

Accessing the epidural space was first described in 1921. The initial reports mostly described lumbar epidural space placement for the thoracic management of situations such as flailed chest, after coronary artery bypass graft, and after thoracotomies. Chronic pain management practitioners have accessed this space for epidural steroid injections, dorsal column stimulation, and so forth.

ANATOMY

The thoracic epidural space extends from the lower margin of the C7 vertebra to the upper margin of L1.[1-5] The vertebral column in the thoracic area normally has a kyphotic curvature, with its apex at approximately T6. Slight scoliosis to the right can occur, even in normal persons. Significant scoliosis is associated with the rotation of the vertebral column, which can produce significant technical difficulty in performing this block. The inclination of the spinous processes is different at different levels of the thoracic vertebral column. The vertebrae from T1 to T4 have very little inclination, whereas those of T5 to T8 tilt significantly downward, making a midline approach to the epidural space practically impossible. The T9 to T12 vertebrae point dorsally without significant inclination, so the midline approach is possible. The ligamentum flavum is not as thick as it is in the lumbar spine, and, occasionally, the epidural space can be entered without encountering much resistance. The attachment of the ligamentum flavum to the lower margin of the lamina on its inner aspect reduces the size of the epidural space, whereas the space is wider at the upper margin of the lamina, because the ligamentum flavum is attached to the outer aspect of the upper margin of the lower lamina (Fig. 24–1). The epidural space is 3 to 4 mm wide in the thoracic area. The thoracic epidural space, just like the rest of the epidural space, contains loose areolar tissue, fat, and vertebral venous plexus.

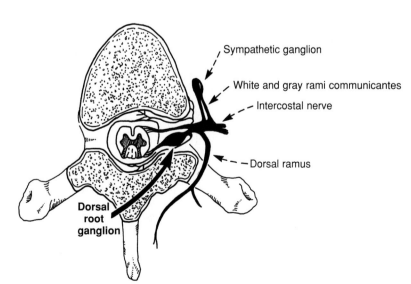

Sympathetic ganglion

White and gray rami communicantes

Intercostal nerve

Dorsal ramus

Dorsal root ganglion

FIGURE 24–1

Coronal cross section of thoracic vertebra that demonstrates the vertebral shape and contents.

INDICATIONS[1-6]

- Surgical
- Postoperative analgesia
- Herpes zoster and postherpetic neuralgia
- Epidural steroids
- Acute pain secondary to trauma
- Angina
- Cancer pain
- Spinal cord stimulation
- Management of acute pancreatitis

CONTRAINDICATIONS

Absolute
- Local infection in the area of needle insertion
- Coagulopathies
- Uncorrected hypovolemia

Relative
- Septicemia
- Distorted anatomy

EQUIPMENT

- Tuohy epidural needle or similar
- When applicable, special needles for epidural and electrical stimulation catheter
- 25-gauge, ¾-inch infiltration needle
- 3-mL syringe
- 10-mL syringe
- Loss-of-resistance (LOR) syringe
- When applicable, epidural catheters and electrodes
- IV T-piece extension

DRUGS

- 1.5% lidocaine
- 2.0% lidocaine
- 0.25% to 0.5% bupivacaine and ropivacaine
- Steroids
- Normal saline, preservative free

PREPARATION OF THE PATIENT

PHYSICAL EXAMINATION

Examine the local area for infections and anatomy-distorting factors such as previous surgery.

LABORATORY

- Complete blood count with platelets
- Prothrombin time and partial thromboplastin time
- Platelet function studies and bleeding times

PREOPERATIVE MEDICATION

For preoperative medication, use the standard American Society of Anesthesiologists' recommendations for conscious sedation.

PROCEDURE

POSITION OF THE PATIENT AND PHYSICIAN

Placement of the thoracic epidural catheter can be done with the patient sitting or in the lateral decubitus position (Fig. 24–2). The sitting position provides better alignment of the skin midline to the spine and facilitates identification of landmarks. The procedure can also be done with the patient prone.

MIDLINE APPROACH

The midline approach (Fig. 24–3) is applicable in the upper part of the thoracic spine between C7 and T5 and

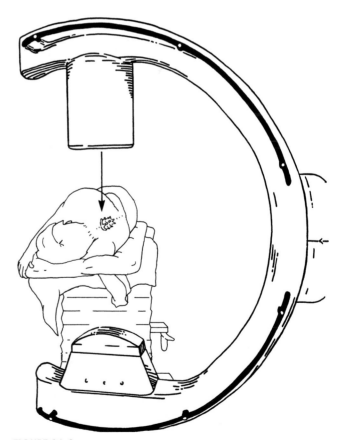

FIGURE 24–2

The patient is in a lateral decubitus position. The fluoroscopy is in position to obtain a lateral image.

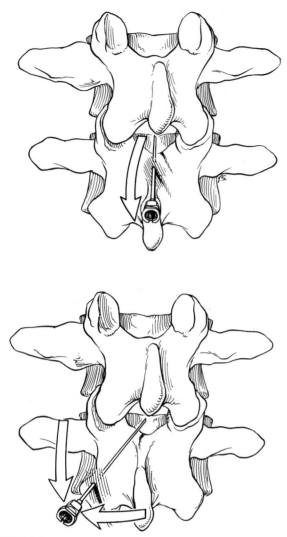

FIGURE 24-3

Angle and the direction of the needle for the median *(A)* and paramedian *(B)* approaches for spinal and epidural techniques. (From Raj PP [ed]: Clinical Practice of Regional Anesthesia. New York, Churchill Livingstone, 1991.)

in the lower part, including T9–L1, since the spinous processes project directly posteriorly and are horizontal. The level of the spinous process corresponds to the level of the vertebra. The epidural technique is similar to that used in the lumbar areas, with a 90-degree approach, starting at the lower part of the interspace, just above the lower spine, so that the needle is angled cephalad. This facilitates insertion and advancement of the catheter. The desired level of entry is determined using fluoroscopy and a radiographic marker in the anteroposterior view. After choosing the desired intralaminar level, the ideal skin entry site is about 1 to 1½ levels more caudal. Dermal infiltration with lidocaine is performed using a short 25-gauge needle. Injection of a local anesthetic with a slightly longer needle, such as 22-gauge, 1.5-inch needle, into the paraspinal muscles on either side of the spine provides significant analgesia for the procedure by blocking the nerve fibers as they come

from lateral areas toward the midline. The 16- or 18-gauge 3½-inch Tuohy needle is advanced with the bevel cephalad so that the smooth part of the needle will bounce off the lamina. The needle is advanced through the skin, subcutaneous tissue, supraspinous ligament, and intraspinous ligament, in the anteroposterior view. As the interlaminar space is approached, the C-arm is switched to a lateral view, posterior to the bony canal (Fig. 24–4).

LOR technique uses an air- or fluid-filled syringe containing a small bubble of air to allow compression (since a liquid is not compressible). If a liquid is used, the author prefers 0.9% saline without preservatives. Hanging-drop technique has been used, especially in the thoracic area, because of the significant negative pressure. Despite a low incidence of dural puncture, the drop is sucked in only 88% of the time. Since both hands are used to slowly advance the needle, entry into the epidural space is recognized even when the drop is not sucked in.

After the epidural space is entered, 1 to 2 mL of nonionic water-soluble radiographic contrast is injected to confirm epidural entry; intravascular or intrathecal injection should be avoided. A mixture consisting of 40 to 80 mg of triamcinolone diacetate or methylprednisolone, 1 mL of 0.25% levobupivacaine, and 2 mL of preservative-free normal saline can be injected. After completion of the bolus injection, the needle is removed and a bandage applied over the skin entry site.

Once entry into the epidural space is confirmed, a catheter is advanced 3 to 4 cm for continuous infusions or phenol injection (Fig. 24–5). As in any epidural technique, the catheter should not be withdrawn after it passes the tip of the needle because the catheter may be sheared off. Needles used for electrode placement in the epidural space are specially designed to allow for gentle withdrawal. Inserting the catheter too far may result in either migration through the intervertebral foramen epidural vein or true knot formation. Tunneling the catheter for 5 cm using another epidural needle reduces the risk of catheter migration in long-term infusions.[7]

The technique described by Raj[8] for taping the catheter using Steri-Strips, Mastisol, and Tegaderm can be employed instead of suturing. This technique reduces the possibility of catheter dislodgment and facilitates maintaining the catheter for a longer period. The catheter is connected to an adapter, a filter, and an injection site and then taped over the infraclavicular area to afford easy access for reinjection.

COMPLICATIONS

The complications of the thoracic epidural technique[9] are similar to those of the lumbar epidural block—infection, epidural hematoma, injury to the nerve roots, intravascular injection, respiratory depression,

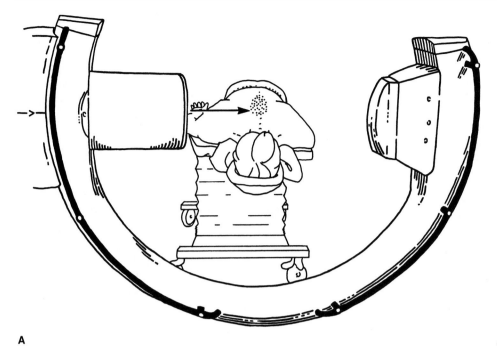

A

FIGURE 24–4

A, Drawing of the C-arm in position for the lateral view. *B,* Drawing of the thoracic spine showing the catheter in place. (*B,* From Raj PP [ed]: Clinical Practice of Regional Anesthesia. New York, Churchill Livingstone, 1991.

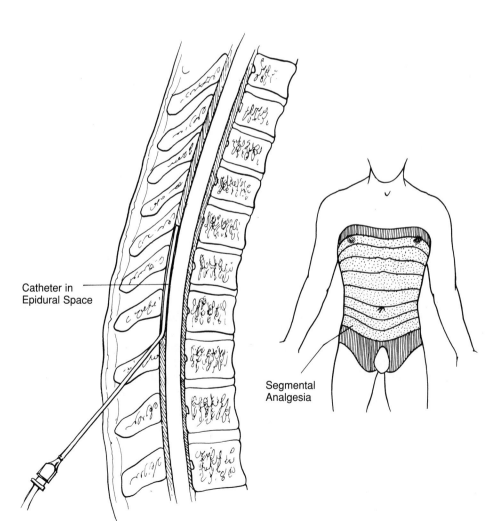

Catheter in
Epidural Space

Segmental
Analgesia

B

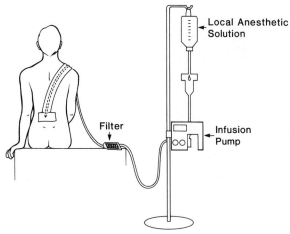

FIGURE 24–5

The diagram shows an arrangement used for continuous epidural analgesia. (From Raj PP [ed]: Clinical Practice of Regional Anesthesia. New York, Churchill Livingstone, 1991.)

and subdural and subarachnoid injection, among others. The presence of the spinal cord in the thoracic vertebral canal brings in the possibility of spinal cord damage. The incidence of spinal cord damage due to attempted thoracic epidural analgesia is not known. There are few reports of this complication. In one series of 1071 postoperative patients, no long-term serious complications were reported. In a study of 4185 patients, absence of serious neurologic complications was documented.[10] A case report of accidental pleural puncture and placement of the catheter in the pleural cavity has been documented.[11, 12] Although uncommon, this complication can be life threatening if not recognized. Many studies document safety and absence of infection.[13]

HELPFUL HINTS

Since the spinal cord is present in the thoracic vertebral level, a thoracic epidural technique should be attempted only by an operator who has extensive experience doing lumbar epidural blocks. Bromage recommended that a person who performs a thoracic epidural block should have done at least 50 consecutive lumbar epidural blocks without a dural puncture or a complication.[4]

Because of the inclination of the spine in the midthoracic area, the technique could be technically difficult, although it can be mastered with some practice.

Because the nerve roots contain the sympathetic nerves to the heart, a block of these fibers can produce significant bradycardia and hypotension.

Intercostal muscle weakness resulting from thoracic epidural block can produce significant difficulty, especially in obese patients and those with respiratory impairment. In a person with impaired function of the diaphragm, chronic obstructive lung disease, or obesity, intercostal paralysis can significantly contribute to the respiratory impairment.

EFFICACY

No random, controlled, double-blind studies can be found. On an individual basis, the thoracic epidural block has shown itself to be useful.

Injection, single cervical or thoracic 62310; daily management of epidural 01996.

REFERENCES

1. Scott D: Central neural blockade. In Scott DB, Hakansson L, Buckhoj P (eds): Techniques of Regional Anesthesia. New York, McGraw-Hill, 1996, pp 178–180.
2. Katz J, Renck H: Lumbar epidural block. In Katz J (ed): Handbook of Thoraco-abdominal Nerve Block. Orlando, Grune & Stratton, 1987, pp 111–113.
3. Anderson JE: The back. In Agur AM (ed): Grant's Atlas of Anatomy, 7th ed. Baltimore, Williams & Wilkins, 1978.
4. Bromage PR: Surgical applications. In Epidural Analgesia. Philadelphia, WB Saunders, 1978, pp 490–492.
5. Cousins MJ, Bridenbaugh PO: Epidural neural blockade. In Cousins MJ, Bridenbaugh PO (eds): Neural Blockade in Clinical Anesthesia and Management of Pain, 2nd ed. Philadelphia, JB Lippincott, 1988, pp 253–360.
6. Lema MJ, Sinha I: Thoracic epidural anesthesia and analgesia. Pain Digest 4:3–11, 1994.
7. Raj P: Postoperative pain. In Raj PP (ed): Handbook of Regional Anesthesia. New York, Churchill Livingstone, 1985, p 106.
8. Kenworthy KL, Hoffman J, Rogers JN: A new dressing technique for temporary percutaneous catheters used for pain management [letter to the editor]. Anesthesiology 76:482–483, 1992.
9. Tanaka K, Watanabe R, Harada T, et al: Extensive application of epidural anesthesia and analgesia in a university hospital: Incidence of complications related to technique. Reg Anesth 18:34–38, 1993.
10. Giebler RM, Scherer RU, Peters J: Incidence of neurologic complications related to thoracic epidural catheterization. Anesthesiology 86:55–63, 1997.
11. Yuste M, Canet J, Garcia M, et al: An epidural abscess due to resistant *Staphylococcus aureus* following epidural catheterization. Anaesthesia 52:163–165, 1997.
12. Strafford MA, Wilder RT, Berde CB: The risk of infection from epidural analgesia in children: A review of 1620 cases. Anesth Analg 80:234–238, 1995.
13. Scherer R, Schmutzler M, Giebler R, et al: Complications related to thoracic epidural analgesia: A prospective study in 1071 surgical patients. Acta Anasthesiol Scand 37:370–374, 1993.

25

Thoracic Discogram

HISTORY

Knut Lindblom, a radiologist in Stockholm, Sweden, first described diagnostic disc puncture and coined the term *discography*.[1] It was Carl Hirsch who employed the procedure to identify painful discs in patients with lumbago and sciatica. The diagnostic parameter of the procedure was the pain response, thus, the concept of provocative discography. Lindblom continued to modify the technique to use the injection of contrast material to visualize the radial ruptures of the discs, and the diagnostic criteria were expanded to include the radiographic appearance of the disc and the patient's response to the injection (i.e., to provocation).

Wise and Weiford were the first in the United States to visualize and study internal disc morphology.[1] Cloward and Busade continued the work and described the technique and indications for discography in their 1952 paper on the evaluation of normal and abnormal discs.[2]

ANATOMY

The gelatinous nucleus pulposus of the thoracic disc is surrounded by a dense, laminated fibroelastic network of fibers known as the *annulus*. The annular fibers are arranged in concentric layers that run obliquely from adjacent vertebrae. It is this annular layer that receives sensory innervation from a variety of sources. Posteriorly, the annulus receives fibers from the sinuvertebral nerves, which also provide sensory innervation to the posterior elements, including portions of the facet joints. Laterally, fibers from the exiting spinal nerve roots provide sensory innervation, and the anterior portion of the disc receives fibers from the sympathetic chain (Fig. 25–1). Each thoracic disc is situated between the cartilaginous end plates of the vertebrae above and below it.

The thoracic nerve roots leave the spinal cord and travel laterally through the intervertebral foramina. If the posterior thoracic disc herniates laterally, it can impinge on the thoracic root as it travels though the intervertebral

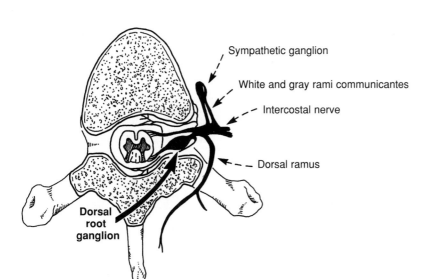

Sympathetic ganglion

White and gray rami communicantes

Intercostal nerve

Dorsal ramus

Dorsal root ganglion

FIGURE 25–1

Coronal cross section of a thoracic vertebra demonstrating the shape and contents.

foramen, producing classic radicular symptoms. If the thoracic disc herniates posteromedially, it may impinge on the spinal cord itself, producing myelopathy that may cause thoracic, lower extremity, and bowel and bladder symptoms. Severe compression of the thoracic spinal cord may result in paraparesis or, rarely, paraplegia.

INDICATIONS

Although thoracic discography is performed less frequently than cervical or lumbar discography, it probably provides the most clinically useful information of the three. The reasons for this paradox are three: (1) less is known about the thoracic disc in health and disease; (2) thoracic disc herniation is less common than lumbar or cervical disc herniation; and (3) clinicians are less comfortable attributing pain symptoms to thoracic discogenic disease. For these reasons, thoracic discography can help the clinician determine whether a damaged thoracic disc is, in fact, the true source of the patient's pain. This information is extremely valuable, given the difficulty and risks associated with surgery on the thoracic discs.

Thoracic discography is indicated as a diagnostic maneuver for a carefully selected subset of patients suffering from thoracic radicular—and occasionally myelopathic—pain. Patients in the following situations may benefit from discography:

1. Patients with persistent thoracic radicular or myelopathic pain, when traditional diagnostic modalities such as magnetic resonance imaging, computed tomography, and electromyography have failed to identify the cause
2. Patients in whom equivocal findings, such as bulging thoracic discs, are identified by traditional diagnostic modalities, to determine whether such abnormalities are in fact responsible for the pain
3. Patients who are to undergo instrumentation and fusion of the thoracic spine, when discography may help identify which levels need to be fused
4. Patients who have previously undergone instrumentation and fusion of the thoracic spine to help identify whether levels above and below the fusion are responsible for persistent pain
5. Patients in whom recurrent disc herniation cannot be distinguished from scar tissue with traditional imaging techniques

CONTRAINDICATIONS

- Local infection
- Coagulopathies
- Inadequate respiratory function
- Distorted anatomy

EQUIPMENT

- 25-gauge, ¾-inch infiltration needle
- 22-gauge, 6-inch spinal needle
- 3-mL syringe
- 5-mL syringe
- IV T-piece extension
- Pressure monitoring system (optional) (Fig. 25–2)

DRUGS

- 1.5% lidocaine
- Iohexol (Omnipaque 240) radiographic contrast medium
- Cephazolin (Kefzol) 5 mg/mL concentration for intradiscal injection
- Ceftriaxone (Rocephin) for IV prophylaxis. May substitute ciprofloxacin (Cipro)
- 0.25% to 0.5% bupivacaine/ropivacaine

PREPARATION OF THE PATIENT

PHYSICAL EXAMINATION

One should superficially examine the area for local infection and distortion of normal anatomy by surgery or masses. Laboratory studies are checked for coagulopathies. Effects of the potential harm from respiratory insufficiencies are considered.

LABORATORY

- Complete blood count with platelets
- Prothrombin time and partial thromboplastin time
- Platelet function studies and bleeding time
- Arterial blood gases (optional)
- Chest radiograph (optional)

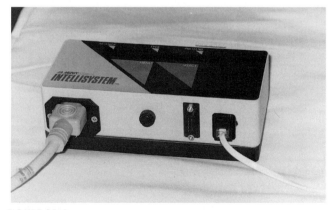

FIGURE 25–2

Pressure monitoring system.

PREOPERATIVE MEDICATION

For preoperative medication, use the standard American Society of Anesthesiologists' recommendations for conscious sedation.

PROCEDURE

POSITION OF THE PATIENT AND PHYSICIAN

The patient is placed prone with a pillow under the lower chest to slightly flex the thoracic spine as if for a thoracic sympathetic block (Fig. 25–3).

TECHNIQUE OF THORACIC DISCOGRAPHY

Computed tomographic (CT) or fluoroscopic views are taken through the discs to be imaged, and the relative positions of the pleural space, lung, ribs, nerve roots, and spinal cord are noted. After antiseptic preparation of the skin, the fluoroscope is rotated laterally and in a caudal and cephalad or cephalad-caudal direction to "open up" the disc. Using a radiodense marker, the skin entry site is found just lateral to the midpoint of the "ear of the Scottie dog" (Fig. 25–4).

A 22-gauge, 13-cm styleted needle is introduced through the skin under CT or fluoroscopic guidance, via "tunnel" view technique, with the middle of the disc being of interest.

The needle is advanced in incremental steps into the central nucleus (Fig. 25–5). A lateral radiographic view is indicated to avoid advancing the needle completely through the disc. Often a "rubbery" sensation of the needle is felt as it passes through the disc.

Water-soluble contrast medium suitable for intrathecal use is then slowly injected through the needle into the disc in a volume of 0.2 to 0.6 mL. The resistance to injection should be noted, because an intact disc offers firm resistance at these volumes. Simultaneously, the patient's pain response during injection is noted. The

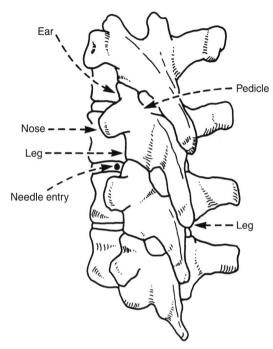

FIGURE 25–4

Oblique view of a thoracic vertebra showing the "Scottie dog" image.

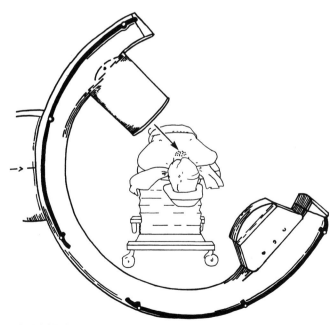

FIGURE 25–3

The patient is placed in the prone position. An oblique "Scottie dog" type view is obtained on the right side to minimize the potential for inadvertent vascular puncture.

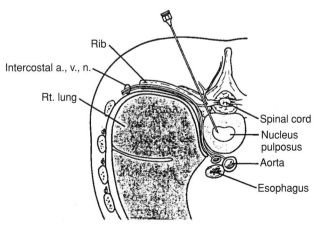

FIGURE 25–5

A drawing that shows the location of the relevant structures in relation to the needle's path into the thoracic disc. (From Waldman SD [ed]: Interventional Pain Management, 2nd ed. Philadelphia, WB Saunders, 2001, p 138.)

site of the patient's pain and its quality and similarity to the ongoing clinical symptoms are evaluated. If multiple levels are involved, it would be helpful to have the patient quantify the amount of pain from each level.

INJECTION OF CONTRAST MEDIUM AND ITS INTERPRETATION

The nucleogram of a normal thoracic disc appears as a lobulated mass with occasional posterolateral clefts, which develop as part of the normal aging process of the disc. In a damaged disc, the contrast material may flow into tears of the inner annulus, producing a characteristic transverse pattern. If the tears in the annulus extend to the outer layer, a radial pattern is produced. Contrast material may also flow between the layers of the annulus, producing a circumferential pattern. Complete disruption of the annulus allows contrast material to flow into the epidural space or into the cartilaginous end plate of the vertebra itself. Although the damage to the annulus is directly proportional to the likelihood that the disc is the source of the patient's pain, the specialist must evaluate all information obtained from discography in the context of the patient's symptoms.

POSTPROCEDURE MONITORING

After injection procedures are completed, the patient is observed for 30 minutes before discharge. The patient should be warned to expect minor postprocedure discomfort, including some soreness of the paraspinous musculature. The patient should be instructed to call immediately if any fever or other systemic symptoms occur that might suggest infection.

COMPLICATIONS

Complications directly related to discography are generally self-limited, although, occasionally, even in the best of hands, serious complications can occur. The most common severe complication of discography is infection of the disc, commonly referred to as *discitis*. Because of the limited blood supply of the disc, such infections can be extremely hard to eradicate. Discitis usually presents as an increase in spine pain several days to a week after discography. At first, there is no change in the patient's neurologic findings as a result of disc infection.

Epidural abscess, which occasionally follows discography, generally presents within 24 to 48 hours. Clinically, the signs and symptoms of epidural abscess are high fever, spine pain, and progressive neurologic deficit. If either discitis or epidural abscess is suspected, blood and urine cultures should be taken, antibiotic treatment started, and emergent magnetic resonance imaging of the spine obtained to allow identification and drainage of any abscess before an irreversible neurologic deficit develops.

In addition to infectious complications, pneumothorax can complicate cervical, thoracic, or lumbar discography. This complication should be rare if radiographic guidance is used during needle placement. A small pneumothorax after discography can often be treated conservatively, and tube thoracostomy can be avoided. Trauma to retroperitoneal structures, including the kidney, may also occur.

Direct trauma to the nerve roots and spinal cord can occur if the needle is allowed to traverse the entire disc or is placed too far lateral. These complications should be rare if serial CT or fluoroscopic views are taken while the needle is advanced. Such needle-induced trauma to the spinal cord and cauda equina can result in devastating neurologic deficits.

HELPFUL HINTS

Analgesic discography is useful in patients whose clinical pain pattern is reproduced or provoked during the injection of contrast medium. If the pain that was provoked during the injection is relieved by a subsequent injection of local anesthetic into the disc, the inference can be drawn that the disc is the likely source of the patient's pain. It must be remembered that, if the annulus is disrupted, the injected local anesthetic may spread into the epidural space and anesthetize somatic and sympathetic nerves that may innervate the disc at adjacent levels. If this occurs, erroneous information may be obtained if discography is then performed on adjacent discs.

EFFICACY

Discography is a straightforward technique that may provide useful clinical information on carefully selected patients. The information obtained from discography must always be analyzed in the context of the clinical presentation. Failure to do so can lead to a variety of clinical misadventures, including additional spine surgeries, which are doomed to failure. CT guidance affords an additional measure of safety, as compared with fluoroscopy, because it allows the pain specialist to clearly identify anatomic structures and monitor the needle position.

REFERENCES

1. Wise RE, Weiford EC: X-ray visualization of the intervertebral disc. Cleve Clin Q 18:127–130, 1951.
2. Cloward RB, Busade LL: Discography: Technique, indications, and evaluation of the normal and abnormal intervertebral disc. AJR Am J Roentgenol 68:552–564, 1952.

26

Lumbar Sleeve and Dorsal Root Ganglion Block

HISTORY

The origin of selective nerve root blockade can be traced back to 1906 when Sellheim performed paravertebral blocks for urological surgery.[1] A few years later, in 1912, Kappis described the blockade of the brachial plexus via the cervical nerve roots. Over the ensuing century, selective root sleeve blocks have become commonplace in the diagnosis and treatment of many painful syndromes. There have been numerous publications on the anatomy and approach to the lumbar nerve root sleeve.[2-4] Kikuchi and associates[5] have described the anatomic variants of the dorsal root ganglia, and Derby and colleagues[6] have reviewed the techniques of blocking the lumbar nerve root sleeve.

ANATOMY

General description of the vertebral structures is given in the thoracic area. The lumbar nerves are five pairs of typical spinal nerves derived from the part of the spinal cord, which is located between the 9th and 11th thoracic vertebrae. On emerging from their respective intervertebral foramina, each nerve gives off a recurrent branch that returns to supply the homologous vertebra and its ligaments and the meninges of the cord. Each of the nerves then divides into a posterior and an anterior primary division (Fig. 26–1).

INDICATIONS

The selective nerve root block (SNRB), when combined with a careful history, physical examination, and quality radiographic studies, is an important tool in the diagnostic evaluation and treatment of patients with predominantly radicular symptoms.[2] It is helpful in patients with multiple level abnormalities and complex postop-

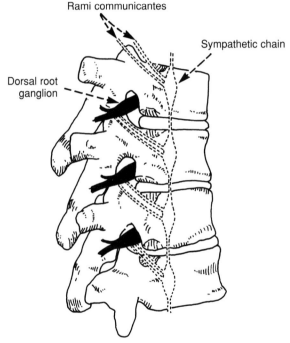

Rami communicantes

Sympathetic chain

Dorsal root ganglion

FIGURE 26–1

Lateral view of the vertebral body showing the nerve roots emerging out of the foramina with their connections to the sympathetic chain.

erative problems and in patients with clearly defined clinical symptoms without significant imaging findings.[3]

More specifically, an SNRB is useful in (1) helping to ascertain the specific nociceptive pathway; (2) helping to define the mechanisms of the chronic pain state; and (3) aiding in the differential diagnosis of the site of the pain.[4] SNRBs are also performed for prognostic and therapeutic purposes. Prognostically, the SNRB aids in predicting the efficacy of the neurolytic or neurosurgical treatment.[4-6]

The prognostic block also affords the patient the opportunity to experience the numbness and other side effects that follow surgical resection or neurolytic block.[4] From this experience, the patient can decide whether or not to undergo the procedure. On a therapeutic basis, SNRBs are useful for treating pain not amenable to other methods of analgesia. This can be on a temporary or permanent basis, depending on the medication used.

Clinical indications include pain secondary to nerve root compression, pain from tumor invasion of a nerve root or in the distribution of a nerve root, vertebral fractures, acute herpetic neuralgia, postherpetic neuralgia, discogenic pain, segmental neuralgia, and postoperative pain.[7, 8, 12, 13]

CONTRAINDICATIONS

- Local infection
- Coagulopathy

EQUIPMENT

Nerve Block

- 25-gauge needle for skin infiltration
- 20-gauge, 10-cm curved-blunt HP needle
- 16-gauge, 1½-inch angiolith
- 3-mL syringe
- 5-mL syringe
- 10-mL syringe
- IV T-piece extension set

Pulsed Electrode Magnetic Field and Radiofrequency Thermocoagulation

- 25 gauge needle for skin infiltration
- 20-gauge 10-cm curved-blunt HP needle
- 16-gauge, 1½-inch angiolith
- 3-mL syringe
- 5-mL syringe
- 10-mL syringe
- IV T-piece extension set
- 10-cm curved-blunt radiofrequency thermocoagulation (RFTC) needle
- RFTC electrode and connecting cables
- Grounding pad

DRUGS

- 1.5% lidocaine
- 2% lidocaine
- 0.5% bupivacaine/ropivacaine
- Steroids (optional)
- Iohexol (Omnipaque 240) radiographic contrast

PREPARATION OF THE PATIENT

PHYSICAL EXAMINATION

Examine for local infection and distorted anatomy that may interfere with performance of the procedure.

LABORATORY

Perform routine laboratory studies as indicated.

PREOPERATIVE MEDICATION

For preoperative medication, use the standard American Society of Anesthesiologists' recommendations for conscious sedation.

PROCEDURE

POSITION OF THE PATIENT

The lumbar nerve roots are approached the same way as the lower thoracic roots, except there is no "4-cm rule." Obtain an anteroposterior fluoroscopic view of the desired level. Oblique the C-arm in the coronal plane until the facet joint is delineated (approximately 20 degrees) (Fig. 26–2). Then oblique the camera 15 degrees in the caudocephalad direction. This gives a clear picture of the superior par articularis.

Insert the angiocatheter and direct the curved-blunt needle toward the tip of the pars (Fig. 26–3). Touch the pars and walk off in the cephalad direction. In the lateral view, ideal placement of the needle is with the tip in the cephalodorsal corner of the neuroforamen (Fig. 26–4). In the anteroposterior plane, the tip of the needle should be the same as described for thoracic nerve roots (Fig. 26–5). Inject contrast medium to visualize the nerve root and then inject the local anesthetic.

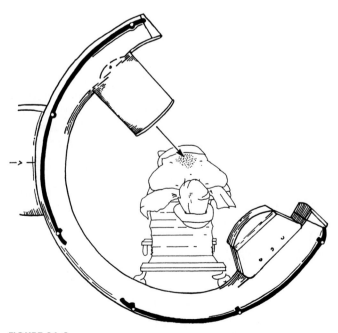

FIGURE 26–2

With the patient in a prone position, oblique the C-arm in the coronal plane until the facet joint is delineated.

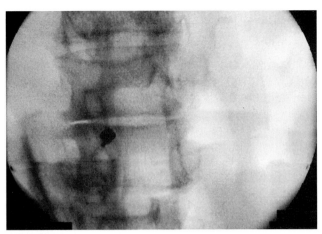

FIGURE 26–3

Fluoroscopic view shows the insertion of the angiocatheter toward the tip of the pars.

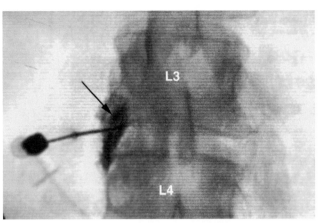

FIGURE 26–5

The AP view shows the needle *(arrow)* on the nerve root; contrast shows the root sleeve.

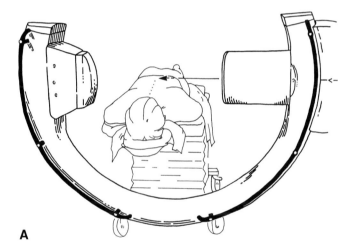

A

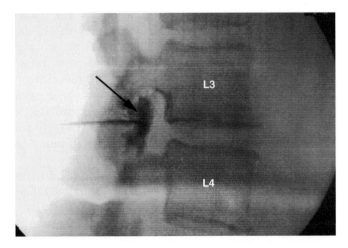

B

FIGURE 26–4

The C-arm position in the lateral view *(A)* to see the needle enter the foramen *(B)*. The arrow indicates the spread of the contrast medium in the epidural space.

A small amount (1 mL) of non-ionic, water-soluble contrast (iohexol 240) is injected slowly to avoid trauma to the nerve root. The spread of the contrast medium should delineate the nerve root only, with no spread in the epidural space or onto the peripheral plexus (see Figs. 26–4*B* and 26–5). If resistance is felt or vascular spread is noted, the needle must be redirected. After negative aspirate, inject 1 to 1.5 mL of local anesthetic (1% to 2% lidocaine or 0.25 to 0.5% bupivacaine) under fluoroscopic guidance. The patient should not feel any pain or paresthesia during injection. Remove the needle and place a sterile bandage.

DORSAL ROOT GANGLIONOSTOMY (PARTIAL RHIZOTOMY)

Only after a successful diagnostic block should a partial rhizotomy of the dorsal root ganglion be attempted. This can be performed using conventional radiofrequency, pulsed electrode magnetic field (pEMF), cryoanalgesia, and neurolytic blocks. Epidural neurolytic blocks have been performed in the past, but with advent of radiofrequency techniques, neurolytics are infrequently used. Only conventional and pulsed radiofrequency, cryoanalgesia, and neurolytics are now recommended. Therefore, only conventional and pulsed radiofrequency are discussed in this section. The current hypothesis on the mechanism of action of EMF is that the membranes of nerves have a capacitor function and that EMF creates a high electric field that punches holes in the capacitor, thus blocking transmission of stimuli through A delta and C fibers.[14]

The goal is to position the tip of the needle directly adjacent to the dorsal root ganglion of the desired nerve root (Fig. 26–6). A sensory paresthesia should be felt in the desired dermatome at less than 1.0 V at 50-Hz stimulation. Ideal stimulation should be felt between 0.4 and 0.6 V. If stimulation is felt at less than 0.4 V, the

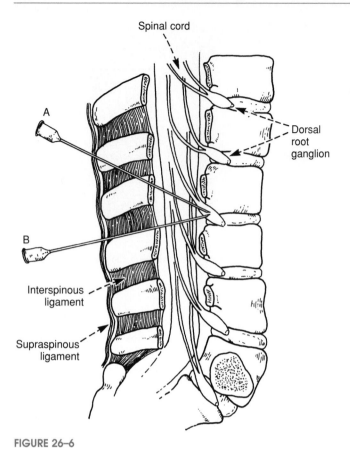

FIGURE 26–6

The drawing shows the position of needles A and B on the dorsal root ganglion as it traverses the foramen close to the disc.

tip of the needle is too close to the dorsal root ganglion, and if stimulation is felt at more than 0.6 V, the tip is too far away from the dorsal root ganglion. Motor stimulation is then performed at 2 Hz. There should be a clear dissociation between motor and sensory stimulation; that is, the voltage required to see motor fasciculations at 2 Hz should be at least two times the voltage that produces sensory stimulation at 50 Hz.[10] Thus, if good sensory stimulation at 50 Hz was noted at 0.5 V, then motor fasciculations at 2 Hz should not be seen at voltages less than 1.0 V.

The point of dissociation defines the position of the dorsal root ganglion. If dissociation between sensory and motor stimulation cannot be obtained, the tip of the needle is not in alignment with the dorsal root ganglion, and lesioning at this point is not recommended.

Once the proper stimulation parameters have been achieved, inject 2 mL of local anesthetic with 40 mg of triamcinolone diacetate. Wait 3 to 5 minutes and then lesion at 65°C for 90 seconds with conventional radiofrequency. With pEMF, local anesthetic is not required since the necessary temperature is just above body temperature. Lesioning is carried out at 42°C for 120 seconds. There has been no reported neuritis with pEMF.

COMPLICATIONS

One of the biggest concerns is damage to the nerve root while positioning the needle. Using a blunt-tip needle can dramatically reduce this complication. Neuritis after radiofrequency lesioning is the other big concern. This is the reason that sensory and motor testing is so important. If the proper parameters are not met, there is an increased incidence (30%)of postprocedure neuritis. Injection of steroid prior to lesioning helps reduce but not completely eliminate the chance of neuritis.

Other complications include intravascular and intrathecal injection of medication, paralysis, bowel and bladder incontinence, bruising, bleeding, increased pain, and infection.[11]

EFFICACY

Krempen and colleagues prospectively evaluated 22 patients with complicated back pathology who presented with sciatica as their chief complaint.[12] Selective nerve root blocks were performed on each patient. Two patients had excellent relief of pain in the immediate postprocedure period but decided against surgery. Sixteen patients had excellent relief of their pain and chose to proceed with surgery. In these 16 patients, intraoperative findings revealed 2 with retained disc material, 13 with scar tissue, and 1 with impingement of the articular process on the nerve root. Four patients received no relief with diagnostic block. No failures were reported at 8- to 24-month follow-up sessions.

Dooley and coworkers retrospectively reviewed 62 patients who had undergone nerve root infiltration (NRI) for lumbosacral radiculopathy and assessed the accuracy and indications for NRI.[13] Group 1 had typical pain reproduced by needle placement and then relieved by NRI. Group 2 had typical pain reproduced by needle placement, but the pain was not relieved by local anesthesia, indicating multiple nerve root involvement. Patients in group 3 or 4 did not have their typical pain reproduced by needle insertion, with or without relief by local anesthesia, and were seldom relieved of the radicular pain. Group 1 (44 patients) was 85% accurate in identifying a single nerve root as the sole cause of radicular symptoms, and these patients proceeded with surgery. Group 2 (4 patients) showed incomplete relief and were felt to have multiple-level root symptoms. In groups 3 and 4, 6 of 14 patients deferred surgery secondary to a negative response to NRI, whereas 5 patients had surgery and were relieved of their radicular symptoms. Supporters of this study proceed with surgery when an NRI successfully abolishes radicular symptoms.

Loeser retrospectively studied 45 patients who had dorsal rhizotomies for relief of chronic pain.[4] The author extensively used nerve blocks in the preoperative evaluation of the patients but thought that the results of the nerve blocks did not enable him to predict the operative results. In the patients with successful preoperative nerve blocks, 20% had a long-term operative success rate, whereas those with an unsuccessful preoperative nerve block had a 27% long-term success rate. In total, 28% of the patients were successfully treated. Thus, the diagnostic blocks done were not helpful in guiding therapy.[11]

Onofrio and Campa retrospectively examined their 12-year experience with dorsal rhizotomy in 286 patients with intractable pain.[15] Of the 286 patients, 112 had pain of unknown etiology and 81 had diagnostic blocks before consideration for surgery. A positive selective root sleeve block was followed by dorsal rhizotomy. Both investigators observed that the blocks were almost always unsuccessful and proved to be an unreliable prognostic indicator of the result to be expected from section of the same root.[16]

North and associates reviewed 13 patients with failed back surgery syndrome who underwent dorsal root ganglionectomy.[17] All preoperative selective root blocks indicated a monoradicular pain syndrome. Nearly all patients reported 100% relief with selective nerve root blockade, whereas 1 reported 95% relief and another 90% relief. The blocks were repeated and reproduced. Most, but not all, patients underwent additional blocks at other levels to confirm the specificity of their responses. Follow-up data were obtained at a mean of 5.5 years following dorsal root ganglionectomy. Follow-up interviews to assess outcome were conducted by a disinterested third party. Treatment "success" (at least 50% sustained relief of pain and patient satisfaction with the result) was recorded in 2 patients at 2 years after surgery and in none at 5.5 years. Equivocal success (at least 50% relief, without clear-cut patient satisfaction) was recorded in 1 patient at 2 and at 5.5 years postoperatively. Improvements in activities of daily living were recorded in a few patients. Loss of sensory and motor function was reported frequently by patients. A few patients had reduced or eliminated analgesic intake. The authors concluded that dorsal root ganglionectomy had a limited role in the management of failed back surgery syndrome.

Transforaminal epidural; lumbar-single level 64483; transforaminal epidural; lumbar, additional levels 64484.

REFERENCES

1. Matas R: Local and regional anesthesia: A retrospect and prospect. Am J Surg 25:189, 1943.
2. Lawen A: Ueber segmentare Schmerzaufhebung durch paravertebrale Novokaininjektionen zur Differential diagnose intra-abdominaler Erkrankungen. Med Wochenschr 69:1423, 1922.
3. Brunn F, Mandl F: Die paravertebrale Injection zur Bekampfung visceraler Schmerzen. Wien Klin Wochenschr 37:511, 1924.
4. von Gaza W: Die Resektion der paravertebralen Nerven and die isolierte Durchschneidung des Ramus communicans. Arch Klin Chir 133:479, 1924.
5. Kikuchi S, Sato K, Konno S, Hasue M: Anatomic and radiographic study of dorsal root ganglia. Spine 19:6–11, 1994.
6. Derby R, Bogduk N, Anat D, et al: Precision percutaneous blocking procedures for localizing spinal pain: I. The posterior lumbar compartment. Pain Digest 3:89–100, 1993.
7. Jain S: Nerve blocks. In Warfield C (ed): Principles and Practice of Pain Management. New York, McGraw-Hill, 1993, pp 379–399.
8. Pang W, Ho S, Huang M: Selective lumbar spinal nerve block: A review. Acta Anaesthesiol Sin 37:21–26, 1999.
9. Sluijter M, van Kleef M: Characteristics and mode of action of radiofrequency lesioning. Curr Rev Pain 2:143–150, 1998.
10. Kline M: Radiofrequency techniques in clinical practice. In Waldman S, Winnie A (eds): Interventional Pain Management. Philadelphia, WB Saunders, 1996, pp 185–218.
11. Botwin K, Gruber R, Bouchlas C, et al: Complications of fluoroscopically guided transforaminal lumbar epidural injections. Arch Phys Med Rehabil 81:1045–1050, 2000.
12. Krempen J, Smith B, DeFreest L: Selective nerve root infiltration for the evaluation of sciatica. Orthop Clin North Am 6:311–315, 1975.
13. Dooley J, McBroom R, Taguchi T, Macnab I: Nerve root infiltration in the diagnosis of radicular pain. Spine 13:79–83, 1988.
14. Loeser J: Dorsal rhizotomy for the relief of chronic pain. J Neurosurg 36:745–750, 1972.
15. Onofrio B, Campa H: Evaluation of rhizotomy: Review of 12 years' experience. J Neurosurg 36:751–755, 1972.
16. Guarino A, Staats P: Diagnostic neural blockade in the management of pain. Pain Digest 7:194–199, 1997.
17. North R, Kidd D, Campbell J, Long D: Dorsal root ganglionectomy for failed back surgery syndrome: A 5-year follow-up study. J Neurosurg 74:236–242, 1991.

Splanchnic Nerve Blocks

27

HISTORY

The first anterior percutaneous approach to splanchnic nerve block was when Kappis introduced splanchnic anesthesia in 1914[1] and followed it up in 1918[2] with the publication of a series of 200 cases. The recognition that splanchnic nerve block may provide relief of pain in a subset of patients who fail to obtain relief from celiac plexus block has led to a renewed interest in this technique.

The technique for splanchnic nerve block differs little from the classic retrocrural approach to the celiac plexus, except that the needles are aimed more cephalad to ultimately rest at the anterolateral margin of the T12 vertebral body.[3] It is imperative that both needles be placed medially against the vertebral body to reduce the incidence of pneumothorax. Abram and Boas[4] described

technique for splanchnic nerve block that used a para-vertebral transthoracic approach. The needle was advanced to rest against the anterolateral aspect of the T11 vertebral body.

ANATOMY

The splanchnic nerves transmit most of the nociceptive information from the viscera. These nerves are contained in a narrow compartment made up by the vertebral body medially and the pleura laterally, the posterior mediastinum ventrally, and the pleural attachment to the vertebra dorsally (Fig. 27–1). This compartment is bounded caudally by the crura of the diaphragm. Abram and Boas[4] have determined that the volume of this compartment is approximately 10 mL on each side.

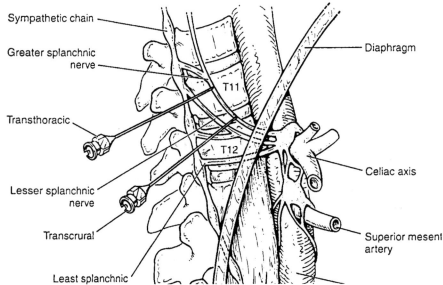

Sympathetic chain

Greater splanchnic nerve

Transthoracic

Lesser splanchnic nerve

Transcrural

Least splanchnic

T11

T12

Diaphragm

Celiac axis

Superior mesent artery

FIGURE 27–1

Drawing of the anatomic origin of the splanchnic nerve and its relation to other structures. (From Waldman SD [ed]: Interventional Pain Management, 2nd ed. Philadelphia, WB Saunders, 2001, p 503.)

INDICATIONS

Celiac plexus and splanchnic nerve local anesthetic blocks have been used as diagnostic tools to determine whether flank, retroperitoneal, or upper abdominal pain is sympathetically mediated with acute pancreatitis in chronic benign abdominal pain syndromes, such as chronic pancreatitis.[5] Most investigators report a lower success rate with this procedure for patients suffering from chronic nonmalignant abdominal pain than when abdominal pain of the neoplastic origin is treated.[6]

CONTRAINDICATIONS

Absolute
- Local infection
- Coagulopathy

Relative
- Tumor-distorting anatomy
- Abdominal aortic aneurysm
- Respiratory insufficiency, for example, if unilateral pneumothorax adversely affects sustaining life

EQUIPMENT

- Radiofrequency (RF) machine
- 15-cm long-curved RF needle with a 15-mm electrode tip
- 14-gauge, 4-cm extracath (for skin entry prior to RF needle insertion)
- Extension set to help manipulate the needle and ease injection of solutions

DRUGS

- Two 10-ml plastic syringes with local anesthetic
- 10-mL syringe with iohexol (contrast solution) to confirm the correct placement of the needle tip
- 2-mL syringe with local anesthetic for skin infiltration

PREPARATION OF THE PATIENT

LABORATORY

- Complete blood count with platelets
- Prothrombin time, partial thromboplastin time
- Platelet function test or bleeding time
- Urinalysis
- Laxative to clear bowels
- Plain anteroposterior chest radiographs

PREOPERATIVE MEDICATION

For preoperative medication, use the standard American Society of Anesthesiologists' recommendations for conscious sedation.

All patients should have an intravenous catheter inserted in a large vein and securely anchored. A 500-mL solution of dextrose-Ringer's lactate should be started, with at least 200 mL of solution infused prior to the lesion. Vital signs should be monitored throughout the procedure. Intravenous analgesic drugs should be available for use as needed. Sedation is used to relax the patient on an as-needed basis, taking into account the physical status of the patient. The patient needs to be kept awake and should be able to answer reliably during the testing of sensory and motor stimulation.

PROCEDURE

POSITION OF THE PATIENT

The patient lies prone in a comfortable position, taking care of the head and feet in particular. The position on the table should be such that the C-arm could be rotated to visualize the T10 to L3 level without difficulty (Fig. 27–2).

SITE OF NEEDLE ENTRY

In the prone position, the T12 vertebral body is identified in the posteroanterior view of the fluoroscope. Keeping a mark on the T12 or T11 vertebra, the

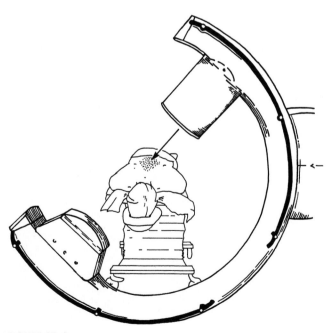

FIGURE 27–2

Drawing shows the fluoroscopic C-arm in oblique view for "tunnel" placement of the needle at the T12 vertebral level.

C-arm is moved to an oblique position (about 45 degrees) (Fig. 27–3). The edge of the diaphragm lateral to the vertebral body is viewed. Its movement during inspiration and expiration is noted. If the diaphragm shadows T12 vertebra and its rib, then the T11 rib is identified. The point of entry for both levels is at the junction of the rib and vertebra. Skin infiltration is made at this point.

TECHNIQUE OF NEEDLE ENTRY

With the oblique fluoroscopic view still in place, a 14-gauge, 5-cm extracath is inserted, such that the catheter traverses toward the target as a pinhead. When two thirds of the extracath is inserted, the stylet is removed and the RF needle is inserted. The oblique view of the fluoroscope is maintained. An extension tubing is attached to the needle. With short thrusts of 0.5 cm at a time, the tip of the needle is advanced anteriorly, keeping in mind that the needle stays hugging the lateral aspect of the T11 or T12 vertebral body, close to the costovertebral angle (Fig. 27–4; see also Fig. 27–3). After advancing 1 to 1.5 cm anteriorly, the lateral fluoroscopic view is taken. In the lateral view, the needle is advanced until it reaches the junction of anterior one third and posterior two thirds of the vertebral body. Then aspirate for blood or cerebrospinal fluid. Lateral views are taken to confirm the final position of the curved needle on the vertebral body. Eight milliliters of iohexol is injected to note that the solutions in anteroposterior and lateral views hug the spine (Fig. 27–5).

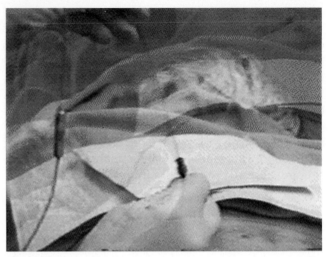

FIGURE 27–4

An oblique radiographic view when an angiocatheter is inserted using a "tunnel" approach.

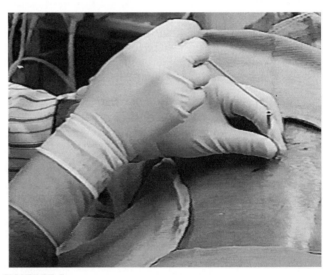

FIGURE 27–5

Insertion of a radiofrequency needle through the angiocatheter.

NEUROLYTIC BLOCKS

Smaller volumes (12 to 15 mL) of absolute alcohol are recommended for single-needle procedures.[7] Many investigators believe that alcohol, as a neurolytic agent, is superior to phenol in duration of neural blockade; however, alcohol has the disadvantage of producing transient severe pain on injection.[8]

Some clinicians have recommended the use of 6% to 10% phenol for splanchnic nerve block.[9] An advantage of phenol over alcohol is that it can be combined with contrast solution. The combination allows radiographic documentation of the distribution of the neurolytic solution. Mixtures of 10% phenol and iodinated contrast medium (iohexol) remain stable for as long as 3 months.[9] The fact that phenol is not commercially avail-

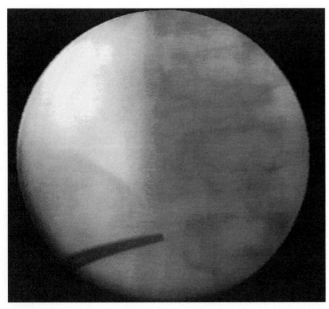

FIGURE 27–3

Radiographic oblique image shows the marking of the skin entry site for the "tunnel" view approach.

able and must be prepared for each patient by a pharmacist is a disadvantage. The apparent greater affinity of phenol for vascular rather than neurologic tissue also represents a theoretical disadvantage, in view of the vascularity of the region surrounding the celiac plexus and splanchnic nerves.[10] Some investigators believe that phenol produces a block of shorter duration than alcohol, making it a less desirable agent for the intractable and progressive pain of malignant origin. Comparative studies between alcohol and phenol are not available.

RADIOFREQUENCY LESIONING

Because splanchnic nerves are contained in a narrow compartment, they are accessible for RF lesioning. To produce a lesion of the splanchnic nerve, the needle needs to lie on the mid-third portion of the lateral side of the T11 or T12 vertebral body (Figs. 27–6 to 27–10). To approach this region, a curved 15-cm long needle with a 15-mm lesion tip is recommended. The needle should remain retrocrural and posterior to the descending aorta, safely away from the aorta. Theoretically then, it is possible to produce a safe and reliable RF lesion of splanchnic nerves.

TEST STIMULATION

Once the needle is in place, a 15-cm electrode is introduced through the RF needle. The electrical circuit is tested and the impedance is noted. It should be lower

than 250 Ω. At 50 Hz, the sensory stimulation is conducted up to 1 V. The patient may report that he or she feels stimulation in the epigastric region. This is typical and satisfactory. If the stimulation is in a girdle-like fashion around the intercostal spaces, the needle needs to be pushed anteriorly. At 2 Hz, motor stimulation is

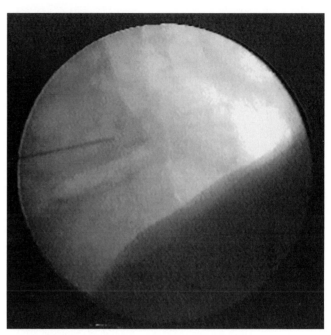

FIGURE 27–7

Step 2. Lateral radiographic view of the needle should show the needle at the junction of the anterior one third and posterior two thirds against the T12 vertebral body.

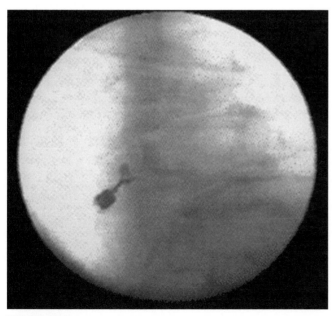

FIGURE 27–6

Step 1. Oblique radiographic image of the radiofrequency needle in position is obtained.

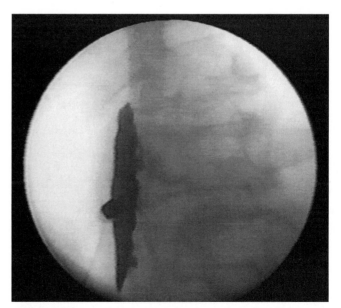

FIGURE 27–8

Step 3. In the anteroposterior radiographic view with the needle in position, contrast medium shows the spread hugging the adjacent vertebral bodies.

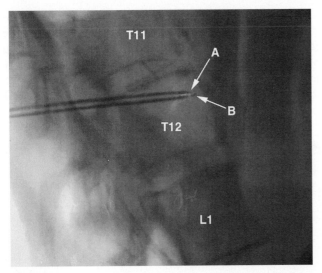

FIGURE 27-9

Step 4. Lateral radiographic view should confirm for bilateral T12-level radiofrequency thermocoagulation with correct needle placement. *Arrows A* and *B* indicate the radiofrequency needle tips.

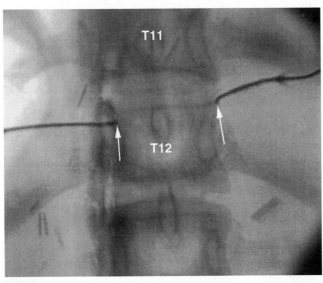

FIGURE 27-10

Step 5. An anteroposterior view of the radiofrequency thermocoagulation needles against the vertebral body confirms its correct position. Arrows indicate the tips of the RF needles.

done up to 3 V. One tries to palpate or see the intercostal muscle contraction. If this is negative, then the test stimulation is satisfactory. The next step is to produce the RF lesioning. Through the RF needle, 2 to 5 mL of local anesthetic (ropivacaine 0.5%) with steroid (40 mg of triamcinolone) is injected.

After waiting 1 to 2 minutes, the physician creates an RF lesion with settings set for 90 seconds at 80°C. The second lesion at the same setting is done turning the RF needle 180 degrees. If the procedure is for the bilateral neurolysis, then the same procedure of testing and lesioning is done on the opposite site.

COMPLICATIONS

Complications of splanchnic and celiac plexus blocks can be regarded as minor, moderate, or severe. Those that are relatively common (e.g., hypotension, diarrhea) are of minor significance and are readily reversible. Complications of moderate nature (e.g., pneumothorax) occur infrequently, and, although generally reversible, entail management that is more demanding, in that they may require hospitalization and additional procedures. Complications of the most severe nature (e.g., paraplegia) are rare and are rarely associated with recovery. The risks of the splanchnic nerve block are similar to those of the celiac plexus block. Apart from the common risks associated with celiac and splanchnic nerve blocks, the rates of pneumothorax, thoracic duct injury, and inadvertent spread of the injected drug to the somatic nerve roots are higher for the splanchnic nerve block than for the celiac plexus block. Serious complications rarely occur from either nerve block. Because of the close proximity of vital structures coupled with the use of large volumes of neurolytic drugs, side effects and complications may occur.

HELPFUL HINTS

The tip of the curved RF needle should face laterally initially until it passes the foramen. Then the tip can be turned medially once it reaches the lateral surface of the vertebral body. This ensures that the needle remains medial to the interpleural surface and in close contact with the vertebral body. Watch for spread and dispersion of contrast material, especially in a blood vessel. A fluoroscopic oblique view ensures medial direction of the needle. A lateral view ensures that the needle stays posterior to the aorta and anterior to the foramen.

Prior to lesioning, the injection of a local anesthetic helps reduce the discomfort owing to the RF lesioning and decreases pain immediately after the procedure. Steroids help in treating the occasional occurrence of neuritis by reducing edema and inflammation of the lesioned structures.

EFFICACY

Neither morbidity (which was minor) nor efficacy (70% to 80% immediate success and 60% to 75% persistence of effect until death) correlated with anatomic technique. Splanchnic nerve block maintains a deservedly meaningful role in the armamentarium of the contemporary pain specialist. Despite a dearth of scientifically determined outcome data, even the most critical observer is nearly certain to acknowledge the therapeutic value of these techniques in patients with viscerally mediated abdominal and/or back pain of neoplastic origin, especially early in the course of established disease. For patients with longer life expectancies, the role of celiac/splanchnic neural blockade is increasingly recognized as modest, on other than a diagnostic basis. Despite daunting logistic and ethical methodologic barriers, there is a pressing need to design and undertake collaborative controlled trials aimed at better determining the relative value of various technical approaches.

Splanchnic nerve 64999; RFTC other nerve 64640.

REFERENCES

1. Kappis M: Erfahrungen mit lokalanästhesie bei bauchoperationen. Verhandl d Deutsch Gesellsch f Cir 43:87, 1914.
2. Kappis M: Die Anästhesierung des Nervus splanchnicus. Zentralbl 45:709, 1918.
3. Parkinson SK, Mueller JB, Little WL: A new and simple technique for splanchnic nerve block using a paramedian approach and 3½-inch needles. Reg Anesth 14(Suppl):41, 1989.
4. Abram SE, Boas RA: Sympathetic and visceral nerve blocks. In Benumof JL (ed): Clinical Procedures in Anesthesia and Intensive Care. Philadelphia, JB Lippincott, 1993, pp 787–805.
5. Malfertheiner P, Dominquez-Munoz JE, Buchler MW: Chronic pancreatitis: Management of pain. Digestion 55(Suppl 1):29–34, 1994.
6. Jacox A, Carr DB, Payne R, et al: Management of cancer pain. Clinical Practice Guideline No. 9. AHCPR Publication No. 94-0592. Rockville, MD, Department of Health and Human Services, 1994.
7. Singler RC: An improved technique for alcohol neurolysis of the celiac plexus. Anesthesiology 56:137, 1982.
8. Prasanna A: Unilateral celiac plexus block. J Pain Symptom Manage 11:154–157, 1996.
9. Boas RA: Sympathetic blocks in clinical practice. Int Anesthesiol Clin 16:149, 1978.
10. Nour-Eldin F: Preliminary report: Uptake of phenol by vascular and brain tissue. Microvasc Res 2:224, 1970.

28 Celiac Plexus Block and Neurolysis

HISTORY

In 1914, Kappis[1] introduced the percutaneous technique for block of the splanchnic nerves and celiac plexus with local anesthetic. He described a posterior approach intended to be used primarily for a surgical anesthesia that used two needles, the tips of which were placed into the retroperitoneum via a retrocrural approach. He rapidly gained experience with this technique and reported on it in a series of 200 patients in 1918.[2]

The same year, Wendling[3] described a method of blocking the celiac plexus and splanchnic nerves using a single needle placed anteriorly through the liver. Judged to be riskier than Kappis's posterior approach, it rapidly fell into disfavor.

Labat, Farr, and others introduced modifications of the Kappis technique over the ensuing 30 years.[4-6] Because of the technical demands and variable results of celiac plexus and splanchnic nerve block as a surgical anesthetic, over time this technique was supplanted by spinal anesthesia and segmental blockade of the somatic paravertebral nerves.[7]

As celiac plexus and splanchnic nerve blocks were falling into disuse for surgical anesthesia, the clinical utility of these techniques was becoming apparent in the new specialty of pain management. Recognizing the difficulty in distinguishing the somatic and visceral components of abdominal pain, Popper[8] recommended the use of splanchnic nerve block with local anesthetic as a diagnostic tool.

Alcohol neurolysis of the splanchnic nerves and celiac plexus for long-lasting relief of abdominal pain was first described by Jones,[9] in 1957. Bridenbaugh and colleagues[10] reported on the role of neurolytic celiac plexus block to treat the pain of upper abdominal malignancy.

In spite of these modifications, Kappis's classic posterior approach to the celiac plexus and splanchnic nerves continues to serve as the basis for contemporary techniques. There is renewed interest in the anterior approach to celiac plexus block, using computed tomography (CT) or ultrasonography to allow more accurate needle placement.[11, 12]

ANATOMY

Innervation of the abdominal viscera originates in the anterolateral horn of the spinal cord with the ventral spinal routes to join the white communicating rami en route to the sympathetic chain. In contradistinction to other preganglionic sympathetic nerves, these axons do not synapse in the sympathetic chain; rather, they pass through the chain to synapse at distal sites, including the celiac, aortic renal, and superior mesenteric ganglia. Postganglionic nerves accompany blood vessels to their respective visceral structures.

Preganglionic nerves from T5 to T9 and occasionally T4 and T10 travel caudally from the sympathetic chain along the lateral and anterolateral aspects of the vertebral bodies. At the level of T9 and T10, the axons coalesce to form the greater splanchnic nerve, course through the diaphragm, and end as numerous terminal endings in the celiac plexus. Most travel ipsilaterally, but a few cross and synapse with contralateral postganglionic cell bodies.

Sympathetic nerves from T10–T11 and, occasionally, T12, combine to form the lesser splanchnic nerve. Their course parallels the greater splanchnic nerve in a posterolateral position and ends in either the celiac plexus or aorticorenal ganglion. The least splanchnic nerves arise from T12, parallel posteriorly the lesser splanchnic nerve, and synapse in the aorticorenal ganglion (Fig. 28–1).

Nociception from abdominal viscera is carried by afferent nerves that are part of the spinal nerves but accompany the sympathetic nerves. Cell bodies exist in the posterior roots of the spinal nerves, with proximal axons synapsing in the dorsal horn of the spinal cord.

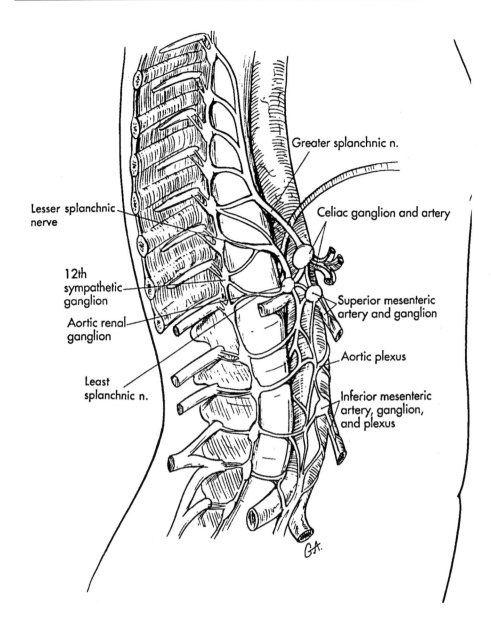

Lesser splanchnic nerve

12th sympathetic ganglion

Aortic renal ganglion

Least splanchnic n.

Greater splanchnic n.

Celiac ganglion and artery

Superior mesenteric artery and ganglion

Aortic plexus

Inferior mesenteric artery, ganglion, and plexus

GA.

FIGURE 28–1

Splanchnic nerves: greater, lesser, and least. Formation of the respective abdominal plexuses is shown. (From Raj PP [ed]: Practical Management of Pain, 3rd ed. St. Louis, Mosby, 2000, p 666.)

The celiac plexus lies anterior to the aorta and epigastrium. It is also located just anterior to the crus of the diaphragm and becomes an important consideration in selection of the approach for blockade. The plexus extends for several centimeters in front of the aorta and laterally around the aorta (Fig. 28–2). Fibers within the plexus arise from preganglionic splanchnic nerves, parasympathetic preganglionic nerves from the vagus, some sensory nerves from the phrenic and vagus nerves, and sympathetic postganglionic fibers. Afferent fibers concerned with nociception pass diffusely through the celiac plexus and represent the main target of celiac plexus blockade.

These fibers coalesce to form a dense, intertwining network of autonomic nerves. Three pairs of ganglia exist within the plexus: (1) the celiac ganglia, (2) the superior mesenteric ganglia, and (3) the aortic renal ganglia. Postganglionic nerves from these ganglia innervate all the abdominal viscera with the exception of part of the transverse colon, the left colon, the rectum, and the pelvic viscera. Pelvic viscera ultimately have nociceptive synapse from T10–L1 spinal levels and include the uterus and cervix.[13]

INDICATIONS

Any pain originating from visceral structures and innervated by the celiac plexus can be effectively alleviated by block of the plexus. These structures include the pancreas, liver, gallbladder, omentum, mesentery, and alimentary tract from the stomach to the transverse portion of the large colon.

An additional benefit in these patients may be the effect of celiac plexus block on gastric motility. Complete sympathetic denervation of the gastroin-

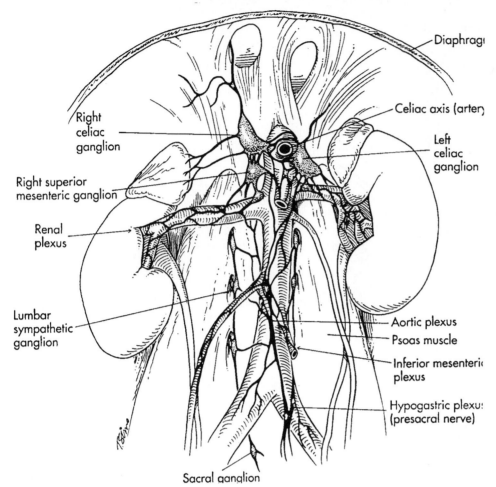

FIGURE 28–2

Anterior view of the celiac plexus. The relationship to nearby structures is shown. Note the dense, diffuse intertwining network of nerves that form the plexus. (From Raj PP [ed]: Practical Management of Pain, 3rd ed. St. Louis, Mosby, 2000, p 667.)

testinal tract allows unopposed parasympathetic activity and increases peristalsis. Diarrhea has been reported in a few patients, and a concomitant decrease in the incidence of nausea and vomiting has also been reported. The presence of severe nausea and vomiting may be a primary indication in patients with pancreatic cancer.

CONTRAINDICATIONS

Owing to the proximity to vascular structures, celiac plexus block is contraindicated in patients who are on anticoagulant therapy or suffer from congenital abnormalities of coagulopathy, antiblastic cancer therapies, or liver abnormalities associated with ethanol abuse.[13, 14] Local or intra-abdominal infection and sepsis represent absolute contraindications to celiac plexus block.

Because blockade of the celiac plexus results in greater bowel motility, the technique should be avoided in patents with bowel obstruction.[15] Neurolytic celiac plexus block should probably be deferred in patients who suffer from chronic abdominal pain, who are chemically dependent, or who exhibit drug-seeking

behavior until these relative contraindications have been adequately addressed.[16] The use of alcohol as a neurolytic agent should be avoided in patients on disulfiram therapy for alcohol abuse.

EQUIPMENT

- 25-gauge skin infiltration needle
- 22-gauge, 1½-inch needle for deep infiltration
- 16-gauge, 2-inch angiocatheter
- Curved-blunt needle
- 10 or 15 cm (10- or 15-mm tip)

DRUGS

Local Anesthesia Block
- 0.5% ropivacaine/0.5% bupivacaine equal parts = 40 mL *or*
- 2% lidocaine
- Steroids (water soluble)
   Dexamethasone
   Depot methylprednisolone (Medrol) or triamcinolone diacetate or equivalent

Neurolytic Block
- 6% to 10% phenol in iohexol (Omnipaque)
- Absolute alcohol
   97% alcohol
   50% alcohol in saline
- Radiofrequency thermocoagulation (RFTC) machine

PREPARATION OF THE PATIENT

PHYSICAL EXAMINATION
Clinical studies should include a chest radiograph and magnetic resonance imaging for cancer in the area of the block and detection of aneurysms.

LABORATORY

- Complete blood count with platelets
- Prothrombin time, partial thromboplastin time, bleeding time, or platelet function

PREOPERATIVE MEDICATION

For preoperative medication, use the standard American Society of Anesthesiologists' recommendations for conscious sedation.

PROCEDURE

POSTERIOR APPROACH—BLIND TECHNIQUE

The patient is placed in the prone position with a pillow beneath the abdomen to reverse the thoracolumbar lordosis (Fig. 28–3). This position increases the distance between the costal margins and the iliac crests and between the transverse processes of adjacent vertebral bodies. For comfort, the patient's head is turned to the side, and the arms are permitted to hang freely off each side of the table. The operative field is prepared and draped in a standard aseptic manner.

Some clinicians find it beneficial to delineate the pertinent landmarks on the skin with a sterile marker. The landmarks include the iliac crests, 12th ribs, dorsal midline, vertebral bodies, and lateral borders of the paraspinal (sacrospinalis) muscles (Fig. 28–4). Moore[17] recommended that the intersection of the 12th rib and the lateral border of the paraspinal muscles on each side (which corresponds to L2) be marked and connected with lines to each other and to the cephalic portion of the L1 spine, forming an isosceles triangle, the sides of which serve as an additional guide to needle positioning.

The skin and underlying subcutaneous tissues and musculature are infiltrated with 1.0% lidocaine at the points of needle entry, which is about four fingerbreadths (7.5 cm) lateral to the midline, just beneath the 12th ribs.

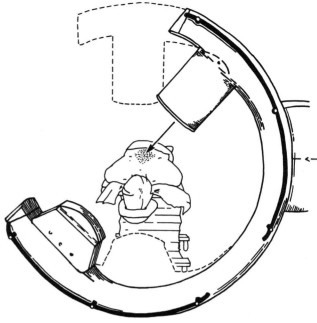

FIGURE 28–3
The patient is placed is prone position with the fluoroscopic C-arm in an oblique position at T12.

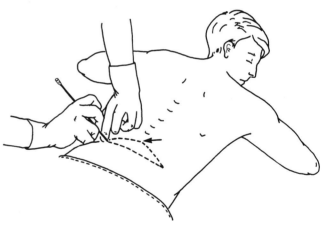

FIGURE 28–4
Surface landmarks for celiac plexus block. The diagram drawn resembles a flat isosceles triangle.

Either 20- or 22-gauge, 13-cm styleted needles are inserted bilaterally through the previously anesthetized areas. The needles are initially oriented 45 degrees toward the midline and about 15 degrees cephalad to ensure contact with the L1 vertebral body (Fig. 28–5). Once contact with the vertebral body has been verified, the depth at which bone contact occurred is noted. (Some clinicians find it useful to actually mark this measurement on the shaft of the needle with a sterile gentian violet marker after the needle is withdrawn.)

After bony contact is made and the depth is noted, the needles are withdrawn to the level of the subcuta-

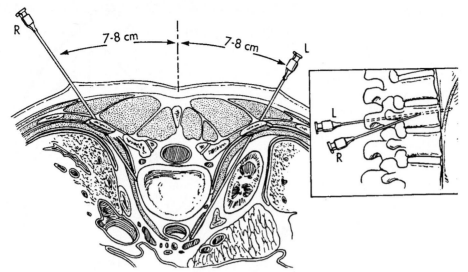

FIGURE 28–5

Retrocrural and transcrural needle placement for celiac plexus block. *Inset,* The left needle (L) is retrocrural and results in solution spreading and blocking the splanchnic nerves. The right needle (R) is transcrural and blocks the celiac plexus directly. (From Raj PP [ed]: Practical Management of Pain, 3rd ed. St. Louis, Mosby, 2000, p 669.)

neous tissue and redirected slightly lateral (about 60 degrees from the midline) so as to "walk off" the lateral surface of the L1 vertebral body. The needles are reinserted to the depth at which contact with the vertebral body was first noted. At this point, if no contact with bone is made, the left-sided needle is gradually advanced 1.5 to 2 cm or until the pulsations emanating from the aorta and transmitted to the advancing needle are felt (Fig. 28–5).[18, 19] The right-sided needle is then advanced slightly farther (i.e., 3 to 4 cm past contact with the ver-

tebral body) (Fig. 28–6). Ultimately, the tips of the needles should be just posterior to the aorta on the left and to the anterolateral aspect of the aorta on the right. It is essential that anteroposterior and lateral images are taken to confirm the correct position (Fig. 28–7).

The stylets are removed, once the needles are in good position and the needle hubs are inspected for blood, cerebrospinal fluid, thoracic fluid, and urine. A small volume of contrast material is injected bilaterally, and its spread is observed radiographically.

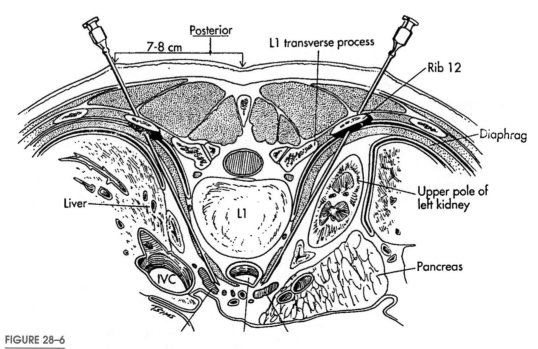

FIGURE 28–6

Cross section of a celiac plexus block. The proximity of renal parenchymal tissue necessitates placing needles no farther than 7 to 8 cm from the midline. IVC, inferior vena cava. (From Raj PP [ed]: Practical Management of Pain, 3rd ed. St. Louis, Mosby, 2000, p 669.)

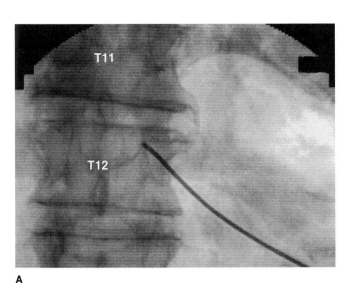

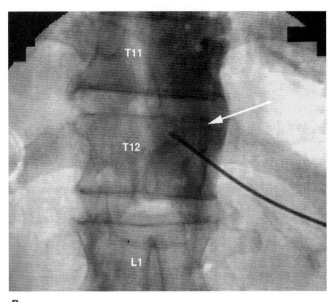

A   **B**

FIGURE 28–7

A, Anteroposterior view shows the needle at T12, which is the correct placement for celiac plexus. *B*, Radiographic image in the lateral position showing the needle tip at the anterior border of the T12 vertebral body.

Ideally, on the fluoroscopic anteroposterior view, contrast material is confined to the midline and concentrated near the T12–L1 vertebral body (Figs. 28–7 and 28–9). A smooth posterior contour can be observed on the lateral view, in front of the vertebral body (Fig. 28–8).

Alternatively, if CT guidance is used, contrast material should appear lateral to and behind the aorta (Fig. 28–9). If contrast material is confined entirely to the retrocrural space, the needles should be advanced to the retrocrural space to minimize the risk of posterior spread of local anesthetic or neurolytic agent to the somatic nerve roots (see later).[20]

INTRADISCAL APPROACH

The intradiscal procedure is performed under fluoroscopy. The patient is placed in the prone position with a pillow beneath the iliac crest to facilitate the opening of the interdiscal space as much as possible. The T12–L1 level is identified under flouroscopy. The fluoroscope is turned oblique at an angle of 15 to 20 degrees (Fig. 28–10). It is important to align the inferior end plates with a cephalocaudal projection (Fig. 28–11).

PARASPINOUS POSTERIOR APPROACH

The paraspinous posterior approach is similar to the approach described for splanchnic nerve block. The differences are that the needle is diverted at the lower posterior of T12–L1 vertebra and anterior to the vertebral body (see Chapter 27 for details).

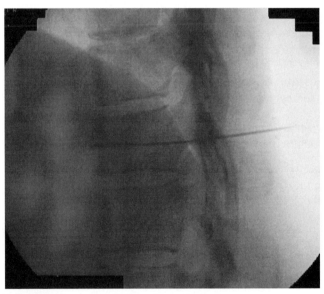

FIGURE 28–8

Anteroposterior view of the celiac plexus with contrast medium.

For diagnostic and prognostic block using the retrocrural technique, 12 to 15 mL of 1.0% lidocaine or 0.25% ropivacaine is administered through each needle.[16] For therapeutic local anesthetic toxicity, all local anesthetics should be administered in incremental doses.[21] For treatment of the pain of acute pancreatitis, an 80-mg dose of depot methylprednisolone is advocated for the initial celiac plexus block, and 40 mg for subsequent blocks.[22]

Most investigators suggest that 10 to 12 mL of 50% ethyl alcohol or 6.0% aqueous phenol be injected

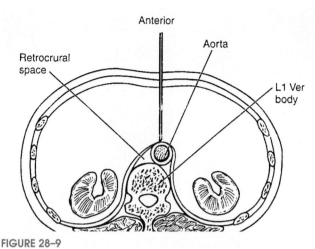

FIGURE 28–9

The CT scan at T12 with the needle on the celiac plexus from the posterior approach. Note the contrast spreading in the retrocrural space.

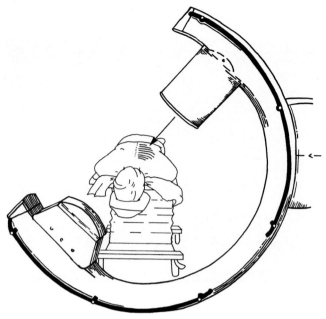

FIGURE 28–10

C-arm in a position to take the oblique view for the celiac plexus paraspinous (intradiscal) approach.

through each needle for celiac plexus neurolytic block. Thomson and colleagues,[19] however, strongly recommend that 25 mL of 50% ethyl alcohol be injected via each needle.

After the neurolytic solution has been injected, each needle should be flushed with sterile saline solution. (There have been anecdotal reports of neurolytic solution being tracked posteriorly along with the needles, as they are withdrawn.) Radiographic guidance, in particular CT guidance, offers the pain specialist an added margin of safety when performing neurolytic celiac plexus block and thus is recommended.

Catheter Placement

Patients with nonmalignant abdominal pain often fare poorly after neurolytic blockade of the celiac plexus, yet many derive temporary benefit from local anesthetic blockade. Because this pain is sympathetically mediated, continuous denervation of the plexus by local anesthetic infusion may provide prolonged analgesia.

The technique for placement is similar to that described previously.[23] Instead of 22-gauge needles, use a 6-or 8-inch catheter system (e.g., Longdwel, Becton-Dickinson) placed bilaterally. Once they are placed, secure the catheters at the skin with either a 2-cm silk skin suture or benzoin and Steri-Strips. Place a sterile, clear dressing over the catheters, which are connected to local anesthetic solutions of bupivacaine 0.1% or 0.125% ropivacaine given at 6 to 8 mL/hr. These catheters can be maintained for 4 to 7 days if placed in a sterile fashion and if the sites are checked daily.

ANTERIOR APPROACHES TO CELIAC PLEXUS BLOCK

A percutaneous anterior approach to the celiac plexus was advocated early in this century, only to be abandoned because of the high incidence of complications.[3, 24] The advent of fine needles, improvements in radiologic guidance technology, and the maturation of the specialty of interventional radiology have since led to renewed interest in the anterior approach to blockade of the celiac plexus.

Extensive experience with transabdominal fine-needle aspiration biopsy has confirmed the relative safety of this approach and provides the rationale and method for the modification of this radiologic technique for anterior celiac plexus block. The anterior approach to the celiac plexus necessarily involves the passage of a fine needle through the liver, stomach, intestine, vessels, and pancreas. Surprisingly, it is associated with very low rates of complications.[23, 25–27]

Advantages of the anterior approach to blocking the celiac plexus include its relative ease, speed, and reduced periprocedural discomfort as compared with posterior techniques.[12, 14] Perhaps the greatest advantage of the anterior approach is the fact that patients are spared having to remain prone for long, which can be a significant problem for patients suffering from intra-abdominal pain. The supine position is also advantageous for patients with ileostomies and colostomies.

The anterior approach is probably associated with less discomfort because only one needle is used. Furthermore, the needle does not impinge on either periosteum or nerve roots or pass through the bulky paraspinous musculature. Because needle placement is precrural, there is less risk of accidental neurologic injury related to retrocrural spread of drug to somatic nerve roots or epidural and subarachnoid spaces.

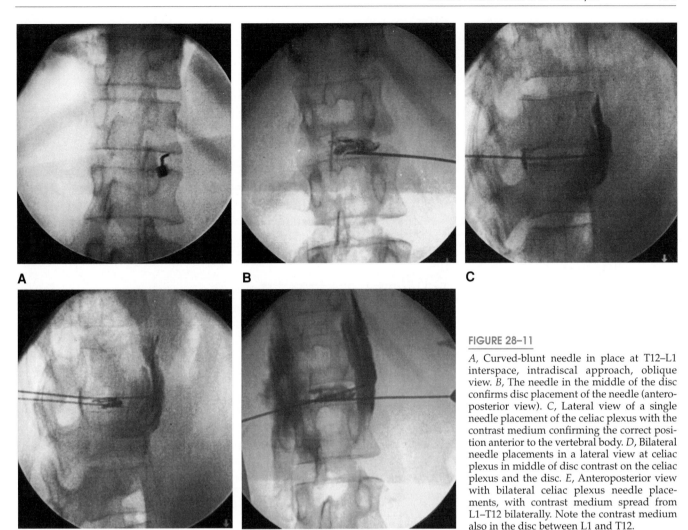

A **B** **C**

D **E**

FIGURE 28–11

A, Curved-blunt needle in place at T12–L1 interspace, intradiscal approach, oblique view. *B*, The needle in the middle of the disc confirms disc placement of the needle (anteroposterior view). *C*, Lateral view of a single needle placement of the celiac plexus with the contrast medium confirming the correct position anterior to the vertebral body. *D*, Bilateral needle placements in a lateral view at celiac plexus in middle of disc contrast on the celiac plexus and the disc. *E*, Anteroposterior view with bilateral celiac plexus needle placements, with contrast medium spread from L1–T12 bilaterally. Note the contrast medium also in the disc between L1 and T12.

Potential disadvantages of the anterior approach to celiac plexus block include the risks of infection, abscess, hemorrhage, and fistula formation.[23] Although preliminary findings indicate that these complications are exceedingly rare, further experience is needed to draw a definitive conclusion.

The anterior technique can be carried out under CT or ultrasonographic guidance. Patient preparation is similar to that for posterior approaches to celiac block. The patient is placed in the supine position on the CT or ultrasound table. The skin of the upper abdomen is prepared with antiseptic solution. The needle entry site is identified 1.5 cm below and 1.5 cm to the left of the xiphoid process (Fig. 28–12).[25] At that point, the skin subcutaneous tissues and musculature are anesthetized with 1.0% lidocaine. A 22-gauge, 15-cm needle is introduced through the anesthetized area perpendicular to the skin and advanced to the depth of the anterior wall of the aorta, as calculated using CT or ultrasonographic guidance (Fig. 28–13).

If CT guidance is being used, 4 mL of water-soluble contrast in solution with an equal volume of 1.0% lido-caine is injected to confirm needle placement. If ultrasonographic guidance is being used, 10 to 12 mL of sterile saline can be injected to help confirm needle position (Fig. 28–14*B*).[12] After satisfactory needle placement is confirmed, diagnostic and prognostic block is carried out using 15 mL of 1.5% lidocaine or 0.25% ropivacaine. Owing to the potential for local anesthetic toxicity, all local anesthetics should be administered in incremental doses.

Matamala and associates[12] recommended 35 to 40 mL of 50% ethyl alcohol for neurolytic blocks of the celiac plexus via the anterior approach. Other investigators have had equally good results using 15 to 20 mL of absolute alcohol.

An alternative technique uses fluoroscopy to guide the passage of a single needle just to the right of the center of the L1 vertebral body, after which it is withdrawn 1 to 3 cm.[24] Important precautions for the anterior approach to celiac plexus block include the administration of prophylactic antibiotics and the use of needles no larger than 22 gauge to minimize the risks of infection and trauma to the vasculature and viscera.

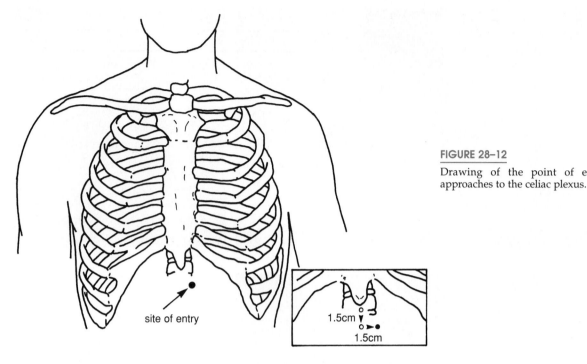

FIGURE 28–12

Drawing of the point of entry for anterior approaches to the celiac plexus.

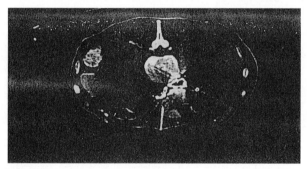

FIGURE 28–13

Note the retrocrural spread of contrast agent around the aorta. (From Waldman SD [ed]: Interventional Pain Management, 2nd ed. Philadelphia, WB Saunders, 2001.)

COMPLICATIONS

In the hands of the skilled clinician, serious complications should rarely occur from celiac plexus and splanchnic nerve block. Because of the proximity of other vital structures, however, coupled with the use of large volumes of neurolytic drugs, side effects and complications may be seen, as listed in Table 28–1.

The main side effect from celiac plexus block is backache, which usually results from the passage of needles through the back muscles. This result can be minimized by gentle positioning of the needles, minimal repositioning, and adequate local infiltration. Although self-limiting, back pain can be a significant complaint and can require use of a nonsteroidal anti-inflammatory drug, muscle relaxant, or heating pad. Celiac catheter placement and subsequent maintenance

can be distressing enough to require the ongoing treatments listed previously.

EFFICACY

Despite general agreement that celiac plexus block is indeed efficacious, significant controversy persists regarding (1) its efficacy relative to opioid therapy; (2) the relative efficacy among different approaches and techniques; and (3) whether even a remote risk of paraplegia warrants a commitment to neurolysis, especially when treatment with analgesics usually provides adequate relief. Regrettably, despite the legacy of a richly descriptive literature, these questions remain largely unresolved because of persisting scientific inadequacies.

A survey of the literature reviewed data from 23 studies on celiac neurolysis performed on 1126 patients, 64% of whom had pancreatic cancer pain and 36% of whom had pain caused by other intra-abdominal malignancies.[26] Good to excellent pain relief was achieved in 90% of available patients during the first 2 weeks after treatment, only 6% of whom required a repeated procedure for inadequate analgesia. Partial or complete pain relief was observed in 95% of patients alive at the time of last follow-up and 87% of patients at the time of death. In another review that addressed the treatment of pain due to intra-abdominal malignancy independent of the site of primary tumor, significant relief of pain and persistence of effect until death were reported in 62% to 100% and 35% to 100%, respectively, with most studies reporting favorable outcomes in the higher ranges.[27]

Another carefully conducted survey of the available literature draws similar conclusions. In this paper, Mercadante and Nicosia[28] conclude that favorable results are achieved in 85% and 73% of patients with pain caused by pancreatic and other malignancies, respectively, independent of the technique used. Such results include a low incidence of serious side effects, dose eduction in most patients, and a half-life for pain relief in excess of 4 weeks, with the likelihood of pain relief receding with increased survival time. In a small, prospective, randomized, controlled trial comparing celiac plexus neurolysis in 12 patients with medical management alone in 12 patients, all of whom suffered from pain caused by pancreatic cancer, neurolysis was associated with significant benefit, although this benefit was ultimately not as dramatic as the older literature would predict.[29] Patients treated with neural blockade had much greater initial pain relief and similar long-term results for pain but used reduced drug doses and differed significantly from untreated patients on the basis of drug-related adverse effects. Complications were limited to transient hypotension and diarrhea in treated patients, whereas control patients experienced more constipation (12 of 12 vs. 5 of 12), nausea and vomiting (4 of 12 vs. 1 of 120), and other events, including a gastric ulcer and a gluteal abscess.

A carefully conducted randomized, prospective evaluation of quality of life in patients with pancreatic cancer treated with celiac neurolysis versus pharmacotherapy reported on 10 and 11 patients, respectively.[30] Patients given neural blockade had less pain for the first 4 weeks after treatment and used less morphine through week 7, after which lower doses persisted but not at a statistically significant level. Whereas performance status improved only transiently after celiac block, the most striking observation was that of a profound deterioration of performance status noted in pharmacologically treated patients that appeared to have been prevented in patients treated with neural blockade.

Using a similar design in 20 patients with pancreatic cancer pain, Mercadante[31] also achieved similar pain scores in patients randomized to pharmacotherapy alone and celiac block with pharmacotherapy but only as a consequence of a significantly greater opioid burden and attendant side effects. Factors influencing efficacy are uncertain but may include plexus invasion by tumor, which, in one study, was found in 70% of patients with pancreatic cancer and was independent of tumor size and histopathology.[32]

Time to maximal pain relief is variable. In most patients, relief is immediate and complete; in others, it will accrue over a few days.[33, 34] In addition, pain relief is often re-established with repetition. If the interval of comfort is extremely short, repetition by an alternate route may be warranted.

Celiac plexus 64530.

▽ TABLE 28–1 Complications of Celiac Ganglion Block

- Hypotension
- Paresthesia of lumbar somatic nerve
- Intravascular injection (venous or arterial)
- Deficit of lumbar somatic nerve
- Subarachnoid or epidural injection
- Diarrhea
- Renal injury
- Paraplegia
- Pneumothorax
- Chylothorax
- Vascular thrombosis or embolism
- Vascular trauma
- Perforation of cysts of tumors
- Injection of the psoas muscle
- Intradiscal injection
- Abscess
- Peritonitis
- Retroperitoneal hematoma
- Urinary tract abnormalities
- Failure of ejaculation
- Pain during and after procedure
- Failure to relieve pain

REFERENCES

1. Kappis M: Erfahrungen mit Lokalansthesia bei Bauchoperationen. Verh Dtsch Ges Circ 43:87, 1914.
2. Kappis M: Die Ansthesierung des Nervus splanchnicus. Zentralbl Chir 45:709, 1918.
3. Wendling H: Ausschaltung der Nervi splanchnici durch Leitungsanesthesie bei Magenoperationen und anderen Eingriffen in der oberen Bauchule. Beitr Klin Chir 110:517, 1918.
4. Braun H: Ein Hilfsinstrument zur Ausfuhrung der splanchnicusanesthesie. Zentralbl Chir 48:1544, 1921.
5. Labat G: L'anesthesie splanchnique dans les interventions chirugicales et dans les affections douloureuses de la cavite abdominale. Gaz d'Hop 93:662, 1920.
6. Roussiel M: Anesthesie des nerfs splanchniques et des plexus mesenteriques superieur et inferieurs enchirurgie abdominale. Presse Med 31:4, 1923.
7. De Takats G: Splanchnic anesthesia: A critical review of the theory and practice of this method. Surg Gynecol Obstet 44:501, 1927.
8. Popper HL: Acute pancreatitis: An evaluation of the classification, symptomatology, diagnosis, and therapy. Am J Digest Dis 15:1, 1948.
9. Jones RR: A technique of injection of the splanchnic nerves with alcohol. Anesth Analg 36:75, 1957.
10. Bridenbaugh LD, Moore DC, Campbell DD: Management of upper abdominal cancer pain: Treatment with celiac plexus block with alcohol. JAMA 190:877, 1964.
11. Matamala AM, Lopez FV, Martinez LI: Percutaneous approach to the celiac plexus using CT guidance. Pain 34:285, 1988.
12. Matamala AM, Sanchez JL, Lopez FV: Percutaneous anterior and posterior approach to the celiac plexus: A comparative study using four different techniques. Pain Clin 5:21–28, 1992.
13. Waldman SD: Celiac plexus block. In RS Weiner (ed): Innovations in Pain Management. Orlando, PMD Press, 1990, pp 10–15.
14. Patt RB: Neurolytic blocks of the sympathetic axis. In Patt RB (ed): Cancer Pain. Philadelphia, JB Lippincott, 1993, pp 393–411.
15. Raj PP: Chronic pain. In Raj PP (ed): Handbook of Regional Anesthesia. New York, Churchill Livingstone, 1985, pp 113–115.
16. Waldman SD: Management of acute pain. Postgrad Med 87:15–17, 1992.
17. Moore DC: Regional Block, 4th ed. Springfield, IL, Charles C Thomas, 1965, pp 137–143.
18. Moore DC, Bush WH, Burnett LL: Celiac plexus block: A roentgenographic, anatomic study of technique and spread of solution in patients and corpses. Anesth Analg 60:369, 1981.
19. Thomson GE, Moore DC, Bridenbaugh PO, et al: Abdominal pain and celiac plexus nerve block. Anesth Analg 56:1, 1987.

20. Jain S: The role of celiac plexus block in intractable upper abdominal pain. In Racz GB (ed): Techniques of Neurolysis. Boston, Kluwer Academic, 1989, p 161.

21. Waldman SD, Portenoy RK: Recent advances in the management of cancer pain: II. Pain Manage 4:19, 1991.

22. Waldman SD: Acute and postoperative pain management. In RS Weiner (ed): Innovations in Pain Management. Orlando, PMD Press, 1993, pp 28–29.

23. Mueller PR, van Sonnenberg E, Casola G: Radiographically guided alcohol block of the celiac ganglion. Semin Intervent Radiol 4:195, 1987.

24. Labat G: Splanchnic analgesia. In Labat G (ed): Regional Anesthesia: Its Technique and Clinical Application, 2nd ed. Philadelphia, WB Saunders, 1928, p 398.

25. Lieberman RP, Nance PN, Cuka DJ: Anterior approach to the celiac plexus during interventional biliary procedures. Radiology 167:562, 1988.

26. Eisenberg E, Carr DB, Chalmers TC: Neurolytic celiac plexus block for treatment of cancer pain: A meta-analysis. Anesth Analg 80:290–295, 1995.

27. Patt RB, Cousins MJ: Techniques for neurolytic neural blockade. In Cousins MJ, Bridenbaugh PO (eds): Neural Blockade in Clinical Anesthesia and Management of Pain, 3rd ed. Philadelphia, JB Lippincott, 1998, pp 1007–1061.

28. Mercadante S, Nicosia F: Celiac plexus block: A reappraisal. Reg Anesth Pain Med 23:37–48, 1998.

29. Polati E, Finco G, Gottin L, et al: Prospective randomized double-blind trial of neurolytic coeliac plexus block in patients with pancreatic cancer. Br J Surg 85:199–201, 1998.

30. Kawamata M, Ishitani K, Ishikawa K, et al: Comparison between celiac plexus block and morphine treatment on quality of life in patients with pancreatic cancer pain. Pain 64:597–602, 1996.

31. Mercadante S: Celiac plexus block versus analgesics in pancreatic cancer pain. Pain 52:187–92, 1993.

32. Ihse I: Pancreatic pain. Br J Surg 77:121–122, 1990.

33. Jain S, Hirsh R, Shah N, et al: Blood ethanol levels following celiac plexus block with 50% ethanol. Anesth Analg 68:S135, 1989.

34. Staats PS, Kost-Byerly S: Celiac plexus blockade in a 7-year-old child with neuroblastoma. J Pain Symptom Manage 10:321–324, 1995.

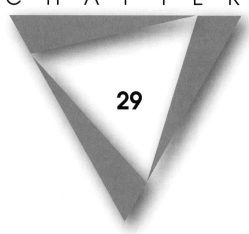

Lumbar Sympathetic Block and Neurolysis

HISTORY

Historically, the first report of lumbar sympathetic block seems to be by Brunn and Mandl, who in 1924 described Sellheim's technique of injecting the lumbar sympathetic nerves as a component of his paravertebral approach to blocking the mixed spinal outflow in the lumbar region.[1] Kappis also described the technique of lumbar sympathetic block and surgical resection of the lumbar sympathetic nerves about this time.[2] Others associated with the technique are von Gaza,[3] Mandl,[4] and Lawen[5] in Germany; Jonnesco[6] and Leriche and Fountain[7] in France; and White[8] in the United States. During the 1950s, Bonica,[9] Moore,[10] and Arnulf[11] described in detail the importance of lumbar sympathetic blockade, particularly its relationship to the treatment of causalgia and post-traumatic reflex dystrophies in military servicemen after World War II. Although the technique described by Mandl[4] in 1926 remains one of the most popular approaches to the lumbar sympathetic trunk, Reid and colleagues,[12] in a large series published in 1970, described a more lateral approach that avoids contact with the transverse process. Two techniques are described in this chapter: (1) the "classic" technique first described by Kappis[2] and Mandl[4] and (2) the lateral technique first described by Mandl and redefined by Reid and colleagues.[12]

Techniques for neurolysis of the lumbar sympathetic chain appeared after 1924, when Royle[13] in Australia attempted to modify skeletal muscle tone in patients with spastic paralysis. Physiologic effects such as increased skin blood flow and dryness were observed and used to treat Raynaud's disease in 1929.[14] In the latter half of the 20th century, arterial reconstructive surgery largely supplanted the use of sympathectomy for peripheral vascular disease, with the possible exception of vascular ulcers. Lumbar sympathetic block continues to be advocated for hyperhidrosis with some justification. Percutaneous and endoscopic techniques have become the methods of choice, as with the cervicothoracic chain.

ANATOMY

Peripherally, the sympathetic nervous system consists of preganglionic and postganglionic efferent fibers that innervate deep somatic structures, skin, and viscera. The two-paravertebral sympathetic trunks are connected segmentally by preganglionic neurons, whose cell bodies are situated in the lateral horn, intermediate nucleus, and paracentral nuclei of the thoracolumbar spinal cord. The cell bodies responsible for vasoconstriction in the lower limbs are in the lower three thoracic and first three lumbar segments. The preganglionic fibers pass by way of their corresponding nerves as white rami communicantes, which communicantes with considerable convergence in the paravertebral ganglia with postganglionic efferents and in the prevertebral ganglia by postganglionic efferents to the pelvic viscera (Fig. 29–1A). A small percentage of postganglionic fibers pass directly to ganglia in the aortic plexus and the superior and inferior hypogastric plexuses (Fig. 29–1B). The postganglionic fibers leave the sympathetic trunk as gray rami communicantes, some passing to the L1 nerve to contribute to the iliohypogastric and genitofemoral nerve territories, some to the L2–L5 nerves, and some to the upper three sacral nerves, where they pass on to their respective destinations in the lumbosacral plexus.

Intermediate ganglia found in the psoas and iliacus muscles also communicate with postganglionic fibers that pass through the segmental lumbar and sacral nerves. The S1 and S2 nerves contain the largest numbers of postganglionic fibers. Most of these represent gray rami communicantes that serve vasomotor, pilomotor, and sudomotor functions. It has been determined that although each root of the lumbosacral

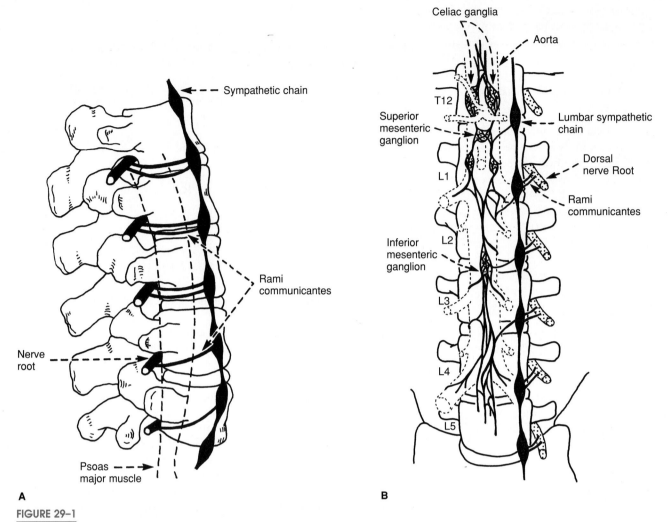

A

B

FIGURE 29–1

A, This drawing shows the sympathetic chain as it courses the lordotic curve of the lumbar vertebrae. *B,* This drawing shows the course of sympathetic chain and its connection to the celiac and aortic plexus.

plexus receives one group of gray rami communicantes, the S1–S3 nerves contain several (i.e., a large convergence), because they innervate the blood vessels in the lower extremity.[14]

Each lumbar sympathetic chain enters the retroperitoneal space under the right and left crura, continuing inferiorly in the interval between the anterolateral aspect of the vertebral bodies and the origin of the psoas muscle to enter the pelvis and the L5–S1 disc. Posteriorly, the periosteum overlies the vertebral bodies and the fibroaponeurotic origin of the psoas muscles and their fascial coverings. Anterior is the parietal reflection of the peritoneum, the aorta lying anteromedial to the left trunk and the vena cava anterior to the right trunk. The white and gray rami communicantes pass to their respective ganglia beneath the fibrous arcades of the psoas attachments to each vertebral body. They also tend to pass alongside the middle of the vertebral body.

The sympathetic ganglia of the lumbar sympathetic chain are variable in both numbers and position. Rarely are five ganglia found on each side in the same individual.[15] In most cases, only four are found. There tends to be fusion of L1 and L2 ganglia in most patients, and ganglia are aggregated at the L2–L3 and L4–L5 discs. Considerable variability is noted in the size of the ganglia, some being fusiform and as long as 10 to 15 mm, others being round and approximately 5-mm long.[16] Because of this aggregation and the fact that the right crus extends to L3 and the left crus to L2, lumbar sympathetic blockade is more efficacious.

INDICATIONS

The indications for lumbar sympathetic block may be divided into three broad categories:

1. Circulatory insufficiency in the leg, including arteriosclerotic vascular disease, diabetic gangrene, Buerger's disease, Raynaud's phenomenon and disease, and reconstructive vascular surgery after arterial embolic occlusion

2. Pain from renal colic, complex regional pain syndrome (CRPS) types I and II, intractable urogenital pain, postamputation stump pain, phantom pain, and frostbite

3. Other conditions, such as hyperhidrosis, phlegmasia alba dolens, erythromelalgia, acrocyanosis, and trench foot

The rationale for sympathetic blocks, particularly in treatment of pain, is based on the observation that pain under certain conditions is potentiated or mediated by sympathetic hyperactivity. Laboratory evidence has demonstrated that the sympathetic postganglionic neuron may act not only at the effector terminal but also on the primary afferent (PA) in certain pathologic conditions; it may communicate with the PA neuron at other sites (direct and indirect coupling).[17] Although the mechanism remains unclear, blocks of the sympathetic nervous system may have two actions: (1) interruption of preganglionic and postganglionic sympathetic efferents may influence function of the PA neuron[19, 20] or (2) visceral afferents from deep visceral structures in the leg that travel with the sympathetic nerves may be blocked.[18-20]

As a diagnostic and prognostic procedure, sympathetic blocks are helpful in determining the nature of the pain (i.e., whether it is sympathetically maintained or whether it is independent of sympathetic function). Such procedures are always used to test the effects of destructive (neurolytic or surgical) sympatholysis.

CONTRAINDICATIONS

Contraindications to sympathetic blocks are a bleeding diathesis, local infection, and certain anatomic anomalies, which may be considered relative contraindications if they are likely to render the procedure difficult or hazardous.

EQUIPMENT

- 25-gauge skin infiltration needle
- 22-gauge, 1½-inch needle for deep infiltration
- 20-gauge, 8- to 10-cm (6-inch) block needle *or*
- 16-gauge, 2-inch angiocatheter
- 10- or 15-cm (with a 10- or 15-mm active tip) curved-blunt needle
- Radiofrequency generator with cables and electrodes

DRUGS

Diagnostic and Therapeutic Block
- 0.5% ropivacaine or 0.5% bupivacaine: equal parts = 40 mL
- 2% lidocaine

- Dexamethasone 4 mg/mL
- Methylprednisolone (Depo-Medrol) 80 mg *or* triamcinolone diacetate 40 mg/mL

Neurolytic Block
- Phenol neurolysis
  6% to 10% phenol in iohexol (Omnipaque) 10 mL
- Absolute alcohol
  97% alcohol
  50% alcohol in saline

PREPARATION OF THE PATIENT

PHYSICAL EXAMINATION

Examine for local infection and distorted anatomy that may interfere with performance of the procedure.

PREOPERATIVE MEDICATION

Follow the standard American Society of Anesthesiologists' recommendations for conscious sedation.

PROCEDURE

The prone position is most convenient for lumbar sympathetic blockade, but pain or anatomic deformity may make it necessary to place the patient in the left or right lateral decubitus position (Fig. 29–2).

PARAMEDIAN (CLASSIC (MANDL'S)) APPROACH

Skin wheals are made 5 to 8 cm lateral to the spinous processes of L2–L4. With the spinal needle held perpendicular to the skin, a track of local anesthetic is infiltrated down to the transverse process at each level. The sympathectomy needle is then directed to the same point, and the depth is noted, after which the needle is withdrawn to the subcutaneous tissue. The needle is then redirected so as to pass below and slightly medial to the inferior border of the transverse process, at an angle of about 10 degrees to the sagittal plane (Fig. 29–3). It is advanced about 2 cm deep to the transverse process, where it should contact the side of the vertebral body. A slight decrease in the angle is made so as to allow the needle to slip past at a tangent to the lateral aspect of the vertebral body. Fluoroscopy at this point will confirm both the needle position and the distance to the anterolateral surface of the vertebral body. A small amount (1 to 2 mL) of iohexol is injected through each needle. The contrast medium hugs the contour of each vertebral body if the needle tips are in the correct tissue plane.

For diagnostic or prognostic blocks, a local anesthetic is used, whereas for neurolytic blocks, one can use a mixture of iohexol and phenol or radiofrequency (Fig. 29–4).

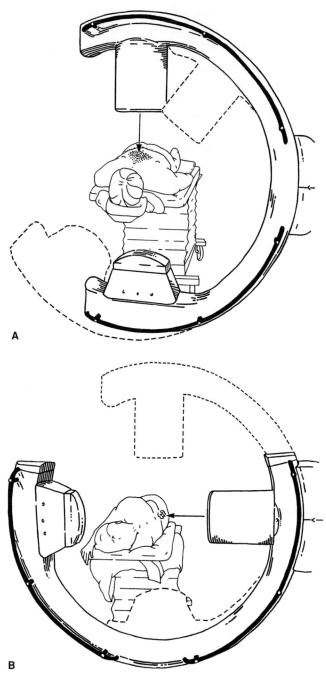

A

B

FIGURE 29–2

A, The position of the patient in prone and C-arm first in the anteroposterior position is used to locate the lumbar vertebrae and then rotated oblique to identify the site of entry. A lateral fluoroscopic view is used to monitor the depth of advancement. *B,* The drawing shows the position of the patient and C-arm when the lateral technique is employed.

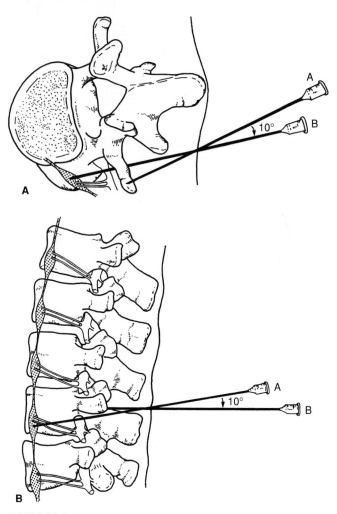

A

B

FIGURE 29–3

A and *B,* Drawing of the classic technique to perform lumbar sympathetic block.

introduced and advanced until it contacts the vertebral body. Fluoroscopy in two planes will confirm its position and the angle to assume for redirection of the needle to its final position at the anterolateral aspect of the vertebral body (Fig. 29–5). With the fluoroscopy positioned laterally, any final adjustments can be made to ensure that the needle tip lies exactly at the anterolateral edge of the vertebral body. A small amount of contrast material identifies the correct tissue plane just beyond the psoas muscle. If necessary, this procedure may then be repeated with the second needle at the L4 vertebral body. The dye should spread to form a line conforming to the anterolateral margin of the vertebral bodies (L2–L4).

LATERAL (REID'S) APPROACH

With the patient in a prone position, a skin wheal is made 10 to 14 cm lateral to the superior border of the spinous processes of L3 and L4. Using the spinal needle as before, tracks of local anesthetic are infiltrated at an angle of 60 degrees to the sagittal plane toward the body of L3 of these vertebrae. The sympathectomy needle is then

INJECTION OF TEST SOLUTION

A short-acting local anesthetic is commonly used for diagnostic sympathetic blocks. A long-acting agent such as bupivacaine or ropivacaine is advantageous for both therapy and prognosis, because it provides the patient a longer time to evaluate the effects of sympatholysis and

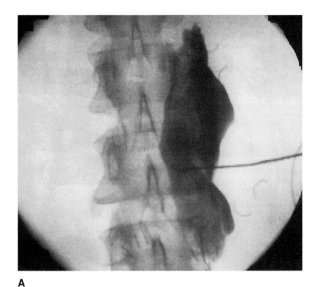

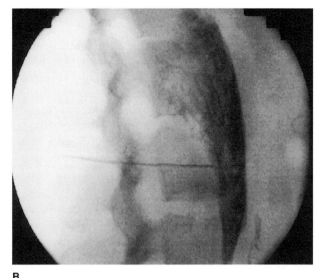

A   **B**

FIGURE 29–4

A, The radiographic image of the lumbar area shows the needle in position and the flow of contrast solution at L2–L4 in an antero-posterior view (correct placement). *B,* The lateral view shows the correct flow of the contrast solution.

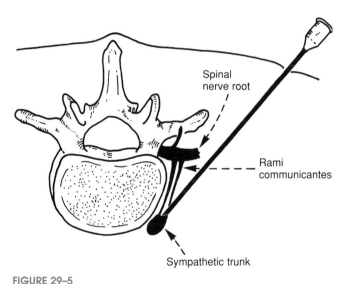

Spinal
nerve root

Rami
communicantes

Sympathetic trunk

FIGURE 29–5

Drawing of the needle inserted with the lateral (Reid's) technique.

any effect this might have on the pain. A concentration of 0.375% bupivacaine or 0.5% ropivacaine gives optimal duration without the need for an added vasoconstrictor.

NEUROLYTIC BLOCK

Neurolysis of the lumbar sympathetic chain is easily performed and is one of the most useful procedures.[21] It can be indicated for recalcitrant CRPS I or II peripheral vascular disease, pelvic malignancies, and deafferentation pain syndromes. Neurolysis should be considered only after local anesthetic blocks of the lumbar sympathetic chain have documented efficacy but have failed to produce long-lasting relief.

Needle placement for neurolysis does not differ from that for a local anesthetic lumbar sympathetic block. Image intensification, in particular, fluoroscopy, greatly facilitates placement, allows real-time visualization of drug diffusion and helps prevent possible complications by ill-placed needles or neurolytic solution. When a single-needle technique is used, fluoroscopy can document adequate cephalad spread to the upper limits of L2 and caudal diffusion of drug to L4.

Significant longitudinal spread of drug along the sympathetic chain is required for adequate neurolysis. When spread cannot be reliably achieved with a single needle, use a two- or three-needle approach. One needle is positioned at the inferior one-third aspect of L2, and the second needle is positioned at the superior one-third aspect of L3. The third needle can be placed at the L4 vertebral body. No comparative studies have reported any difference in efficacy with the use of one, two, or three needles. Check needle placement before injecting contrast material in both the anteroposterior and the lateral views. C-arm fluoroscopy is ideal and allows real-time visualization.

Monitor distal skin temperatures during neurolysis for further documentation of the block. Inject a local anesthetic solution before neurolysis, and evaluate the efficacy by a temperature rise and relief of symptoms.

The spread of contrast agent is characteristic and reproducible. The dye confines itself to the anterolateral border of the vertebral body in a tight, linear fashion (see Fig. 29–4). Movement of contrast agent is cephalad and caudal, with no lateral diffusion of drug to the vertebral bodies. Contrast material that diffuses laterally is usually deposited either in the psoas muscle or on the fascia; the effect appears either as a roundish, poorly circumscribed picture or bandlike with muscular striations visibly present. In neither situation should neurolytic agents be injected.

Phenol is the agent of choice for neurolysis. It produces a lower incidence of neuralgia than that with equivalent injections with alcohol.[22] Although volumes as small as 2 mL through each of three needles have been used, larger volumes (15 mL) through a single needle have been equally efficacious.[23] Concentrations of 6% phenol have been replaced with 10% and 12% solutions, with evidence in cat sciatic nerves that higher concentrations provide prolonged neurologic destruction.[24] After the neurolytic agent has been injected, place 1 mL of saline solution through the needle to prevent any neurolytic agent from spilling onto the somatic nerve during withdrawal.

RADIOFREQUENCY OF LUMBAR SYMPATHETIC CHAIN

In radiofrequency of the lumber sympathetic chain, the position of the patient is similar to that described for other procedures in prone positions. A curved-blunt radiofrequency needle is used for this technique. The lesion should be at the inferior one third of L2, upper one third of L3, and middle of L4 vertebral bodies (Fig. 29–6).

Technique

Oblique the C-arm is turned 15 to 20 degrees until the vertebral body "covers" the transverse apophysis (Fig. 29–7). Mark the point of entry of the needle below

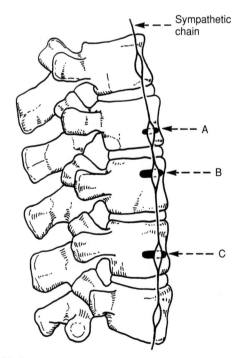

FIGURE 29–6

The drawing showing the anatomic location of the lumbar sympathetic chain and sites of lesion (arrows A, B, and C) with radiofrequency.

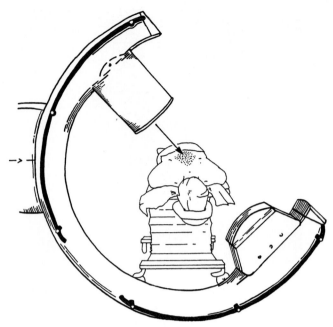

FIGURE 29–7

Drawing of the patient in the prone position and the C-arm in the oblique position prior to performing lumbar sympathetic radiofrequency.

the transverse process and in line with the lateral edge of the vertebral body (Fig. 29–8A). A 16-gauge angiocatheter is then introduced at the appropriate levels at L2, or L3 or L4 (Fig. 29–8B). A curved-blunt needle is then introduced through the angiocatheter with the tip directed laterally (Fig. 29–8C). The C-arm then should be rotated laterally. The needle should be advanced to the anterior edge of the lumbar body (Fig. 29–8D and E).

In the lateral position the needle tip should stay at the anterior edge of the vertebral body. In the anteroposterior view the needle tip should be at the pedicle (Fig. 29–8F). Correct needle position will show that the tip is at the facetal line while in bone contact with the vertebral body. Verify the position with 1 or 2 mL of contrast material. If it spreads into the psoas muscle, the tip is posterior or lateral and should be repositioned more anteriorly or medial. There should be no resistance on injection of the contrast medium.

Stimulation Parameters

Once the needle tip is in the correct position, the following tests should be done for radiofrequency neurolysis:

- Sensory stimulation at 50 Hz. Vague discomfort may be felt in the back with 0.2 to 0.5 V. If necessary, stimulate up to 1 V. If paresthesia exists in the groin at the L2 and L3 level, one should reposition the needle owing to its proximity to the genitofemoral nerve
- Motor stimulation at 2 Hz. There should not be fasciculation when tested up to 3 V in the lower extremity

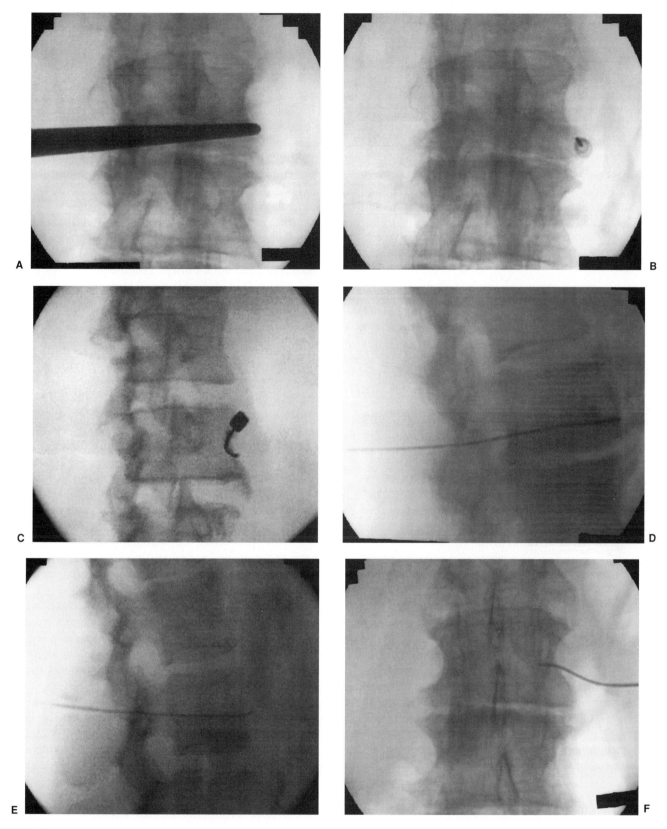

FIGURE 29–8

A, The radiographic image shows the place of entry of the needle at the L2 vertebra for lumbar sympathetic block. *B*, The 16-gauge angiocatheter insertion at that side after local anesthetic infiltration at that site (note the "tunnel" view). *C*, Insertion of a 15-cm, curved-blunt radiofrequency (RF) needle through the angiocatheter with the tunnel view. The curved needle should be inserted with the tip directed laterally. *D*, The lateral view of the RF needle tip at the anterior border of the L2 vertebral body in correct position. *E*, The RF needle at the L4 vertebral body level slightly in front of the anterior border of the vertebral body. This position avoids the lesion of the lumbar plexus in the psoas muscle. *F*, The RF needle position of L4 (anteroposterior view) correctly placed at the waist and pedicle.

- To minimize patient discomfort, prior to lesioning 1 to 2 mL of local anesthetic and/or steroid should be injected.
- Wait for 45 seconds, then insert the electrode and lesion at 80°C for 60 to 90 seconds. The lesion should be done with a 10-mm needle tip on L2–L4 and sometimes at L5.

Postblock Monitoring

After the lesion, the patient should be monitored for 30 to 45 minutes. After a normal neurologic examination, the patient should be discharged home with an escort.

COMPLICATIONS

Potential complications of lumbar sympathetic block and neurolysis include the following:

- Intravascular or subarachnoid injection, neuralgia, and muscular spasm
- Retrograde ejaculation is rare (do not perform bilateral sympathectomy)
- Postoperative discomfort for approximately 5 days
- Neuralgia may occur owing to spread of the neurolytic material onto a somatic nerve root; the most susceptible nerve to this complication is the genitofemoral nerve[25]

The list of possible complications is significant, but these complications can be largely avoided if meticulous attention is paid to the approach track of the needle and cannula, the final position of the tip, and the spread of contrast agent.[26] The postprocedural discomfort felt in the groin, particularly after chemical sympathectomy, is thought to represent a chemical irritation of the genitofemoral nerve. It is suggested that the more discrete lesion of radiofrequency reduces the incidence of neuralgic pain. An alternative explanation might lie in convergence phenomena as sympathetic afferents pass to the central nervous system through the nerve roots of L1–L2.[27] The tracking of neurolytic agents to components of the lumbar plexus or contents of the spinal canal can lead to significant neurologic deficit. Although this can be largely avoided by careful technique, such rare occurrences are inherently more likely with the uncontrolled spread of neurolytic solutions.

HELPFUL HINTS

The location of the lesion is correlated such that L2 is involved if there is lumbar pain, L3 if the pain is axial in the spine, L4 if the pain is in the lower limb, and L4 and L5 if the pain is in the ankle or foot. Several lesions may be performed at different levels.

It is advisable to perform a previous diagnostic blockade with 1% lidocaine or 0.25% bupivacaine to avoid false-positive results (impregnation of somatic nerves). The blockade should be performed in L2–L4, and if the foot is involved, block L3–L5. No sensory or motor blockade should be produced.

The most common side effect after a lumbar sympathetic block is backache, which results from the placement of the needles through the paravertebral muscles of the back. This possibility should be carefully explained to patient before the blockade, and the use of a heating pad and ice packs, along with rest and occasional muscle relaxants, may be necessary.

Intravascular injections of larger volumes of local anesthetics can produce serious, systemic toxic reactions. These are best avoided by the use of test doses, repeated aspiration, and epinephrine-containing solutions in combination with electrocardiographic monitoring.

Inadvertent subarachnoid injections occur rarely if the needle is mistakenly repositioned from bone into a dural cuff. The length of the needle and its small diameter hinder the free flow of cerebrospinal fluid (CSF). The high pressure generated during aspiration of the small, 22-gauge needle often sucks the arachnoid membrane against the bevel, resulting in no flow of CSF. An initial small injection of local anesthetic followed by testing for spinal anesthesia avoids the subsequent total spinal block seen if 15 mL of local anesthetic is injected into the subarachnoid space.

Occasionally, the needle passes through the intervertebral disc. The sensation of passing through Swiss cheese is easily noted, necessitating removal of the needle and repositioning. Medication cannot be easily injected into a disc. No sequelae have been reported from this occurrence, and any extrusion of disc material would be lateral, away from the spinal canal, and not of any clinical significance.

Renal trauma or puncture of a ureter can occur if proper technique is not followed. Most important, the needle should not be inserted more than 7 to 8 cm from the midline. Sequelae are minimal unless neurolytic agent is injected, resulting in possible ureteral stricture or extravasation of urine.

Blockade of the genitofemoral nerve or lumbar plexus within the psoas muscle can occur if the needle is placed too far laterally or posteriorly. If a local anesthetic solution is used, a resulting numbness or weakness can occur in the groin, anterior thigh, or quadriceps. To avoid the 18- to 24-hour weakness seen with bupivacaine, a short-duration agent (1% lidocaine) can be injected initially and the strength of the quadriceps tested.

Lateral spread of neurolytic solution from the lumbar sympathetic chain can result in genitofemoral neuralgia and, less often, lumbar plexus involvement.[22, 28, 29]

Boas[30] reported a 6% incidence of genitofemoral neuralgia in one study. Cousins and associates[22] reported on 35 patients receiving 100% alcohol using a technique without image intensification. Mild neuralgia (<1 week) occurred in 14% and severe neuralgia (>1 week) occurred in 26%. Use of a similar technique with phenol resulted in a respective incidence of 6% and 16%. Sensory loss was reported in 5% of patients, and motor weakness occurred in 6%.[22]

The genitofemoral nerve is most susceptible at the L4–5 vertebral level, after it has emerged from the psoas major muscle, and lies anterior to the fascia in close proximity to the sympathetic chain. Most mild neuralgias can be treated with non-narcotic analgesics and reassurance that this complication is transient. For severe cases, Boas[30] reported success using intravenous lidocaine 1 to 2 mg/kg over 2 to 3 minutes, sufficient to produce light toxicity symptoms. The pain will disappear and normal cutaneous sensation will return. In refractory cases, transcutaneous electrical nerve stimulation, tricyclic antidepressants, and antiepileptic agents may be necessary. Similarly, intravenous lidocaine may be used in a dose of 1 to 2 mL/kg.

EFFICACY

INTERPRETATION OF AND RESPONSES TO LUMBAR SYMPATHETIC BLOCK

It is important to understand the patient's personality when interpreting the subsequent effects of sympatholysis. Although evidence of sympatholysis (vasodilation, increased temperature, and reduction of edema) is important, it is the qualitative effect on the preexisting symptoms, manifested by continuous pain, hyperalgesia, or touch-evoked pain such as allodynia, that requires careful assessment after sympatholysis. Technical failure might be the cause of therapeutic failure, even on repeated occasions. A placebo response is normal and may merely be the response of a grateful patient to the fact that something fundamental has been done to unravel a particular medical condition. The amount of local anesthetic used for sympatholysis may, as the result of its own uptake, have an effect on multisynaptic pathways in the central nervous system, producing central inhibition of nociception, an effect that may erroneously be attributed to sympatholysis.[31]

Some have questioned the efficacy and reproducibility of sympathetic block, particularly in relation to pain relief, as a response. Nevertheless, carefully performed, sympathetic block is a useful and important therapeutic diagnostic procedure.[32]

EVALUATION OF COMPLETENESS OF BLOCKADE

Whenever possible, monitor the effectiveness of a sympathetic block. Many tests have been reported to monitor sympathetic activity. Unfortunately, many such tests lack applicability for the practicing clinician secondary to their intricate apparatus involved, cost, and time for setup. The test described here can be performed at the bedside, and one or two should be used to monitor all blocks.

Surface Temperature Monitoring

Skin temperature recording represents the easiest and fastest way to test sympathetic blockade. New temperature monitors have two or three channels combined with very sensitive sensors and easily read digital displays. For the upper extremity, monitor the shoulder, the flexor surface of the forearm, the dorsum of the hand, and one of the digits, preferable the thumb. Measure lower extremity temperature of the anterior thigh, the medial aspect of the leg, the dorsum of the foot, and the great toe.

Measure skin temperatures 15 to 20 minutes before the block to allow for equilibration with the ambient surrounding. Wrapping of the extremities subjects them to less environmental change. Monitor both affected and unaffected sides.

Thermography has been advocated for documentation of sympathetic blockade. It records skin temperature either by an infrared technique or by liquid crystals. Both methods effectively demonstrate changes in skin temperature.

Look for a minimum positive change of 2ºC after sympathetic block. At times, this may not occur despite appropriate blockade. A fixed proximal blockage and a larger artery may prevent enhanced distal flow if collateral circulation is insufficient. This is seen most commonly in the elderly population. Some patients with reflex sympathetic dystrophy also present with a very warm extremity that does not become warmer with sympathetic blockade. If a skin temperature change cannot be evoked or further documentation is deemed necessary, record the sympathogalvanic reflex. Initially described by Lewis[33] in 1955, this reflex is also known as *skin conductance response, galvanic skin reaction, electrodermal reaction,* and *psychogalvanic reflex.*

To measure the sympathogalvanic reflex, place standard electrodes on the dorsal and plantar surfaces of the distal extremity (i.e., foot or hand), with a third grounding electrode remotely located. The skin should be free of epithelial cells before electrode placement. The patient is allowed to rest in silence for several minutes to permit the tracing to return to baseline. A short deep breath, loud noise, or pinch of the skin usually suffices to elicit the response, which is recorded as a deflection on the electrocardiographic paper. The deflection lasts 4 to 5 seconds, and changes of 1 to 3 mV are normal. Measure both blocked and unblocked extremities. The blocked side should have an absent sympathogalvanic reflex 20 to 30 minutes after the procedure.

The presence of the sympathogalvanic reflex varies among patients, with younger patients having much greater deflections and unstable baseline patterns. Not all patients have an obtainable sympathogalvanic reflex, particularly older, diabetic, or significantly depressed individuals. Furthermore, patients receiving drugs such as opiates, barbiturates, atropine, or other centrally acting agents exhibit minimized or absent sympathogalvanic reflex. Marked habituation can also occur, with smaller deflections occurring with succeeding stimuli.

Sweat Test

Three methods of sweat testing have been used clinically to test sympathetic blockade.

1. The *Ninhydrin test* relies on the protein in sweat to change the color to yellow.[34] A blocked extremity cannot sweat and shows no color change. The test is considered accurate but requires a lot of time and cannot produce immediate results for clinical use.

2. The *cobalt blue test* involves filter papers that are saturated with cobalt blue, then dried and stored in a desiccator. When needed, the papers are removed from the desiccator and placed on a clean, dry surface; the blocked and unblocked extremity is pressed onto the respective paper. The presence of sweat changes the paper from blue to pink. An extremity that has been sympathetically denervated shows no color change.

3. The *starch-iodine test* also relies on color change. Its major drawback concerns the length of clean-up time involved after the starch-iodine application.

Pain Assessment

The assessment of preblock and postblock pain also provides some indication of sympathetic blockade. Pain relief can be reported almost immediately after a block or can be delayed for several hours in some patients. The long-lasting neurolytic effect of phenol is often delayed, but its local anesthetic action is usually more immediate. If narcotics or sedative drugs have been employed, pain assessment scores are rendered meaningless in the immediate postblock period. Patients should be instructed to keep pain diaries after each block to aid in assessment of effectiveness.

Lumbar/thoracic sympathetic 64520; RFTC other nerve 64640.

REFERENCES

1. Brunn F, Mandl F: Die paravertebral Injektion zur Bekampfung visceraler Schmerzen. Wien Klin Aschsch 37:511, 1924.
2. Kappis M: Weitere Erfahrungen mit der Sympathektomie. Klin Wochenschr 2:1441, 1923.
3. von Gaza W: Die Resektion der paravertebralen Nerven und die isolierte Durchschneidung des Ramus communicans. Arch Lkin Chir 133:479, 1924.
4. Mandl F: Die Paravertebrale Injektion. Vienna, J Springer, 1926.
5. Lawen A: Uber segmentare Schmerzaufhegungen durch paravertebrale Novokaininjektion zur differential Diagnose intraabdominaler Erkrankungen. Munchen Med Wochenschr 69:1423, 1922.
6. Jonnesco R: Angine de poitrien guerie par le resection du sympathique cervico-thoradique. Bull Acad Med 84:93, 1920.
7. Leriche R, Fountain R: L'Anesthesie isolee du ganglion etoile: Sa technique, ses indications, ses resultats. Presse Med 42:849, 1934.
8. White JC: Diagnostic Novocain block of the sensory and sympathetic nerves. Am J Surg 9:264, 1930.
9. Bonica JJ: The Management of Pain. Philadelphia, Lea & Febiger, 1953.
10. Moore DC: Stellate Ganglion Block. Springfield, IL, Charles C Thomas, 1954.
11. Arnulf G: Practique des Infiltrations Sympathetiques. Lyon, Camgli, 1954.
12. Reid W, Watt JK, Gray RG: Phenol injection of the sympathetic chain. Br J Surg 57:45, 1970.
13. Royle ND: The treatment of spastic paralysis by sympathetic ramisection. Surg Gynecol Obstet 39:701–704, 1924.
14. Gabella G: Structure of the Autonomic Nervous System. London, Chapman & Hall, 1976.
15. Hovelacque A: Anatomie des Nerfs Craniens et Rachidens et du Systeme Grand Sympathique chez 1'Homme. Paris, G Doin, 1927.
16. Rocco AG, Palomgi D, Raeke D: Anatomy of the lumbar sympathetic chain. Reg Anesth 20:13–19, 1995.
17. Bonica JJ: Autonomic innervation of the viscera in relation to nerve block. Anesthesiology 29:793–813, 1968.
18. White JC, Sweet W: Pain: Its Mechanisms and Neurosurgical Treatment. Springfield, IL, Charles C Thomas, 1955.
19. Bonica JJ: Sympathetic Nerve Blocks for Pain Diagnosis and Therapy. New York, Breon Laboratories, 1984.
20. Brunn F, Mandl F: Die paravertebral Injektion zur Bekampfung visceraler Schmerzen. Wien Klin Aschsch 37:511, 1924.
21. Boas RA, Hatangdi VS, Richards EG: Lumbar sympathectomy: A percutaneous chemical technique. Adv Pain Res Ther 1:685, 1976.
22. Cousins MJ, Reeve TS, Glynn CJ, et al: Neurolytic lumbar sympathetic blockade: Duration of denervation and relief of rest pain. Anaesth Intensive Care 7:121–135, 1979.
23. Shihabi ZK, Rauch RL: Plasma phenol determination by HPLC. J Liquid Chromatogr 14:1691–1697, 1991.
24. Gregg R, Costantin CH, Ford DJ, et al: Electrophysiologic and histopathologic investigation of phenol in Renografin as a neurolytic agent [Abstract]. Anesthesiology 63:A239, 1985.
25. Umeda S, Arai T, Halano Y, et al: Cadaver anatomic analysis of the best site for chemical lumbar sympathectomy. Anesth Analg 66:643–646, 1987.
26. Sri Kantha K: Radiofrequency percutaneous lumbar sympathectomy: Technique and review of indications. In Racz G (ed): Techniques of Neurolysis. Boston, Kluwer Academic, 1989, pp 171–183.
27. Nakamura S, Takahashi K, Takahashi Y, et al: The afferent pathways of discogenic low-back pain: Evaluation of L2 spinal nerve infiltration. J Bone Joint Surg Br 78:606–612, 1996.
28. Dam WH: Therapeutic blockades. Acta Chir Scand 343(Suppl):89–101, 1965.
29. Raskin NH, Levinson SA, Hoffman PM, et al: Post-sympathectomy neuralgia amelioration with diphenylhydantoin and carbamazepine. Am J Surg 128:75–78, 1974.
30. Boas RA: Sympathetic blocks in clinical practice. Int Anesthesiol Clin 16:149–182, 1978.
31. Woolf CJ, Wiesenfeld-Hallin Z: The systemic administration of local anesthetics produces a selective depression of C-afferent fibre-evoked activity in the spinal cord. Pain 23:361–374, 1985.
32. Treede RD, David KD, Campbell JN, Rajc SN: The plasticity of cutaneous hyperalgesia during sympathetic ganglionic blockade in patients with neuropathic pain. Brain 115:607–621, 1992.
33. Lewis LW: Evaluation of sympathetic activity following chemical or surgical sympathectomy. Curr Res Anesth Analg 34:334–345, 1955.
34. Dhuner KG, Edshage S, Wilhelm A: Ninhydrin test: Objective method for testing local anesthetic drugs. Acta Anaesthesiol Scand 4:189–198, 1960.

C H A P T E R

30

Lumbar Facet and Median Branch Blocks

HISTORY

In 1941, Badgley[1] focused his attention on the facets to explain the large numbers of patients with low back pain whose symptoms were not due to a ruptured disc. He showed that facet joint pathology could cause symptoms, including radiation of pain into the lower extremity. Badgley was the first clinician to associate facet arthritis with nerve root irritation as a cause of low back pain and sciatica. Hirsch and colleagues,[2] in 1963, were the first to demonstrate that low back pain distributed along the sacroiliac and gluteal areas with radiation to the greater trochanter could be induced by injecting hypertonic saline in the region of the facet joints. These findings were confirmed by Mooney and Robertson,[3] who in 1976 performed intra-articular facet injections with hypertonic saline and noted that the pain produced could be relieved by intra-articular injection of local anesthetics. In addition Pawl[4] reported the reproduction of pain in patients after injecting hypertonic saline into their cervical facet joints.[5]

No specific therapeutic approach to facet syndrome emerged until the 1970s. Credit for advancing the concept of facet joint denervation as a therapy goes to the Australian physician W. E. S. Rees,[6] who proposed a surgical approach to serving the posterior sensory nerve.[7, 8] Subsequent dissections established the anatomy of dorsal face intervention more precisely and thus paved the way for the more accurate and simpler percutaneous denervation techniques described by Shealy.[9] In fact, Shealy was the first to report the use of fluoroscopic localization of the facet joint in an attempt to specifically treat facet syndrome.[9, 10] Since then, much work has been done, particularly by Bogduk and colleagues, to delineate the anatomy, incidence, and techniques for blocking spinal facet pain.

ANATOMY

As Ghormley stated, "the facet joints are the only true joints of the vertebral column."[11] They are the only joints that permit movement of two intimately related cartilaginous articular surfaces in the axial skeleton. As bilateral, paired, diarthrodial articulations, facet joints are composed of the inferior articular process of the vertebra above and the superior articular process of the vertebra below (Fig. 30–1). The superior pars (articular process) are large, concave, and face posteromedially. The inferior pars are smaller and face anterolaterally.[12, 13] The facet joints in the lumbar vertebral column form the posterior aspect of the neural foramen.[14] A capsule that is lined by a synovial membrane surrounds each joint. This capsule is approximately 1 mm thick, inserts 2 mm below the articular margin, and encloses a space with a maximal volume capacity of 1 to 2 mL of synovial fluid.[15–17] The posterolateral aspect of this membrane is thick, tough, and fibrous. Additionally, the ventromedial aspect is contiguous with the ligamentum flavum. The adipose tissue overlying the ligamentum flavum in the superior aspect of the facet joint is intimately related to the neural root sleeve.[5, 14, 18] This relationship explains why the nerve root can be compromised in some instances of severe arthritis and joint deformity.[19] In the superior and inferior recesses of the facet joints, the capsule appears to be redundant, forming two meniscoid structures: one superior and one inferior.[14, 18, 19] In addition to containing synovial fluid, this capsule may contribute to limiting the joint's range of motion. Finally, the articular surfaces are covered with cartilage that is relatively thick and prone to degeneration with advances in age.

The poor localization of facet joint pain is explained in part by the pattern of profuse overlapping of sensory innervation of these joints. Initially, the posterior and anterior primary rami of a nerve root diverge at the

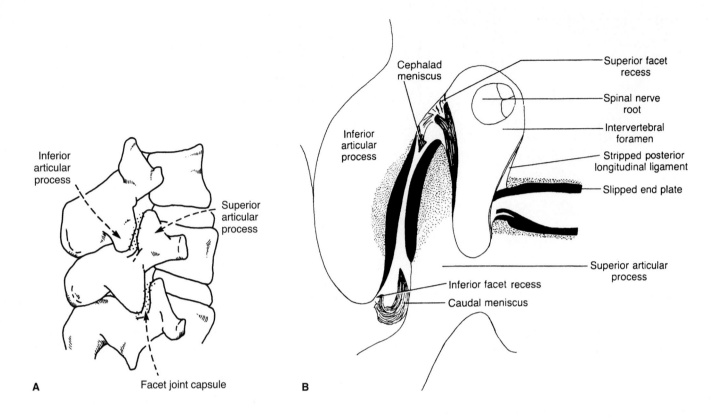

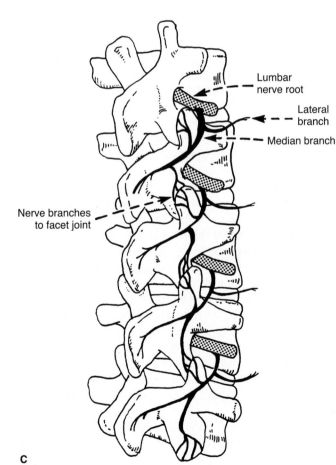

FIGURE 30–1

A, Drawing of the lumbar spine in an oblique view identifying the "Scottie dog" in a radiographic image and the relationship of inferior and superior articular processes. Note the facet joint capsule stippling. *B,* A cross section of the facet joints shows the details of the facet joint. *C,* Drawing of the oblique view of the lumbar spine that shows the lumbar nerve root and the formation of the lateral and median branches of the posterior primary rami. Note the innervation of the facet joint by the median branch. (*B,* From Waldman SD [ed]: Interventional Pain Management, 2nd ed. Philadelphia, WB Saunders, 2001, p 447.)

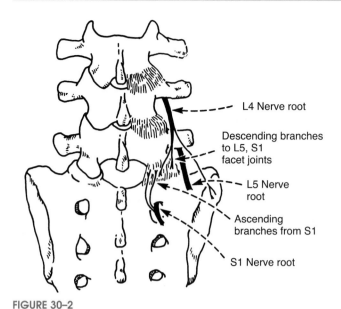

FIGURE 30–2

Innervation of the facet joints at L5–S1 from the L4–L5 nerve root.

intervertebral foramen. The posterior ramus passes dorsally and caudally through a foramen in the intertransverse ligament.[20] At a point 5 mm from its origin, it divides into medial, lateral, and intermediate branches. The medial branch supplies the lower pole of the facet joint at its own level and the upper pole of the facet joint below.[21, 22] Therefore, each of the facet joints receives its innervation from a medial branch nerve of two posterior primary rami. One branch arises from the nerve at the same level as the joint and the other arises from the segmental level above.[23] For example, the facet joint between the L4 and L5 vertebral bodies is innervated by the medial branch nerves from the L3 and L4 nerve roots.

In the lumbar region, the medial branch of the posterior ramus lies in a groove on the base of the superior articular facet, where it lies in direct contact with the base of the superior surface of the transverse process, passing between the mammillary and accessory processes. The nerve actually passes under the mammilloaccessory ligament, and this is the most reliable site for locating the nerve in the lumbar spine. This ligament can become calcified, especially at the L3, L4, and L5 levels (20% at the L5 level).[24] It is suspected that this could even lead to entrapment of the medial branch nerve at this location. The medial branch nerve then progresses posteriorly and inferiorly, first sending fibers cephalad to innervate the caudad-capsular margin of the adjacent superior joint capsule before sending fibers to the next lower level at its cephalad-capsular margin.[25] The course of the L5 medial branch is somewhat modified, because the transverse process is replaced by the ala of the sacrum (Fig. 30–2). An additional abnormality at the lumbosacral junction is the proposal that a branch from the posterior opening of the S1 nerve root in the sacrum

runs cephalad to supply the L5–L1 facet joint.[26, 27] This would result in the L5–L1 facet joint's being innervated by three nerves, and this third nerve would also need to be blocked to completely anesthetize this joint.

Each medial branch of the posterior primary ramus also supplies the multifidus, interspinales, and intertransversarii mediales muscles and the ligaments and periosteum of the neural arch.[28–30] However, there is considerable segmental overlap of this sensory innervation. Therefore, blockade of the two medial branch nerves, which have been shown to be the main source of nociceptive signals from an individual facet joint, can reasonably be expected to be specific for the facet joint.

Therefore, each joint has dual segmental innervation, and each segmental nerve supplies two facet joints plus the soft tissues overlying them. Because of the duality of segmental innervation, each joint must be denervated at two segmental levels (and perhaps three for the L5–S1 joint), both at and above the level of the involved joint (see Fig. 30–2).

Controversy once surrounded the question of whether there is innervation from a third ascending branch that arises from the mixed spinal nerve just anterior to the intertransverse fascia (ligament). The proposed nerve branch apparently ascends, well clear of the transverse process, through the soft tissue into the posterior aspect of the facet above (Fig. 30–3).[25, 27, 31, 32] Although this has been proposed, more recent anatomic studies have failed to find such an ascending nerve. It likely does not exist, and even if it actually does exist, it appears to be small and inconsistent and likely clinically insignificant. Additional articular branches to the

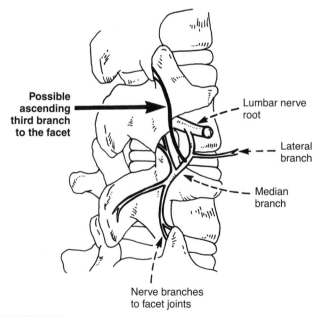

FIGURE 30–3

This illustration shows that there is a possibility of three median nerve branches innervating the one facet joint. Note the ascending branch from the median nerve supplying the nerve above.

ventral aspect of the facet joints from the dorsal ramus have also been described, but subsequent studies also failed to locate them.[29] If these branches actually exist, they seem likewise to be small and inconsistent and likely are not clinically significant.

There is evidence in rats and humans of multilevel innervation of the lumbar facet joints, which includes not only the posterior primary ramus but also the sympathetic and parasympathetic ganglia.[29, 33] The sympathetic fibers innervating the lumbar facet joints have been found to pass through the dorsal root ganglion and to go directly into rami communicantes, on their way to the paravertebral sympathetic trunk. The origins of these nerves have been found to be several segmental levels away from the innervated facet joint. The sympathetic fibers have been reported to regulate the activity of sensory neurons, and this is compatible with some reports that the sympathetic trunk contributes to low back pain.

INDICATIONS

The major indications for facet joint injection include (1) focal tenderness over a facet joint, (2) chronic low back pain with or without radiation but with a normal radiographic evaluation, (3) back pain with evidence of disc disease and facet arthritis, and (4) postlaminectomy syndrome without arachnoiditis or recurrent disc disease.[13, 34]

CONTRAINDICATIONS

The only absolute contraindication to facet joint block is infection in the overlying soft tissues. A relative contraindication is allergy to injecting agents. Facet joint block can be accomplished, however, without injection of contrast material, and the newer non-ionic contrast agents also decrease the risk in allergic individuals.

EQUIPMENT

- 25-gauge needle for skin infiltration
- 22-gauge, 8½-inch spinal needle

Radiofrequency Thermocoagulation
- 16-gauge, 1½-inch angiocatheter
- 20-gauge, 10 cm (with 10-mm tip) radiofrequency needle
- Radiofrequency machine with electrode

DRUGS

- 0.5% bupivacaine or 0.5% ropivacaine
- 2% lidocaine
- Triamcinolone diacetate or equivalent

PREPARATION OF THE PATIENT

Clinicians do not have consensus regarding specific, nonradicular pain referral patterns for the lumbar facet joints. The pain originating in a single lumbar facet joint is usually described as a unilateral, dull ache in the paraspinal region, occasionally radiating to the buttocks and proximal lower extremity.[2, 3, 11, 35] Pain from a lumbar facet joint rarely radiates below the knee, but this is not absolute. Intra-articular injections of hypertonic saline were performed in normal individuals as well as individuals with low back pain to map the characteristics of observed referral patterns.[3] In general, lumbar facet joint pain has a nonradicular pattern and the presence of arthropathy can make the referral different than in individuals in whom no arthropathy is seen. A composite of the results is in Figure 30–4.

The diagnosis of lumbar facet joint pain on clinical grounds is a challenging feat. Historically, a patient who presented with low back pain and a normal neurologic examination was diagnosed with an arthropathy of a

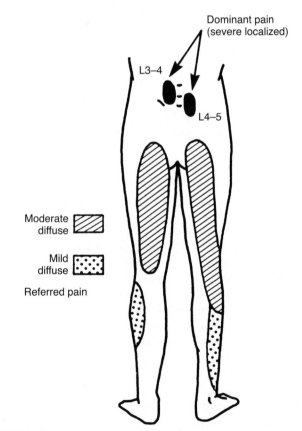

FIGURE 30–4

Pain distribution in the facet syndrome. Referred pain patterns from facet joints reflect the distribution of the segmental nerve supply at each level involved. Distal reference to the buttocks relates to the caudad migration of posterior branches, whereas limb distribution mimicking root pain results from pain reference in the anterior division of each segmental nerve. (Adapted from Boas RA: Facet joint injections. In Stanton-Hicks M, Boas RA [eds]: Chronic Low Back Pain. New York, Raven, 1982, pp 199–211.)

lumbar zygapophyseal joint. However, provocative electrical stimulation of any structure within the posterior column of the lumbar spine can essentially produce an identical clinical picture.[36]

Another study that attempted to elucidate the referral patterns of the lumbar zygapophyseal joints was performed by Fukui and associates[37] in 1997. Several intra-articular injections were performed with contrast material followed by radiofrequency thermocoagulation after stimulation of the medial branches. Noteworthy is the lower incidence of referred pain down the lower extremities in comparison to Mooney's study. The most common referral patterns are seen in Figure 30–4. Characteristically the referral pattern for the high lumbar facet joints (L1–L2 and L2–L3) were more frequently observed in the lumbar area, whereas the lower lumbar joints referred pain into the gluteal region, groin area, and posterolateral thigh.

Usually, the patient's clinical picture is absent of any neurological deficit, and if a deficit is detected, other causes of back pain have to be ruled out before arriving at the diagnosis of facet joint pain. Physical examination can reveal paraspinal pain to palpation in the lower back. Spasm of the paravertebral muscles overlying the affected joint may also be detected. Patients suffering from lumbar facet chondropathy experience less pain with movement and posturing in the flexion direction. Pain is reduced in the morning and worsens as the day progresses. During the examination, the greatest pain is produced during three-dimensional movements that lock the facets (combined movements, e.g., extension, side bending, and ipsilateral rotation). Conversely, patients with synovial irritation experience less pain in extension owing to the increased stability invested in the joint in the extended position. These patients experience increased pain in the evening and will experience the greatest provocation during coupled movements because of the maximized stress imposed on the capsule and synovial lining (e.g., extension, side bending, and contralateral rotation).

LABORATORY

One again, the clinical neurologic examination is crucial. Any evidence of radiculopathy should prompt imaging studies to rule out any other etiology of the pain, such as the more common primary disc affliction (prolapse or extrusion). As mentioned previously, facet joint pathology typically follows intervertebral disc disease. One investigation demonstrated the presence of degenerative disc disease on computed tomography (CT) in virtually all cases exhibiting facet joint degenerative changes. This creates confusion for diagnosing radiculopathy and requires differentiating between the facet joint and the intervertebral disc as the source of the referred pain.

The importance of imaging studies in the lumbar facet syndrome rests on the elimination of other diagnostic possibilities. Conventional radiologic studies may identify severe changes in the facet joint, but the more subtle changes go undetected. CT and magnetic resonance imaging (MRI) studies are able to detect less obvious changes such as articular cartilage wear and subchondral bone cysts.[38] To understand that these are only anatomic findings and should be interpreted as such is paramount to effective clinical diagnosis. Additionally, the correlation of these findings and clinical manifestations is very tenuous. One investigation demonstrated the presence of arthritic changes in 10.4% of asymptomatic patients.[39] Furthermore, arthritic joint changes detectable by CT or MRI appear in more than 50% of persons older than 40 years of age and without low back pain. Because of the highly elusive value of radiologically appreciable changes in the facet joint and the poor correlation of these changes with symptomatology, a facet block should be undertaken if the diagnosis of lumbar facet joint pain is likely and conclusive evidence of intervertebral disc pathology is not available. Of importance to mention is the understated value of the radionuclide bone scan. Although its value is undetermined in clinical trials, if positive findings are obtained, it may direct one's attention to a specific pain-producing facet joint.

PREOPERATIVE MEDICATION

For preoperative medication, use the standard American Society of Anesthesiologists' recommendations for conscious sedation.

PROCEDURE

Lumbar facet block has the same purpose as its cervical counterpart. The most commonly used technique is with the patient lying prone on the fluoroscopy table (Fig. 30–5). The patient's lower back is prepared in a sterile fashion and draped. The level chosen to be blocked is identified under fluoroscopic view in the posteroanterior projection (Fig. 30–5A). Once the level is identified, the fluoroscopy ray is rotated in an oblique fashion toward the lateral projection slowly until a view of the "Scottie dog" is obtained in Fig. 30–5B. This view is basically described as the projection that allows visualization of the facet joint space as well as the superior and inferior articular processes that form the joint. The "Scottie dog" is formed by the superior as well as the inferior pars of the same vertebra. The "ear" of the dog is the superior articular process (pars) and the "front legs" of the dog are formed by the inferior articular process (pars) (Fig. 30–6). Once this view has been obtained, the

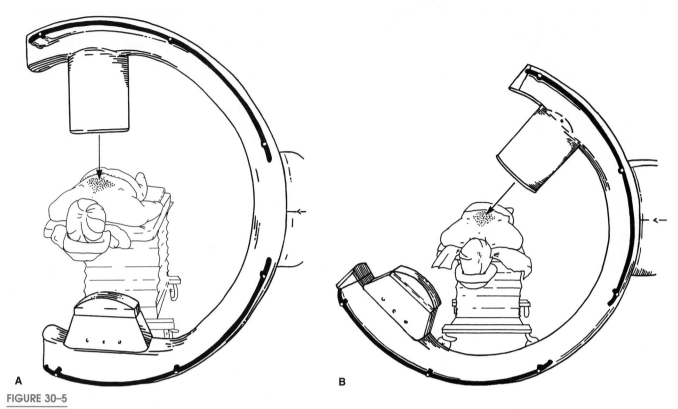

FIGURE 30–5

A, C-arm for the anteroposterior view of the lumbar spine as a first step toward identifying the facet joints. *B*, In Step 2, the C-arm turns to an oblique view to identify the "Scottie dog" in the radiographic imaging.

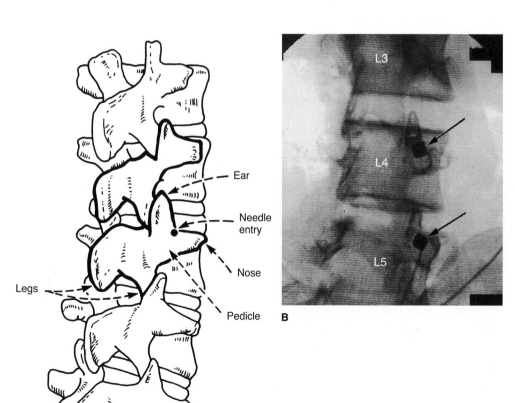

FIGURE 30–6

A, Drawing of the lumbar spine that shows the "Scottie dog" in the oblique view. The site of entry for median branch block and radiofrequency is shown. *B*, Radiographic imaging of the lumbosacral spine shows the correct placement of the radiofrequency needle (curved blunt) *(arrow)* at the eye of the "Scottie dog" at L4–L5.

optimal point of contact with the bone by the needle should be the "eye of the dog" (Fig. 30–6).

SITE OF NEEDLE ENTRY

The skin is prepared and draped in a sterile fashion. After the skin is anesthetized, the 22-gauge spinal needle is directed vertically toward the facet joint. Local anesthesia is achieved in the soft tissues overlying the facet joint by injection of lidocaine through the spinal needle while it is advanced. Care should be taken to pass the tip of the needle directly to the facet joint by observing its tip frequently with fluoroscopy. Sometimes puncture of the joint capsule can be felt. More often, however, the bone prevents further advance of the needle after entering the joint.

When the tip of the needle is superimposed on the facet joint and the needle cannot be advanced any further, the needle tip should be in or very near the facet joint (see Fig. 30–7). Small adjustments can be made in needle position by retracting the needle 1 to 2 cm and readvancing. To prevent having to work around already-positioned needles, it is most convenient, for injection of multiple joints, to start with the most cephalad joint and work caudally.

When the needle tip is positioned within the joint, the anesthetist attempts aspiration to ensure that the needle has not entered the subarachnoid space. If there is no return of cerebrospinal fluid, the extension tubing with contrast agent is attached, and 1 mL of iodinated contrast medium is injected. A spot film is exposed, with each facet injection to document the intra-articular position of the needle tip. Once the needle position has been documented, 1.5 mL of 0.5% bupivacaine and 20

mg of methylprednisolone acetate are injected into each joint, and the needles are removed.

MEDIAN BRANCH BLOCK

After a skin weal is raised and the skin is properly anesthetized, then in a gun-barrel fashion a spinal needle is advanced toward the eye of the "Scottie dog" (see Fig. 30–6). It should be emphasized that there should always be bone in front of the needle to avoid complications. Once bone contact is made, then the needle position should be confirmed by the lateral projection, at which point the needle should be seen at the level of the facet line and not beyond this point, posterior to the foraminal opening, and finally below the level of the intervertebral disc (Fig. 30–8). If desired, an anteroposterior view can also be used to confirm the position of the needle (Fig. 30–9). In this view the needle should be seen at the junction of the superior articular process and the medial-most aspect of the transverse process. At this point then, after careful aspiration, the local anesthetic solution is to be injected. This should be repeated at the level corresponding to the medial branch innervating the facet joint targeted.

When performing a block of the medial branch of L5, a somewhat different approach is used. The medial branch at this level lies in the groove formed by the superior articular process of the sacrum and the ala of this bone. To obtain this view, the fluoroscope may need to be rotated in a cephalocaudad fashion to remove the iliac crest from the view (Fig. 30–10). Once the view is obtained, the needle is directed in a gun-barrel fashion to the most superior aspect of the "valley" formed by the ala of the sacrum and its superior articular process.

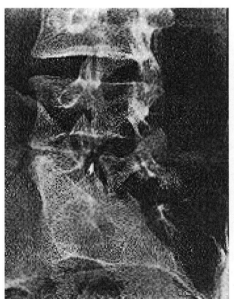

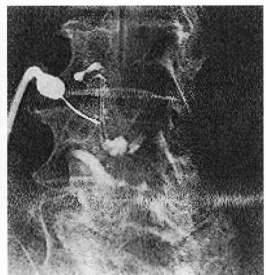

A   **B**

FIGURE 30–7

A, Oblique radiograph of the lower spine shows spondylolysis with bilateral defects in the pars interarticularis at L5 *(arrow).* Note the "Scottie dog" at L4 and the facet joint. *B,* Facet arthrogram showing the S-shaped contour with filling of the smaller superior recess and larger inferior recess. (From Raj PP [ed]: Practical Management of Pain, 3rd ed. St. Louis, Mosby, 2000, pp 747, 748.)

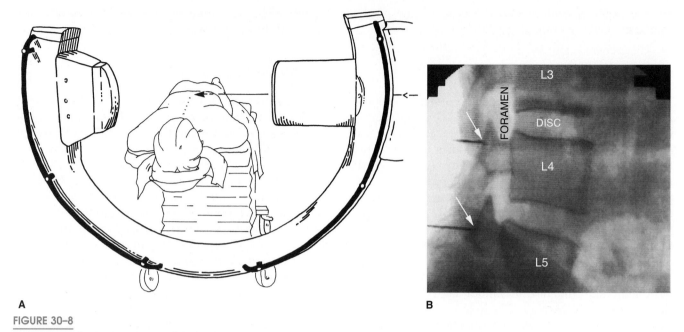

A

B

FIGURE 30–8

A, C-arm to take the lateral view of the lumbar spine. *B,* Lateral radiographic image shows the correct placement of the junction of the superior articular process and transfer position of the needle tip *(arrow)* is below the disc and at the level of the facet joint.

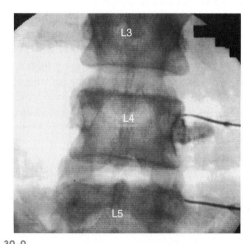

FIGURE 30–9

Anteroposterior view of the correct needle placement of radiofrequency at L4–L5.

In the lateral view, the needle should be seen outside and posterior to the neural foramen (see Fig. 30–10).

COMPLICATIONS

These include bruising, backache, muscle spasm, neuritis, and numbness of the leg. Treat infections with antibiotics. Expectant treatment should be sufficient, but patient should be followed closely.

HELPFUL HINTS

In the upper lumbar spine, approximately 80% of the facet joints are curved and 20% are flat. In the lower lumbar spine, the situation is reversed and approximately 80% of the facet joints are flat.[40] The upper lumbar facets are more oriented in the sagittal plane, and by the L5–S1 level they have rotated to a more oblique angle. The facet joints are oriented lateral to the sagittal plane from the midline posteriorly as follows: the L1–L2 joint 30 degrees or less, the L2–L3 joint 15 to 45 degrees, and the L3–L4 joints 30 to 75 degrees.[32, 40–44] The lumbar facets are all almost vertically oriented, being tipped approximately 10 degrees with the cephalad end of the joint farther anterior than the caudad end of the joint.[44] Because of the curvature of the upper lumbar facet joints, the posterior opening is usually more in the sagittal plan than the overall angle of the joint. This usually means that the accessible posterior joint space opening is usually 5 to 10 degrees less oblique than the best fluoroscopic image, which shows the angle of the joint overall.

EFFICACY

As mentioned before, one cannot find any conclusive evidence in the literature showing the superiority of medial branch blocks over intra-articular injections. One of the most complete revisions of the literature regarding the efficacy of cervical medial branch radiofrequency was done by Lord and associates in 1995.[45] Seven series were included in this revision. The results demonstrated that all studies reported a percentage of patients between 37% to 89%, who experienced more than 40% relief for more than 2 months. Even though these studies were flawed due to technical and anatomic errors, these results show encouraging evidence that medial branch

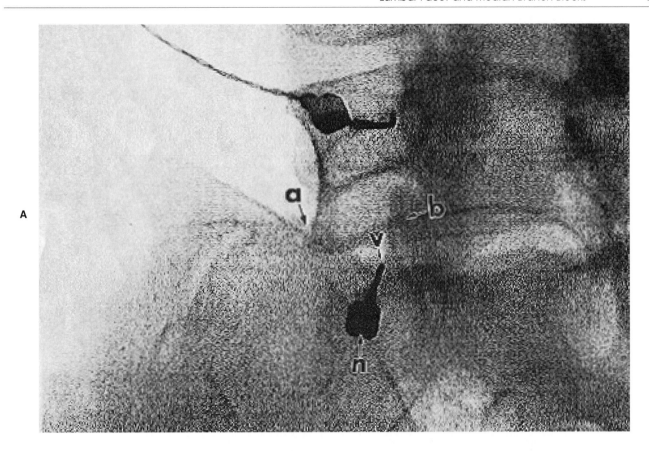

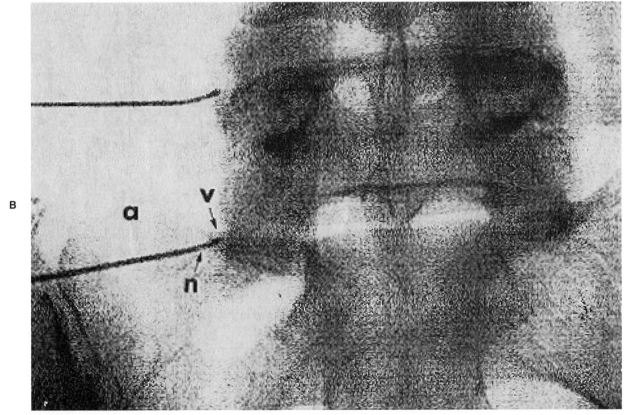

FIGURE 30–10

Oblique *(A)*, anteroposterior *(B)*, and lateral *(C)* views of the needle placement at L5–S1. a, median border of the ilium; b, inferior plate of L5, the tip of the needle at L5–S1 junction; n, needle; v, vertebra; NF, neuroforamen. (From Raj PP [ed]: Textbook of Regional Anesthesia. St. Louis, Mosby, 2000.)

Continued

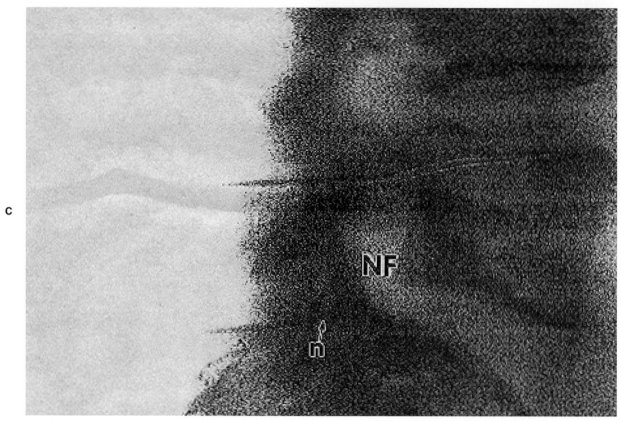

FIGURE 30–10

Continued

radiofrequency could be beneficial in well-selected patients. In another study by the same authors in 1996,[46] they compared a group of control patients to a radiofrequency group and concluded that the radiofrequency group had significantly longer pain relief (median time 263 days) compared to the control group. It has also been concluded that 71% of patients undergoing denervation by radiofrequency had a good response when they were chosen by double diagnostic blocks. On the other hand Barnsley and colleagues[47] has calculated a 27% false-positive rate when double diagnostic blocks are used. With these results, it is safe to say that there is some benefit to facet denervation when the patients are chosen appropriately, but this still has to be proven by evidence stemming from large prospective, randomized trials with a control population.

For lumbar medial branch blocks Schwarzer and coworkers[48] have calculated single diagnostic blocks as having a false-positive rate of 38%. Other studies[49, 50] have advocated comparative blocks to decrease this false-positive rate. The analgesia following these medial branch blocks has been used as the selection criteria for radiofrequency thermocoagulation neurotomy. Several studies, including Lora,[51] Ogsbury,[52] Silvers,[7] and their colleagues have reported long-term relief rates by neurotomy from 32% to 75%. Patients who have had previ-

ous surgery experienced prolonged relief between 26% and 50% compared to those without previous surgery at 75%. Another study with mixed results was by Mehta and Sluijter.[53] This study reported good results at 1 month in 45% of patients, with a steep decline to 28% at 1 year with 50% at 1 year with poor results.

In contrast with the earlier studies, we have other studies that somewhat justify lumbar medial branch radiofrequency. North and associates[54] published a retrospective review of 82 patients. Of these 82, 42 patients went on to have a medial branch neurotomy, of which 45% had approximately 50% relief with a mean duration of 3.2 years. Rashbaum[55] published results of 82% of patients with good pain relief (>50%) at 3 and 6 months and 68% with good relief remaining at 3 years. It is clear by looking at these results that the studies, which had more strict selection criteria (clinical evidence and positive response to medial branch blocks), had the better long-term results. In conclusion, a more specific means of diagnosing facet arthropathy is needed, combined with clinical evidence via controlled trials that medial branch neurotomy is effective in this scenario.

Lumbar facet, single level 64475; lumbar, each additional level 64476; RFTC lumbar facet, single level 64622; RFTC lumbar facet, additional levels 64623.

REFERENCES

1. Badgley CE: The articular facets in relation to low back pain and sciatic radiation. J Bone Joint Surg Am 23:481–496, 1941.
2. Hirsch C, Inglemark B, Miller M: The anatomical basis for low back pain. Acta Orthop Scand 33:1, 1963.
3. Mooney V, Robertson J: The facet syndrome. Clin Orthop 115:149–156, 1976.
4. Pawl RP: Headache, cervical spondylosis, and anterior cervical fusion. Surg Annu 9:391, 1971.
5. Bogduk N: Back pain: Zygapophysial blocks and epidural steroids. In Cousins MJ, Bridenbaugh PO (eds): Neural Blockade in Clinical Anesthesia and Management of Pain, 2nd ed. Philadelphia, JB Lippincott, 1988, pp 935–946.
6. Rees WES: Multiple bilateral subcutaneous rhizolysis of segmental nerves in the treatment of the intervertebral disk syndrome. Ann Gen Pract 16:126, 1971.
7. Silvers RH: Lumbar percutaneous facet rhizotomy. Spine 15:36–40, 1990.
8. Raymond J, Dumas J: Intra-articular facet block: Diagnostic test or therapeutic procedure? Radiology 151:333–336, 1984.
9. Shealy CN: Percutaneous radiofrequency denervation of spinal facets: Treatment for chronic back pain and sciatica. J Neurosurg 43:448–451, 1975.
10. Mooney V: Facet syndrome: Clinical entities. In Weinstein JN Wiesel SW (eds): The Lumbar Spine (The International Society for the Study of the Lumbar Spine). Philadelphia, WB Saunders 1990, pp 422–441.
11. Ghormley RK: Low back pain with special reference to the articular facet, with presentation of an operative procedure. JAMA 101:1773–1777, 1993.
12. Lewin T, Moffet B, Viidik A: The morphology of the lumbar synovial intervertebral joints. Acta Morphol Nerland Scand 4:299–319, 1962.
13. Bogduk N, Twomey LT (eds): Clinical Anatomy of the Lumbar Spine, 2nd ed. London, Churchill Livingstone, 1991.
14. Paris SV: Anatomy as related to function and pain. Orthop Clin North Am 14:475–489, 1983.
15. Moran R, O'Connell D, Walsh M: The diagnostic value of facet joint injection. Spine 13:1407–1410, 1988.
16. Cyron BM, Hutton WC: The tensile strength of the capsular ligaments of the apophyseal joints. J Anat 132:145–150, 1981.
17. Yahia LH, Garzon S: Structure on the capsula ligaments of the facet joints. Ann Anat 175:185–188, 1993.
18. Derby R, Bogduk N, Schwarzer A: Precision percutaneous blocking procedures for localizing spinal pain: I. The posterior lumbar compartment. Pain Digest 3:89–100, 1993.
19. Bogduk N, Engel R: The menisci of the lumbar zygapophysial joints: A review of their anatomy and clinical significance. Spine 9:454–460, 1984.
20. Gray DP, Bajwa ZH, Warfield C: Facet block and neurolysis. In Waldman SD (ed): Interventional Pain Management, 2nd ed. Philadelphia, WB Saunders, 2001, pp 446–483.
21. Taren JA, Kahn EA: Anatomic pathways related to pain in face and neck. J Neurosurg 19:116, 1948.
22. Bovim G, Berg R, Gunnar DL: Cervicogenic headache: Anesthetic blockades of cervical nerves and facet joint (C2/C3). Pain 49:315–320, 1992.
23. Barnsley L, Bogduk N: Medial branch blocks are specific for the diagnosis of cervical zygapophyseal joint pain. Reg Anesth 18:343–350, 1993.
24. Barnsley L, Lord SM, Wallis BJ, et al: The prevalence of chronic cervical zygapophyseal joint pain after whiplash. Spine 20:20–26, 1995.
25. White AA, Southwick WO, DePonte RJ, et al: Relief of pain by anterior cervical spine fusion for spondylosis: A report of 65 patients. J Bone Joint Surg Am 55:525, 1973.
26. Bogduk N, Marsland A: The cervical zygapophyseal joints as a source of neck pain. Spine 13:610–617, 1988.
27. Bous RA: Facet joint injections. In Stanton-Hicks M, Bous R (eds): Chronic Low Back Pain. New York, Raven, 1982, pp 199–211.
28. Glover JR: Arthrography of the joints of the lumbar vertebral arches. Orthop Clin North Am 8:37–42, 1977.
29. Bogduk N, Anat D: The clinical anatomy of the cervical dorsal rami. Spine 7:319–330, 1982.
30. Ebraheim NA, James ST, Xu R, et al: The anatomical location of the dorsal ramus of the cervical nerve and its relation to the superior articular process of the lateral mass. Spine 23:1968–1971, 1998.
31. Tournade A, Patay Z, Krupa P, et al: A comparative study of the anatomical, radiological, and therapeutic features of the lumbar facet joints. Radiology 34:257–261, 1992.
32. Lynch MC, Taylor JF: Facet joint injection for low back pain: A clinical study. J Bone Joint Surg Br 68:138–141, 1986.
33. Maigne J-Y, Maigne R, Guerin-Surville H: The lumbar mamillo-accessory foramen: A study of 203 lumbosacral spines. Surg Radiol Anat 13:29–32, 1991.
34. Hadden SB: Neurologic headache and facial pain. Arch Neurol 43:405, 1940.
35. McCall IW, Park WM, O'Brien JP: Induced pain referral from posterior lumbar elements in normal subjects. Spine 4:441–446, 1979.
36. Destouet JM, Giluaalla LA, Murphy WA, Monsees B: Lumbar facet joint injections: Indication, technique, clinical correlation, and preliminary results. Radiology 145:321–325, 1982.
37. Fukui S, Ohseto K, Shiotani M, et al: Distribution of referred pain from the lumbar zygapopyseal joints and dorsal rami. Clin J Pain 13:303–307, 1997.
38. Carrera GF: Lumbar facet joint injection in low back pain and sciatica. Radiology 137:661–664, 1980.
39. Twomey LT, Taylor JR, Taylor MM: Unsuspected damage to lumbar zygapophyseal (facet) joints after motor vehicle accidents. Med J Aust 151:210, 1989.
40. Horvitz T, Smith RM: An anatomical, pathological, and roentgenological study of the intervertebral joints of the lumbar spine and of the sacroiliac joints. AJR Am J Roentgenol 43:173–186, 1940.
41. Maldjian C, Mesgarzadeh M, Tehranzadeh J: Diagnostic and therapeutic features of facet and sacroiliac joint injection. Radiol Clin North Am 36:497–508, 1998.
42. Malmivaara A, Videman T, Kuosma E, et al: Facet joint orientation, facet and costovertebral joint osteoarthrosis, disc degeneration, vertebral body osteophytosis, and Schmorl's nodes in the thoracolumbar junctional region of cadaveric spines. Spine 12:458–463, 1987.
43. Tulssi RS, Hermanis GM: A study of the angle of inclination and facet curvature of superior lumbar zygapophyseal facets. Spine 18:1311–1317, 1993.
44. Punjabi MM, Oxland T, Takata K, et al: Articular facets of the human spine: Quantitative three-dimensional anatomy. Spine 18:1298–1310, 1993.
45. Lord SM, Barnsley L, Bogduk N: Percutaneous radiofrequency neurotomy in the treatment of cervical zygapophyseal joint pain: A caution. Neurosurgery 36:732–739, 1995.
46. Lord SM, Barnsley L, Wallis BJ, et al: Percutaneous radiofrequency neurotomy for chronic cervical zygapophyseal joint pain. N Engl J Med 335:1721–1726, 1996.
47. Barnsley L, Lord S, Wallis B, Bogduk N: False-positive rates of cervical zygapophyseal joint blocks. Clin J Pain 9:124–130, 1993.
48. Schwarzer AC, Aprill CN, Derby R, et al: The false-positive rate of uncontrolled diagnostic blocks of the lumbar zygapophyseal joints. Pain 58:195–200, 1994.
49. Boas RA: Nerve block in the diagnosis of low back pain. Neurosurg Clin North Am 2:807–816, 1991.
50. Schwarzer A, Scott A, Wang S, et al: The role of bone scintigraphy in chronic low back pain: Comparison of SPECT and planar images and zygapophyseal joint injection [Abstract]. Aust N Z J Med 22:186, 1992.
51. Lora J, Long D: So-called facet denervation in the management of intractable back pain. Spine 1:121–126, 1976.
52. Osgsbury JS, Simon RH, Lehman RAW: Facet "denervation" in the treatment of low back syndrome. Pain 3:257–263, 1977.
53. Mehta M, Sluijer ME: The treatment of chronic back pain: A preliminary survey of the effect of radiofrequency denervation of the posterior vertebral joints. Anesthesia 34:768, 1979.
54. North RB, Hann M, Zahurak M, Kidd DH: Radiofrequency lumbar facet denervation: Analysis of prognostic factors. Pain 57:77, 1994.
55. Rashbaum RF: Radiofrequency facet denervation: A treatment alternative in refractory low back pain with or without leg pain. Orthop Clin North Am 14:569, 1983.

CHAPTER 31

Lumbar Provocative Discography

HISTORY

In 1948 Linblom studied the effects of puncturing the intervertebral discs.[1] Hirsch followed this with a clinical study to determine how the ruptures or tears in the annulus would lead to pathologic processes producing pain. He hypothesized that putting pressure to a ruptured or degenerated disc would reproduce a patient's pain. His technique used saline to pressurize the disc and procaine solution to modulate the pain response generated. He showed reproduction of pain in all cases.[2] The value of the study was that disc puncture could be used to make a clinical diagnosis of a patient's back pain.

Five forms of herniations were identified, and the discs were pressurized to 300 kPa (1 mm Hg = 133.32 Pa = 0.13332 kPa). There were no disc ruptures or herniations reported.[3] Collins thought that discography would be an improvement on computed tomographic (CT) myelogram due to the fact that with a normal myelogram, one cannot be assured that internal disc disruption is absent.[4]

In 1964, Crock[5] advanced the theory of internal disc disruption. He showed that these patients have abnormal discograms and that pain is reproduced by a small volume (0.3 mL) of solution injected, due to hypersensitivity of pain fibers in the disc. Discographic patterns on radiographs were shown to be abnormal.

Bogduk[6] in 1996 described the cardinal component of discography as disc stimulation. The characteristic grade I lesion is a radial fissure extending to the inner third, a grade II to the middle third, and grade III to the outer third. Seventy-five percent of grade III disruptions are associated with exact or similar pain reproduction, and 77% of discs with exact pain reproduction were found to have a grade III tear.[6] Bogduk stated that discography is a diagnostic tool designed only to obtain information about the source of a patient's pain.

ANATOMY

The intervertebral disc is composed of three structures: the annulus fibrosus, the nucleus pulposus, and the end plates (Fig. 31–1). The annulus surrounds the nucleus in a beltlike fashion, and the end plates cover the superior and inferior aspects of the nucleus. Although the end

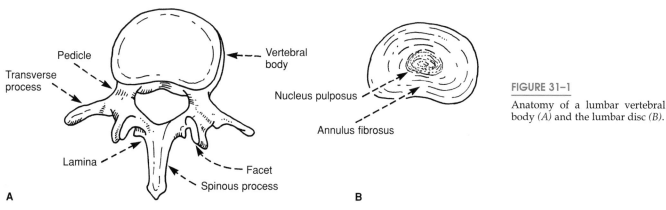

Pedicle

Transverse process

Vertebral body

Nucleus pulposus

Annulus fibrosus

Lamina

Facet

Spinous process

A

B

FIGURE 31–1

Anatomy of a lumbar vertebral body *(A)* and the lumbar disc *(B)*.

plates do not completely cover the annulus, the collagen fibers of the most superficial lamellae of the annulus insert directly into the bone of the vertebral body.[7, 8] These lamellae that join the annulus and consequently the end plates and nucleus run obliquely from one vertebra to another. This arrangement, although allowing some movement between adjacent vertebra, provides a very strong bond between them.[9] Before the degenerative changes associated with aging are seen, the lamellae fully cover the vertebral bodies. Later, they are absorbed secondarily into the bone.[8]

The annulus fibrosus is a concentric lamellae of fibrocartilage made of collagen and fibroblasts that surround the nucleus.[9] Although the concept of the annulus is that of a complete ring or belt, in any given quadrant, 40% of the lamellae are incomplete, and in the posterolateral quadrant, some 50% are incomplete.[8, 10] The lamellae are thicker toward the center of the disc.[10] Similarly, they are thick in the anterior and lateral portions of the annulus. However, posteriorly they are finer and more tightly packed. Consequently, the posterior portion of the annulus fibrosus is thinner than the rest of the annulus.[11–13] This ultimately leads to more tears posteriorly.[9, 14]

The nucleus pulposus consists of a three-dimensional network of collagen fibers, enmeshed in a mucoprotein gel that contains various mucopolysaccharides.[15, 16] The water content of the nucleus pulposus diminishes with increasing age,[15–18] whereas the polysaccharides complex decreases and is replaced by collagen.[16, 19] The proteoglycans of the center allow for absorption and dispersion of forces.[9, 20] This allows the disc to act as a shock absorber for axial forces and like a semifluid ball-bearing during flexion, extension, rotation, and lateral flexion of the vertebral column.[9]

Because of the gelatinous center of the nucleus pulposus, the disc was postulated to act hydrostatically.[21, 22] This was a reasonable assumption because of the high water content of 70% to 90%.[15, 17, 22–26] This was proven in 1960 by Nachemson.[26] However, this fluid content varies with the applied load (i.e., lumbar flexion) and represents an equilibrium between the applied load, which caused fluid to be expelled from the disc, and the swelling pressure of the hydrophilic proteoglycans, which acts to retain the fluid. At equilibrium, there is no net fluid loss or gain. The highest fluid content is thought to be in the morning, after a long period of rest, and the lowest fluid content is in the evening after a long period of sustained loading.[27–30] This was verified in a study by Wilke and associates.[30] This study took a healthy volunteer and measured intradiscal pressure while the subject was performing various activities of daily life. It was discovered during sleeping, intradiscal pressure increased substantially, presumably because of rehydration of the disc. The pressure increased after 7 hours in the lying position to 240% of its pressure at the time of going to bed.[31] This may be due to diurnal variation in fluid flux that in vivo findings indicated to be approximately 20%.[31, 32]

INDICATIONS

Discography has been used as a tool to aid in the diagnosis of low back pain. It is used routinely prior to surgical intervention for a ruptured disc and as a confirmatory procedure prior to spinal fusion.

Gresham and Miller[32] described three groups in which discography is beneficial:

Group I: to help determine the feasibility of fusion at the time of disc removal, either with or without a positive myelogram

Group II: as a diagnostic aid in helping to determine the presence or location of disc pathology or to help clarify any question about the actual need for surgery

Group III: as an excluding diagnostic study in certain litigation compensation cases[32]

Brodsky and Binder[33] described their indications for discography in 1979:

- Negative myelogram where the symptoms and the signs are not localized
- When clinical findings point to one level and myelogram is positive at another level
- In spinal stenosis with single root symptoms or in cases of complete block
- Arachnoiditis obscuring diagnostic myelographic pattern
- Previously operated-on patient with recurrent pain or failure of primary operation
- When fusion is contemplated, to evaluate adjacent discs[33]

Guyer and Ohnmeiss[34] further defined indications for discography in 1995. They contended that discography should be performed only after conservative measures have failed and after noninvasive tests have failed to yield sufficient diagnostic information. Indications as stated were the following:

- For further evaluation of demonstrably abnormal discs to help assess the extent of abnormality, for correlation of the abnormality with the clinical symptoms
- Patients with persistent severe symptoms in whom other diagnostic test have failed to reveal clear confirmation of a suspected disc as a source of pain
- Assessment of failed surgical patients to determine if there is a painful pseudarthrosis or a symptomatic disc in a posteriorly fused segment if the discs adjacent to the segment are normal
- For assessment of minimally invasive surgical candidates to confirm a contained disc herniation or to investigate dye distribution before chemonucleolysis[34]

CONTRAINDICATIONS

Absolute
- Discitis
- Local infection of skin
- Coagulopathies
- Allergies to contrast solutions

Relative
- Allergy to (antibiotic) drugs to be injected
- Pregnancy
- Disc herniation

EQUIPMENT

Needles
- 25-gauge needle for skin wheal
- 20-gauge needle for skin puncture
- 22-gauge, at least 6-inch spinal needle for deep tissue local anesthetic infiltration
- 16-gauge angiocatheter (introducer for the curve blunt needle)
- 20-gauge curved-blunt radiofrequency thermocoagulation needle (optional)
- 18-gauge angiocatheter as introducer (optional) for Chiba needle
- Chiba needle

Syringes
- 10-mL syringe

Audiovisual System
- Video camera
- Color monitor
- Video tape recorder

Special Equipment
- Pressure measurement system
- Intellisystem (Fig. 31–2)

DRUGS

- 20-mL 1.5% lidocaine vial
- 50-mL water-soluble, non-ionic contrast with cefazolin 1 mg/mL in sterile preservative-free saline

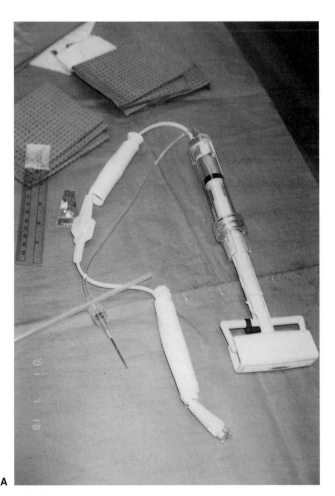
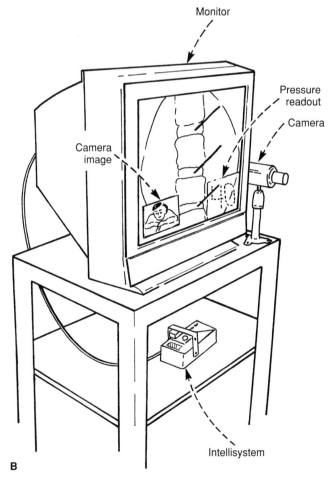

FIGURE 31–2

A, Pressure syringe and attachment for provocative discography. *B,* Drawing of the Intellisystem, with its connection to the camera for provocative discography.

■ Midazolam, and fentanyl for sedation
■ Topical antibiotic ointment for skin injection sites

PREPARATION OF THE PATIENT

PHYSICAL EXAMINATION

All patients for discography should have detailed history and physical examinations in addition to magnetic resononance imaging (MRI) or CT myelogram studies. On MRI scans (T2-weighted images), the high-intensity zone should be visualized. This zone is a high-intensity signal (bright white) located in the substance of the posterior annulus fibrosus, which is clearly dissociated from the signal produced by the nucleus pulposus. It is surrounded by the low-intensity (black) signal of the annulus fibrosus and is brighter than the signal of the nucleus pulposus.[35]

LABORATORY

■ Complete blood count
■ Platelet function test
■ Prothrombin time, partial thromboplastin time

PREOPERATIVE MEDICATION

All patients should receive intravenous sedation, if appropriate (midazolam and fentanyl titrated to effect),

and intravenous antibiotics (ceftriaxone 1 g or ciprofloxacin 400 mg if the patient is allergic to penicillin) or ciprofloxacin 500 mg orally 30 minutes prior to the procedure.

MONITORING

All patients' vital signs should be monitored by American Society of Anesthesiologists' standards.

PROCEDURE

The patient is positioned prone and prepared and draped in a sterile manner (Fig. 31–3A). The C-arm image is turned obliquely, and the inferior end plate is flattened to help visualize the disc space (Fig. 31–3B). After sterilization of the lumbar region and appropriate draping of the patient, the entry site is infiltrated with 1% lidocaine at the selected disc space. The spinal or Chiba needle is introduced just lateral to facet joint (superior pars) in the middle of the disc (Fig. 31–4). After the introduction of the needle into the rubbery substance of the annulus using a tunnel view, a lateral view is taken (Fig. 31–5).

Needle placement is confirmed with posteroanterior and lateral fluoroscopic views. Final needle position should be in the midline without touching the end plate in both views (Figs. 31–6 and 31–7; see also Fig. 31–5). The needle is then attached to an in-line

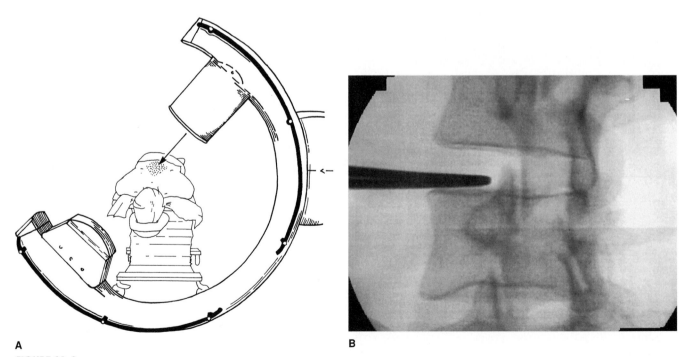

A **B**

FIGURE 31–3

A, This illustration shows the patient in prone position and the C-arm is turned oblique to identify the superior pars. *B,* Identification of the site of entry for needle insertion for discography.

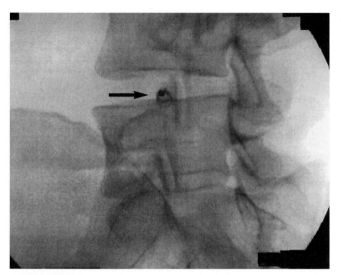

FIGURE 31-4

The spinal or Chiba needle (arrow) is introduced just lateral to the facet joint (superior pars) in the middle of the disc.

pressure transducer monitor with video recording of the patient's face (Fig. 31–8). A known volume of water-soluble, non-ionic contrast material and cefazolin (1 mg/mL) is then injected. The fluoroscopic image shows three needles in position in posteroanterior and lateral views (Figs. 31–9 and 31–10).

INTERPRETATION OF PRESSURE MONITORING

Based on the provocation of pain and the pressure at which that pain is produced, a disc is determined to be symptomatic or not symptomatic. Chemically sensitive discs are defined as reproduction of patient's pain at less than 15 psi. Mechanically sensitive discs are defined as exact reproduction of patient's pain at 15 to 50 psi (Table 31–1). Pressure is increased to 1.5 times standing pressure (75 psi) to a maximum pressure of 120 psi and within 15 psi of opening pressure.

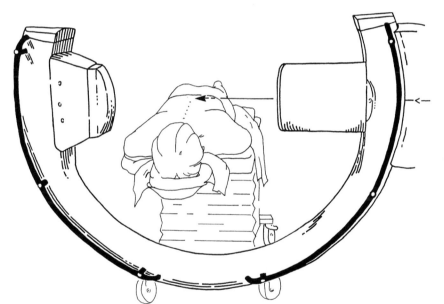

FIGURE 31-5

The fluoroscope is turned to the lateral position.

TABLE 31-1 Manometric Classification of Intervertebral Disc

Disc Classification	Pounds Force per Square Inch (psi) Above Opening Pressure at Which Pain Occurs	Subjective Assessment of Pain	Result
Chemically sensitive	Onset of pain with <15 psi >opening pressure	Replication of patient's usual pain	Positive; may be a candidate for IDET
Mechanically sensitive	Onset of pain between 15 to 50 psi > opening pressure	Replication of patient's usual pain	Positive; may be candidate for LASE or surgical discectomy
Indeterminate	Onset of pain at pressures >50 psi above openingpressure	Pain pattern dissimilar to usual pain	Negative; further investigation for other sources of pain is warranted

psi, pounds-force per square inch; IDET, intradiscal electrothermal Coagulation;
Adapted from Derby R, Howard MW, Grant JM, et al: The ability of pressure-controlled discography to predict surgical and nonsurgical outcomes. Spine 24:364–372, 1999.

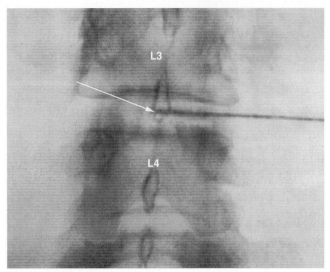

FIGURE 31–6

Anteroposterior view of the needle in the disc *(arrow)*, final view.

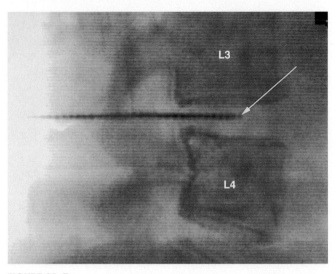

FIGURE 31–7

Lateral view of the needle in the disc *(arrow)*.

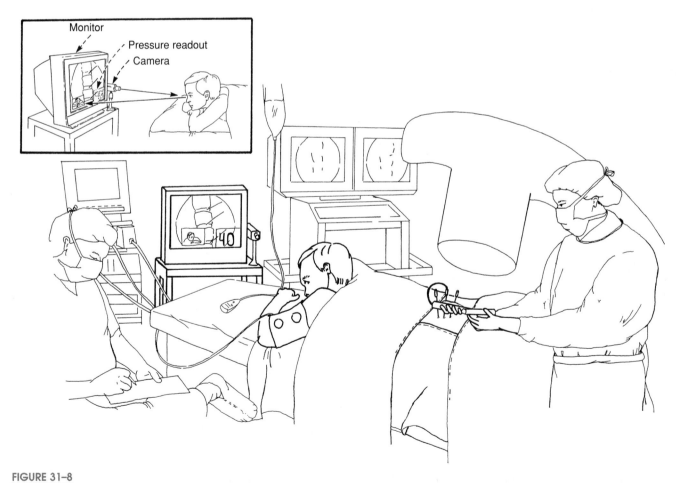

FIGURE 31–8

Drawing of the patient in a position to be monitored when disc pressure is measured with video imaging of his face.

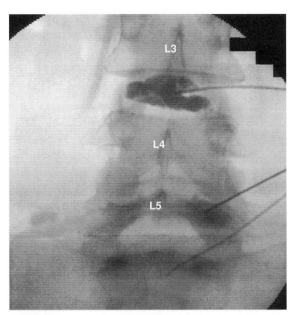

FIGURE 31–9

The fluoroscopic image shows three needles in position in the posteroanterior views.

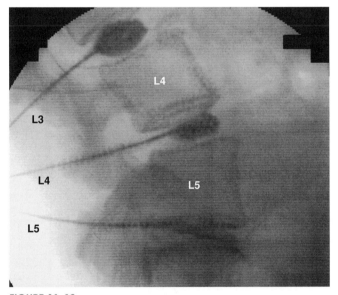

FIGURE 31–10

The needles are shown placed in the lateral view.

Following discography, all patients are sent for CT scan for visualization of the internal disc structure. It should be performed within 2 hours of injection to ensure that the contrast material has not been extravasated from the disc. It is recommended that at least five to seven slices per disc be performed (Figs. 31–11 and 31–12). If the end plate has a defect, thin cuts need to be used. Axial images should be obtained to best visualize the internal disc and associated disruption.[36] Typical imaging patterns in normal and abnormal discograms are shown in Figures 31–13 and 31–14.

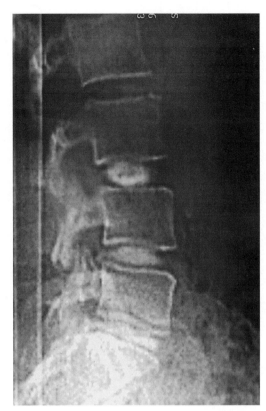

FIGURE 31–11

Lateral view of the contrast material in the discs following discography.

Efficacy is not discussed here because this technique is used only for diagnostic studies.

HELPFUL HINTS

Entry into the disc is facilitated by "squaring up" the inferior end plate of the cephalad vertebrae. Pain may occur 2 to 12 hours after disc puncture and persists for 2 to 3 weeks. Postprocedural recommendations include the following:

- Use a back support, brace, or corset
- Limited lifting is recommended; ask the physician for further recommendations

Anteroposterior and lateral views of discograms should be obtained to confirm the presence of disc leaks because of the two-dimensional limitations of fluoroscopic imaging. If two views are not obtained, a "normal" disc pattern may be found to be "abnormal" in the other view.

COMPLICATIONS

Pease[35] in 1934 discussed pain generation in patients undergoing lumbar puncture. He thought that this was due to inadvertent disc puncture. He demonstrated nar-

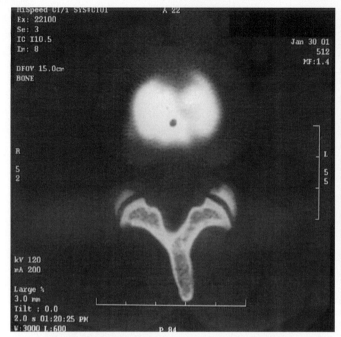

A

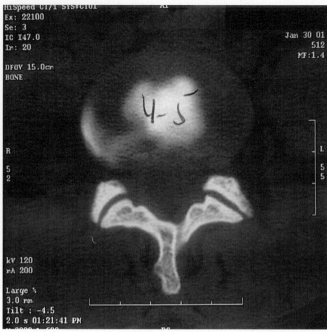

B

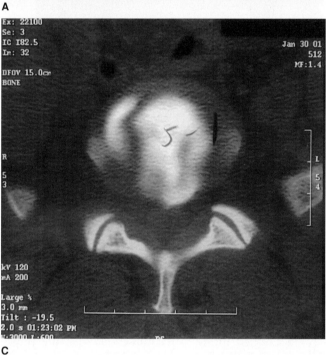

C

FIGURE 31–12

A–C, CT scan of the contrast material in the discs following discography. (*A* = L3, *B* = L4, and *C* = L5.)

rowing of the lumbar disc after introduction of the needle intradiscally in a 2-year-old child. He was also concerned about the possibility of the introduction of organisms into the disc space, setting up the possibility of a localized infection process.[35]

Desezes and Levernieux in 1952 described 55 cases at 12 months postdiscography that had disc necrosis with isolated areas of tissue degradation.[36] Goldie[37] in 1957 studied 122 discs removed at operation, 53 of which had been previously studied with discography. Twenty-eight of 53 discs showed edema, rupture, and the presence of hyaline droplets, which were thought to be a reaction to the contrast material.

Collins[3] in 1975 reported complications in only 5 of more than 2000 cases of discography. These were 1 infected disc space, 1 broken needle, 1 cauda equina syndrome, and 1 diatrizoate (Hypaque) reaction (later determined to be a subarachnoid injection). He also reported headaches, febrile reactions, myalgias, allergic reactions, and increased symptoms.

Johnson[38] in 1988 described two categories for potential side effects: (1) discitis (septic and aseptic) and (2) disc rupture. Goldie reported on sterile discitis in rabbits[37] and Desezes and Levernieux[36] reported on discitis in humans. Johnson described 34 patients undergoing serial discograms at 80 levels and found no evidence of

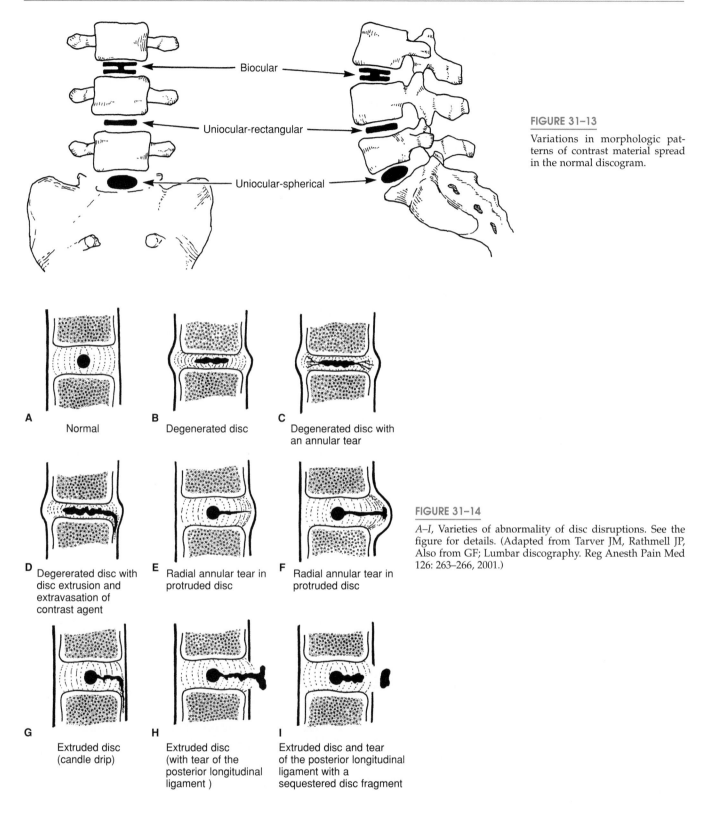

FIGURE 31–13

Variations in morphologic patterns of contrast material spread in the normal discogram.

A Normal

B Degenerated disc

C Degenerated disc with an annular tear

D Degererated disc with disc extrusion and extravasation of contrast agent

E Radial annular tear in protruded disc

F Radial annular tear in protruded disc

G Extruded disc (candle drip)

H Extruded disc (with tear of the posterior longitudinal ligament)

I Extruded disc and tear of the posterior longitudinal ligament with a sequestered disc fragment

FIGURE 31–14

A–I, Varieties of abnormality of disc disruptions. See the figure for details. (Adapted from Tarver JM, Rathmell JP, Also from GF; Lumbar discography. Reg Anesth Pain Med 126: 263–266, 2001.)

damage to a normal disc. He defined parameters such as type and volume of contrast medium, the gauge of needle used, and the frequency of annular puncture as possible causes for disc rupture. Flanagan and Chung[39] in 1986 reported no significant deleterious effects on the lumbar spine despite consistent disc space narrowing associated with chemonucleolysis.

Fraser and associates[40] in 1987 described discitis in sheep discs inoculated with bacteria. They believed that discitis is a common and important complication that is often underestimated. This is due to a latent period between injection and onset of symptoms, a lack of clinical contact by the clinician performing the discogram, and a lack of awareness of complications by the clinician. They reported a 4.9% incidence of discitis without the use of prophylactic antibiotics. Osti and colleagues[41] in 1990 studied the incidence of discitis postdiscography after prophylaxis with antibiotics. Antibiotics given intravenously 30 minutes prior to disc puncture or given intradiscally prevented radiologic, neurologic, and histologic evidence of discitis. They proposed using a styleted needle and a two-needle technique to help decrease the incidence of discitis. An often-unrecognized complication of discography is a delayed pain response. Lehmer and coworkers[42] described a 2.5% incidence of delayed pain response in individuals whose initial discogram failed to elicit a pain response. There may be a delay of 2 to 12 hours lasting as long as 2 weeks.[42] Patients complained of pain of a different character (groin, thigh, and calf pain tenderness). It is believed that this represents leakage of contrast over time and stimulation of the outer third of the annulus in a normal disc.[42] Therefore, close follow-up over 24 hours is recommended.

Diskography, each level; lumbar 62290; interpretation, diskography; lumbar 72295–26.

REFERENCES

1. Linblom K: Diagnostic puncture of intervertebral disks in sciatica. Acta Orthop Scand 17:231, 1948.
2. Hirsch C: An attempt to diagnose the level of a disc lesion clinically by disc puncture. Acta Orthop Scand 18:132, 1948.
3. Collins HR: An evaluation of cervical and lumbar discography. Clin Orthop 107:133–138, 1975.
4. Holt EP Jr: The question of lumbar discography. J Bone Joint Surg Am 50:720–726, 1968.
5. Crock HV: Internal disc disruption: A challenge to disc prolapse fifty years on. Spine 11:650–653, 1986.
6. Bogduk N, Modik MT: Lumbar discography. Spine 21:402–404, 1996.
7. Inoue H: Three-dimensional architecture of lumbar intervertebral discs. Spine 6:138–146, 1981.
8. Bogduk N: The interbody joint and the intervertebral discs. In Bogduk N (ed): Clinical Anatomy of the Lumbar Spine, 3rd ed. New York, Churchill Livingstone, 1997, p 16.
9. Tehranzadeh J: Discography 2000. Radiol Clin North Am 36:463–495, 1998.
10. Marchand F, Ahmed AM: Investigation of the laminate structure of lumbar disc annulus fibrosus. Spine 15:402–410, 1990.
11. Armstrong JR: Lumbar Disc Lesions, 3rd ed. Edinburgh, Churchill Livingstone, 1965, p 13.
12. Jayson MIV, Barks JS: Structural changes in the intervertebral disc. Ann Rheum Dis 32:10–15, 1973.
13. Peacock A: Observations on the prenatal development of the intervertebral disc in man. J Anat 85:260–274, 1951.
14. Moore KL: Clinically Oriented Anatomy, 3rd ed. Baltimore, Williams & Wilkins, 1992, pp 342–343.
15. Hirsch C, Paulson S, Sylven B, Snellman O: Biophysical and physiological investigations on cartilage and other mesenchymal tissues: IV. Characteristic of human nuclei pulposi during aging. Acta Orthop Scand 22:175, 1952.
16. Nachemson A: Measurement of intradiscal pressure. Acta Orthop Scand 28:269–289, 1959.
17. Puschel J: Der Wasserhalt normaler und degenerierter Zwischenwirbelscheiben. Beitr Z Path-Anat Uz Allg Path 84:123, 1930.
18. Keyes DC, Compere EL: The normal and pathological physiology of the nucleus pulposus of the intervertebral disc: An anatomical, clinical, and experimental study. J Bone Joint Surg 14:897, 1932.
19. Sylven B: On the biology of nucleus pulposus. Acta Orthop Scand 20:275, 1950.
20. Fabris G, Lavaroni A, Leonardi M, et al: Discography. Del Centauro Udine, Italy, European Society of Neuroradiology, 1991.
21. Virgin WJ: Experimental investigations into the physical properties of the intervertebral disc. J Bone Joint Surg Br 33:607–611, 1951.
22. Nachemson AL: Disc pressure measurements. Spine 6:93–97, 1981.
23. Beard HK, Stevens RL: Biochemical changes in the intervertebral disc. In Jayson MIV (ed): The Lumbar Spine and Back Pain, 2nd ed. London, Pitman, pp 407–436.
24. Naylor A: Intervertebral discs prolapse and degeneration: The biochemical and biophysical approach. Spine 1:108–114.
25. Naylor A, Shental R: Biochemical aspects of intervertebral discs in aging and disease. In Jayson MIV (ed): The Lumbar Spine and Back Pain. New York, Grune & Stratton, pp 317–326.
26. Nachemson A: Lumbar intradiscal pressure. Acta Orthop Scand Suppl 43:1–104, 1960.
27. Adams MA, Hutton WC: The effect of posture on the fluid content of lumbar intervertebral discs. Spine 8:665–671, 1983.
28. Ohshima H, Tsuji H, Hirano N, et al: Water diffusion pathway, swelling pressure, and biomechanical properties of the intervertebral disc during compression load. Spine 14:1234–1244, 1989.
29. Lu YM, Hutton WC, Gharpuray VM: The effect of fluid loss on the viscoelastic behavior of the lumbar intervertebral disc in compression. J Biomech Engineer 120:48–54, 1998.
30. Wilke HJ, Neef P, Caimi M, et al: New in vivo measurements of pressures in the intervertebral disc in daily life. Spine 24:755–762, 1999.
31. Botsford DJ, Esses SI, Ogilvie-Harris DJ: In vivo diurnal variation in intervertebral disc volume and morphology. Spine 19:935–940, 1994.
32. Gresham J, Miller R: Evaluation of the lumbar spine by discography and its use in selection of proper treatment of the herniated disc syndrome. Clin Orthop 67:29–41, 1969.
33. Brodsky AE, Binder WF: Lumbar discography. Spine 4:110–120, 1979.
34. Guyer RD, Ohnmeiss DD: Contemporary concepts in spine care: Lumbar discography. Spine 20:2048–2059, 1995.
35. Pease CN: Injuries to the vertebrae and intervertebral discs following lumbar puncture. Am J Dis Child 849–860, 1934.
36. Desezes A, Levernieux J. Rev de Rheum 19:1027, 1952.
37. Goldie I: Intervertebral disc changes after discography. Acta Clin Scand 113:438, 1957.
38. Johnson R: Does discography injure normal discs? Analysis of recent discograms. Spine 14:424–426, 1989.
39. Flanagan MN, Chung BU: Roentgenographic changes in 188 patients 10 to 20 years after discography and chemonucleolysis. Spine 11:444–448, 1986.
40. Fraser RD, Osti OL, Vernon-Roberts B: Discitis after discography. J Bone Joint Surg Br 69:26–35, 1987.
41. Osti OL, Fraser RD, Vernon-Roberts B: Discitis after discography: The role of prophylactic antibiotics. J Bone Joint Surg Br 72:271–274, 1990.
42. Lehmer SM, Dawson MH, O'Brien JP: Delayed pain response after lumbar discography. Eur Spine J 3:28–31, 1994.

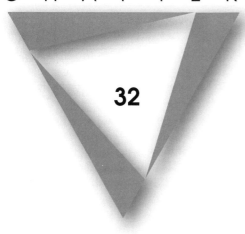

C H A P T E R

32

Intradiscal Electrothermal Coagulation

HISTORY

There is no definitive history of who first used the procedure now known as *intradiscal electrothermal coagulation* (IDET). Van Kleef and Barendse[1] were the first to publish a description of an intradiscal lesioning technique.

ANATOMY

The intervertebral disc is composed of three structures: the annulus fibrosus, the nucleus pulposus, and the end plates (Fig. 32–1). The annulus surrounds the nucleus in a beltlike fashion, and the end plates cover the superior and inferior aspects of the nucleus. Although the end plates do not completely cover the annulus, the collagen fibers of the most superficial lamellae of the annulus insert directly into the bone of the vertebral body.[2, 3] These lamellae that join the annulus, and consequently the end plates and nucleus, run obliquely from one vertebra to another. This arrangement, although allowing some movement between adjacent vertebra, provides a very strong bond between them.[4] Before the degenerative changes associated with aging are seen, the lamel-lae fully cover the vertebral bodies. Later, they are absorbed secondarily into the bone.[5]

The annulus fibrosus is a concentric lamellae of fibrocartilage made of collagen and fibroblasts that surround the nucleus.[4] Although the concept of the annulus is that of a complete ring or belt, in any given quadrant, 40% of the lamellae are incomplete, and in the posterolateral quadrant, some 50% are incomplete.[5, 6] The lamellae are thicker toward the center of the disc.[6] Similarly, they are thick in the anterior and lateral portions of the annulus. However, posteriorly they are finer and more tightly packed. Consequently, the posterior portion of the annulus fibrosus is thinner than the rest of the annulus.[7–9] This ultimately leads to more tears posteriorly.[4, 10]

The nucleus pulposus consists of a three-dimensional network of collagen fibers, enmeshed in a mucoprotein gel that contains various mucopolysaccharides.[11, 12] The water content of the nucleus pulposus diminishes with increasing age,[11–14] whereas the polysaccharides complex decreases and is replaced by collagen.[12, 15] The proteoglycans of the center allow for absorption and dispersion of forces.[4, 16] This allows the disc to act as a shock absorber for axial forces and like a

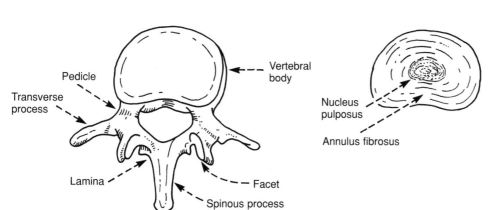

A
Pedicle
Transverse process
Vertebral body
Lamina
Facet
Spinous process

B
Nucleus pulposus
Annulus fibrosus

FIGURE 32–1

Anatomic structure of the lumbar vertebral body *(A)* and the lumbar disc *(B)*.

207

semifluid ball-bearing during flexion, extension, rotation, and lateral flexion of the vertebral column.[4]

It is known that in the healthy back, only the outer third of the annulus fibrosus of the intervertebral disc is innervated. However, in diseased intervertebral discs (such as in internal disc disruption), due to the stimulation of nociceptive fibers in the disc, neovascularization and neural expression of substance P occur. These nerve fibers demonstrate ingrowth into the inner third of the annulus fibrosus and nucleus pulposus. Freemont and associates[16] suggested that the finding of the nerve fibers in the inner third expressing substance P and their association with pain gives credence to the important role for nerve growth into the intervertebral disc in the pathogenesis of chronic low back pain.

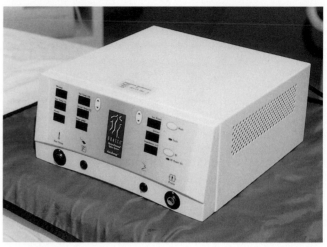

FIGURE 32–2

The Oratec intradiscal electrothermal coagulation lesioning base unit.

INDICATIONS

- Lumbar discogenic pain by provocative discography[17]
- Low back pain from internal disc disruption
- Limited herniation (disc bulge)

CONTRAINDICATIONS

- Local infection
- Coagulopathy
- Discitis
- Nerve root compression[18]

EQUIPMENT

- Thermal navigable catheter (Spine-CATH)
- 17-gauge needle introducer
- Thermal delivery system, including generator and extension cable (Fig. 32–2)
- 25-gauge, 1½-inch needle for subcutaneous infiltration
- 22-gauge, 3½-inch needle for infiltrating deeper tissue
- 18-gauge, ½-inch needle for piercing the skin
- LuerLok syringes (10-, 5-, or 3-mL)
- Sterile drapes (fenestrated) and C-arm drape

DRUGS

- 1.5% lidocaine plain for local infiltration
- Antibiotics for intravenous prophylaxis and intradiscal injection
- Sedatives for intravenous administration

PREPARATION OF THE PATIENT

Pain and guarded movements are the cardinal features of discogenic pain.[18] Otherwise, the condition is characterized by essentially normal radiographic and computed tomographic (CT) images. Provocative discography is the definitive test for this diagnosis.

In 1979, Brodsky and Binder[19] characterized the mechanism for the provocation of pain with discography. Their findings included (1) stretching of the fibers of an abnormal annulus; (2) extravasation of extradurally irritating substances such as glycosaminoglycans, lactic acid, and acidic media; (3) pressure on nerves posteriorly caused by bulging of the annulus; (4) hyperflexion of posterior joints on disc injection[20]; and (5) the presence of vascular granulation tissue, with pain caused by scar distention.[21] Another mechanism speculated was pain generators in the end plates that may be provoked by end plate deflection.[20]

LABORATORY

- Complete blood count with platelets
- Prothrombin time and partial thromboplastin time
- Platelet function study and bleeding time

PREOPERATIVE MEDICATION

For preoperative medication, use the standard American Society of Anesthesiologists' (ASA) recommendations for conscious sedation.

MONITORING

For monitoring, use the standard ASA recommendations for this procedure.

PROCEDURE

Prior to the procedure, the patient is given 1 g of intravenous ceftriaxone (antibiotic).

POSITION OF THE PATIENT

The patient is placed in the prone position on the fluoroscopy table (Fig. 32–3).

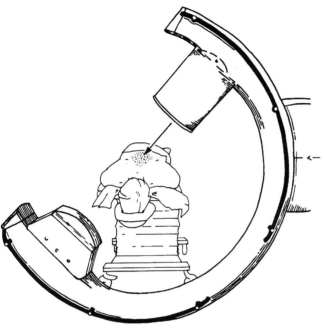

FIGURE 32–3

The drawing shows the patient's position and the C-arm in the oblique position to visualize the disc and its end plates.

TECHNIQUE

The lumbosacral area is prepared and draped in a sterile manner. The patient is lightly sedated with midazolam and fentanyl. The infiltration of the L2 root sleeve (transforaminal epidural) injection is recommended prior to the intradermal electrothermal coagulation procedure. The injection is with local anesthetic only to provide postprocedural pain relief.

For the placement of the introducer needle, the proper disc level is identified under fluoroscopic view. It is important to align the inferior end plates (bringing the superior pars "up" to the disc level). To accomplish this, some cephalocaudal trajectory may be required in the lower lumbar spaces to adjust for lordosis. This trajectory may be as much as 25 to 30 degrees. The fluoroscopic beam is then obliqued to place the spinous processes lateral, and the facet line should appear "midline". This may be referred to as the "Scottie dog" view. It is important to obtain the required amount of oblique view, because less than adequate rotation will cause a lateral placement of the needle.

At the midpoint of the superior articular process, at the lateral edge, a skin wheal is raised with 1 mL of 1.5% preservative-free lidocaine using a 25-gauge needle. It is important to anesthetize not only the skin but also the subcutaneous tissues to the level of the superior pars. Therefore, more anesthetics and a longer needle (25-gauge, 3.5-inch spinal needle) are required (Fig. 32–4A).

A "nick" is made over the targeted site with an 18-gauge needle. The 17-gauge introducer needle is inserted through the opening. A "tunnel" view is maintained and the needle is advanced to the superior pars (Fig. 32–4B). It is important to make contact with the

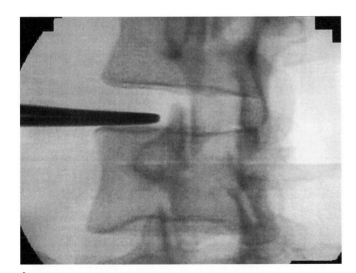

A   **B**

FIGURE 32–4

A, Radiographic marker that identifies the entry point on the skin for approaching the disc. B, "Tunnel" view of the introducer needle (arrow) just lateral to the superior pars articulares.

superior pars at its most lateral aspect. This provides safety: As one barely touches the bone, it will not change the trajectory of the introducer needle causing lateral placement.

Frequent lateral views are taken. This provides the physician with accurate depth of the needle. Keep the introducer needle facing the posterior wall of the discs as it enters the annulus. The annulus will provide resistance and feel "gritty" to the physician as the needle passes. This will be followed by a sudden loss of resistance.[18] The needle should be placed in this transitional zone between the annulus and the nucleus; this should be confirmed in both the posteroanterior and lateral views (Figs. 32–5 and 32–6).

Once the introducer needle is properly placed, the navigable catheter is threaded through the needle hub. When using the Spine-CATH system, the curve at the

tip of the catheter and the white line on the catheter handle should be aligned with the bevel marker on the needle hub and facing to the posterior aspect of the disc.[22]

As the catheter is advanced into the needle, note when the first bold depth marker on the catheter enters the needle hub. This indicates the tip of the catheter has reached the tip of the introducer needle.[22] Using continuous fluoroscopic guidance, in the lateral view the catheter will pass in the transitional zone between the annulus and the nucleus and curl inside the disc at the interface of the nucleus and the interior annular wall.

Ideal placement is the posterior third of the disc, across the midline of the posterior wall, and centered between the plates.[22] Note that the catheter must not be outside of the disc wall. Also note that when the second bold marker of the proximal shaft enters the needle, the heater end has completely exited the tip of the needle into the disc (Figs. 32–7 and 32–8).[22] The fluoroscope is then rotated cephalocaudad to view the catheter from the top of the disc (Fig. 32–9). This should be observed as radiopaque markers of the resistive coil being outside of the introducer needle.

Care must be taken not to force the catheter or kinking will result. If the physician observes significant resistance to movement, especially during withdrawal of the catheter through the introducer needle, both the needle and the catheter should be immediately removed together.

After proper catheter placement, the catheter is heated to 65°C. The temperature is then raised 1°C every 30 seconds until the desired therapy level is reached. Ideally, this is between 80°C and 90°C, 4 to 6 minutes, to thoroughly distribute the heat. The total time for a heating lasts between 14 to 17 minutes. As the temperature increases, the patient is continuously evaluated for back pain and any other signs of nerve root irritation

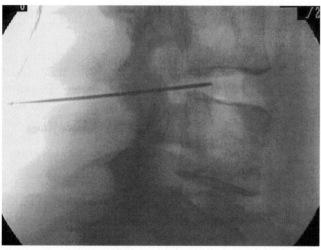

FIGURE 32–5

Lateral view of the introducer needle in the transition zone between the annulus fibrosus and the nucleus pulposus.

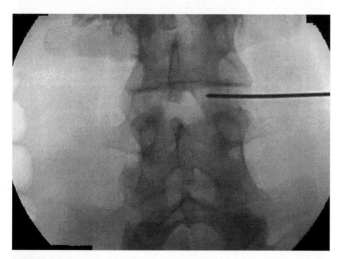

FIGURE 32–6

Anteroposterior view of the introducer needle in the transition zone between the annulus fibrosus and the nucleus pulposus.

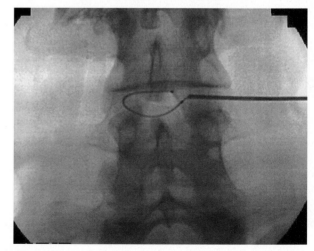

FIGURE 32–7

Anteroposterior view of the lumbar spine with the Spine-CATH in place.

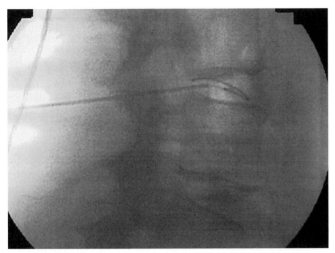

FIGURE 32–8

Lateral view of the lumbar spine with the Spine-CATH in place at L4–L5.

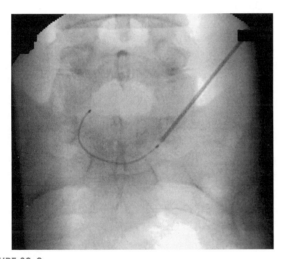

FIGURE 32–9

Cephalocaudal view of the Spine-CATH in the L4–L5 created by the curvature of the lumbosacral spine in an anteroposterior radiographic image.

such as extremity pain. It is expected that there may be reproduction of back or extremity pain concordant with the patient's normal symptoms.[22]

It is important to monitor the impedance. Prior to placement of the catheter, this should be checked and verified that it is within the acceptable range of 120 to 200 Ω. This range should be maintained throughout the thermocoagulation and is an indicator of a functioning power circuit.[22]

After the thermocoagulation is complete, gently remove the catheter. This may require some rotation. Intradiscal antibiotics (1 mL of 5 mg/mL cefazolin) should be administered through the needle. After removal of the introducer needle, the site is covered with antibiotic ointment and a Band-Aid dressing.

COMPLICATIONS

Immediate
- Improper placement of the introducer needle results in trauma to neural structures, vasculature, or retroperitoneal structures, including the kidneys[17]
- Complications from the catheter itself include shearing, kinking, and thermal injuries due to improper placement. Ability to communicate with the patient during the procedure helps prevent complications related to movement

Late
- Infection[18]
- Discitis
- Epidural abscess
- Meningitis[18]
- Increased back pain

HELPFUL HINTS

It is important to educate patients regarding an increase in their typical back pain after the procedure. This usually will subside over the first 1 to 7 days. The patient may require supplemental pain medications during this time. It the pain persists, without tapering, after the first week, an oral prednisone taper may be considered.[9] It is important to not overlook the patients' complaints of back pain, which may be due to infection. Other options for treatment of the back pain during the first month include nonsteroidal anti-inflammatory drugs, ice, and bed rest.

The patient's activities are limited for the first 6 weeks. The patient should be fitted for a lumbar corset to wear immediately postprocedure for the first 6 weeks. The function of the corset is to limit the activity of the back of the patient. While the patients are limited on sitting time (20 to 45 minutes),[22] they are encouraged to begin walking and perform gentle leg stretching. The patient should be in an active physical therapy program from weeks 6 to 12 to gradually increase activity and educate regarding basic lumbar stabilization exercises. Patients may be expected to return to full physical activity (e.g., tennis, golf, and running) in 4 to 6 months.[22]

EFFICACY

In a preliminary report by Saal and Saal,[23] 25 patients with chronic discogenic back pain were treated with IDET and had a mean follow-up of 7 months. Of the 25 patients, 20 (80%) reported a reduction of at least 2 points in visual analog pain scores and 18 (72%) reported an improvement in sitting tolerance as well as reduction or discontinuation of analgesic medication. No significant complications were reported.

In a later prospective outcome study by Saal and Saal,[24] 62 patients were followed for a minimum of 1 year. The mean follow-up in this study was 16 months and the mean preoperative duration of symptoms was 60 months. Baseline and follow-up outcome measures demonstrated a mean change in the visual analog score of 3.0. They also demonstrated a statistically significant clinical improvement.

Karasek and Bogduk[25] used a case-control study to compare 35 patients treated with IDET and 17 patients treated with a physical rehabilitation program. These 52 patients were determined to have internal disc disruption by CT discography. At 3 months, only one control patient obtained any significant degree of relief of pain, compared with 23 in the IDET treatment group. Patients treated with IDET demonstrated sustained relief of pain at 6 and 12 months. They also showed improvement in disability, reduced drug use, and a return to work rate of 53%.[25] IDET was determined to eliminate or dramatically reduce the pain of internal disc disruption in a substantial proportion of patients. It also appeared to be superior to conventional conservative care.[12]

REFERENCES

1. Van Kleef M, Barendse GA: Percutaneous intradiscal radiofrequency thermocoagulation in chronic nonspecific low back pain. Pain Chronic Pain Clin 9:259–268, 1996.
2. Inoue H: Three-dimensional architecture of lumbar intervertebral discs. Spine 6:138–146, 1981.
3. Bogduk N: The interbody joint and the intervertebral discs. In Bogduk N (ed): Clinical Anatomy of the Lumbar Spine, 3rd ed. New York, Churchill Livingstone, 1997, p 16.
4. Tehranzadeh J: Discography 2000. Radiol Clin North Am 36:463–495, 1998.
5. Marchand F, Ahmed AM: Investigation of the laminate structure of lumbar disc annulus fibrosus. Spine 15:402–410, 1990.
6. Armstrong JR: Lumbar Disc Lesions, 3rd ed. Edinburgh, Churchill Livingstone, 1965, p 13.
7. Jayson MIV, Barks JS: Structural changes in the intervertebral disc. Ann Rheum Dis 32:10–15, 1973.
8. Peacock A: Observations on the prenatal development of the intervertebral disc in man. J Anat 85:260–274, 1951.
9. Moore KL: Clinically Oriented Anatomy, 3rd ed. Baltimore, Williams & Wilkins, 1992, pp 342–343.
10. Hirsch C, Paulson S, Sylven B, Snellman O: Biophysical and physiological investigations on cartilage and other mesenchymal tissues: IV. Characteristic of human nuclei pulposi during aging. Acta Orthop Scand 22:175, 1952.
11. Nachemson A: Measurement of intradiscal pressure. Acta Orthop Scand 28:269–289, 1959.
12. Puschel J: Der Wasserhalt normaler und degenerierter Zwischenwirbelscheiben. Beitr Z Path-Anat Uz Allg Path 84:123, 1930.
13. Keyes DC, Compere EL: The normal and pathological physiology of the nucleus pulposus of the intervertebral disc: An anatomical, clinical, and experimental study. J Bone Joint Surg 14:897, 1932.
14. Sylven B: On the biology of nucleus pulposus. Acta Orthop Scand 20:275, 1950.
15. Fabris G, Lavaroni A, Leonardi M, et al: Discography. Del Centauro Udine, Italy, European Society of Neuroradiology, 1991.
16. Freemont AJ, Peacock TE, Goupille P, et al: Nerve ingrowth into diseased intervertebral disc in chronic back pain. Lancet 350:178–181, 1997.
17. Waldman SD, Siwek SM, Waldman KA: Intradiscal electrothermal annuloplasty. In Waldman SD (ed): Interventional Pain Management, 2nd ed. Philadelphia, WB Saunders, 2000, pp 703–706.
18. Schwarzer AC, Aprill CN, Derby R, et al: The prevalence and clinical features of internal disc disruption in patients with chronic low back pain. Spine 20:1878–1883, 1995.
19. Brodsky AE, Binder WF: Lumbar discography. Spine 4:110–120, 1979.
20. Wiley JJ, Macnab I, Wortzman G: Lumbar discography and its clinical applications. Can J Surg 11:280–289, 1986.
21. Heggeness MH, Doherty BJ: Discography causes end plate deflection. Spine 18:1050–1053, 1993.
22. IntraDiscal ElectroThermal Therapy: Training Course Syllabus. Menlo Park, CA, Oratec Interventions, Inc, 1999, pp 11–12.
23. Saal JS, Saal JA: Management of chronic discogenic low back pain with a thermal intradiscal catheter: A preliminary report. Spine 25:382–388, 2000.
24. Saal JA, Saal JS: Intradiscal electrothermal treatment for chronic discogenic low back pain: A prospective outcome study with minimum 1-year follow-up. Spine 25:2622–2627, 2000.
25. Karasek M, Bogduk N: Twelve-month follow-up of a controlled trial of intradiscal thermal anuloplasty for back pain due to internal disc disruption. Spine 25:2601–2607, 2000.

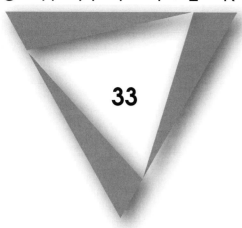

C H A P T E R

33

Vertebroplasty

HISTORY

Vertebroplasty is the percutaneous augmentation of a vertebral body using polymethylmethacrylate (PMMA). PMMA was first introduced in 1970 by Charnley for orthopedic use in total hip replacements.[1, 2] In 1984, Galibert and associates[3] performed percutaneous vertebral augmentation using PMMA in France. They placed the PMMA in a cervical vertebra of a 50-year-old woman with a C2 vertebral hemangioma with a long-term complaint of neck pain. The procedure was then called *percutaneous vertebroplasty*.[3] In 1988, Bascoulergue and colleagues[4] used percutaneous vertebroplasty for treatment of compression fractures caused by osteoporosis or malignancy. In the United States, Mathis[5] and Jensen[6] introduced percutaneous vertebroplasty to treat compression fractures in 1993.

ANATOMY

THORACIC VERTEBRA

The thoracic vertebrae are intermediate in size between those in the cervical region and those in the lumbar region, and they increase in size from above downward, the upper vertebrae in this segment of the spine being much smaller than those in the lower part of the region. The thoracic vertebrae may be at once recognized by the presence on the sides of the body of one or more facets or half-facets for the heads of the ribs (Fig. 33–1A).

- The *bodies* of the thoracic vertebrae resemble those in the cervical and lumbar regions at the respective ends of this portion of the spine; however, in the middle of the dorsal region, their form is very characteristic, being heart

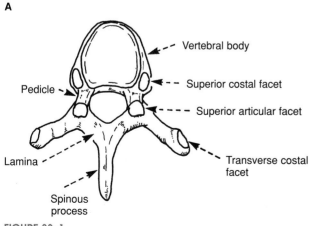

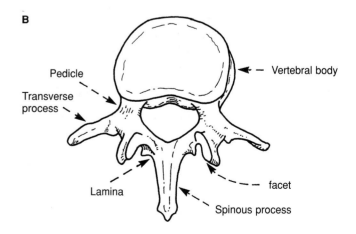

FIGURE 33–1

Anatomic structure of the thoracic *(A)* and lumbar *(B)* vertebrae.

shaped and as broad in the anteroposterior as in the lateral direction. They are thicker behind than in front, flat above and below, convex and prominent in front, deeply concave behind, slightly constricted in front and at the sides, and marked on each side, near the root of the pedicle, by two demi-facets, one above, the other below.

- The *pedicles* are directed backward, and the inferior intervertebral notches are of large size, and deeper than in any other region of the spine.
- The *laminae* are broad, thick, and imbricated, overlapping one another like tiles on a roof.
- The *spinal foramen* is small and circular.
- The *spinous processes* are long, triangular on transverse section, directed obliquely downward, and terminate in a tubercular extremity. They overlap one another from the fifth to the eight but are less oblique in direction above and below.
- The *articular processes* are flat, nearly vertical in direction, and project from the upper and lower part of the pedicles, the superior being directed backward and slightly outward and upward, the inferior forward and a little inward and downward.
- The *transverse processes* arise from the same parts of the arch as the posterior roots of the transverse processes in the neck and are situated behind the articular processes and pedicles; they are thick, strong, and of great length, directed obliquely backward and outward, presenting a clubbed extremity, which is tipped on its anterior part by a small concave surface.

LUMBAR VERTEBRA

The lumbar vertebrae are the largest segments of the vertebral column and can at once be distinguished by the absence of the foramen in the transverse process, the characteristic point of the cervical vertebrae, and any articulating facet on the side of the body, the distinguishing mark of the thoracic vertebrae (Fig. 33–1*B*).

- The *bodies* are large and have a greater diameter from side to side than from front to back, slightly thicker in front than behind, flattened or slightly concave above and below, concave behind, and deeply constricted in front and at the sides, presenting prominent margins, which afford a broad basis for the support of the weight above.
- The *pedicles* are very strong, directed backward from the upper part of the bodies; consequently, the inferior intervertebral notches are of considerable depth.
- The *laminae* are broad, short, and strong, and the spinal foramen is triangular, larger than in the dorsal, smaller than in the cervical, region.

- The *spinous processes* are thick and broad, somewhat quadrilateral, horizontal in direction, thicker below than above, and terminate with a rough, uneven border.
- The *superior articular processes* are concave and look backward and inward; the inferior, convex, look forward and outward; the former are separated by a much wider interval than the latter, embracing the lower articulating processes of the vertebra above.
- The *transverse processes* are long, slender, directed transversely outward in the upper three lumbar vertebrae, slanting a little upward in the lower two. They are situated in front of the articular processes, instead of behind them as in the thoracic vertebrae, and are homologous with the ribs.

INDICATIONS

Vertebroplasty may be used for patients with compression fractures due to osteoporosis, metastatic tumors, or benign tumors such as vertebral angiomas.[7] Osteolytic metastasis and myeloma constitute the main indications for vertebroplasty. Myeloma has painful osteolytic lesions where vertebroplasty provides stabilization and pain relief. The best indication is severe back pain due to vertebral collapse.

Patients with metastasis and myeloma usually experience severe pain and disability.[7] Radiation therapy is indicated whenever pain is caused either directly or indirectly by a malignant lesion because such treatment affords partial or complete pain relief in more than 90% of patients.[7, 8] However, patients do not begin to experience relief until 10 to 14 days after the start of therapy. More important, radiation therapy results in minimal, delayed (2 to 4 months after the start of irradiation) bone strengthening, which is usually more effective in patients with myeloma than in those with metastases.[7, 9] This delay in bone reconstruction increases the risk of vertebral collapse and, consequently, of neural compression.

Vertebroplasty is performed to provide pain relief or to produce bone strengthening and vertebral stabilization when the lesion threatens the stability of the spine.[5, 10–13] Radiation therapy may be performed in conjunction with vertebroplasty when the latter is performed for tumor lesions because cement injection does not prevent tumor growth.[5] Radiation therapy does not interfere with the mechanical properties of bone cement[3] and complements its action with similar but delayed effects on pain and bone strengthening.[4] Vertebroplasty can also be performed after initial radiation therapy when the latter fails to relieve pain or in cases of local recurrence.[5, 7, 12, 14]

Vertebral hemangiomas are common benign lesions of the spine that are often asymptomatic and discovered incidentally during radiologic evaluation. Rarely, they may be painful, and there must be a close correlation between clinical findings and radiologic features to ensure that the patient's pain is due to the vertebral hemangioma. In such cases, vertebroplasty is performed to provide pain relief.[5] The PMMA is injected for pain relief, bone strengthening, and direct embolization of the hemangiomatous body.[3-5, 15-18] Vertebroplasty may be used prior to laminectomies or excision of the epidural hemangioma (when present) in cases of aggressive vertebral hemangiomas that result in spinal cord or nerve root compression.[5] A combination of vertebroplasty with surgery may be preceded by embolization of arteries feeding the vertebral hemangioma or used in conjunction with other percutaneous injections.[3, 5]

Vertebral fractures are the most common complication of osteoporosis.[19, 20] Age-related osteoporotic compression fractures occur in more than 500,000 patients per year in the United States.[21] About 15% of women in the United States older than 50 years of age will suffer one or more vertebra compression fractures related to osteoporosis. The lifetime risk of vertebral fracture for a 50-year-old white man is 5.4%. This number is increasing because of aging of the population and an increase in the age-specific incidence of fractures, and likewise in younger individuals with secondary osteoporosis.[20, 22] Not all patients make a complete and early recovery from stable fractures. About 75% of them were found to be suffering from persistent back pain symptoms.[20, 23] Currently, approximately 13% to 18% of the population or 4.6 million white women in the United States will be affected. It is expected that 50% of white women will have an osteoporotic fracture in her lifetime.

CONTRAINDICATIONS

Absolute
Lack of patient consent and a coagulopathy are absolute contraindications for almost any procedure, including vertebroplasty. Local infection at skin entry site is another absolute contraindication.

Relative
Extensive vertebral destruction and significant vertebral collapse (i.e., vertebra reduced to less than one third of its original height) may lead to a technically difficult procedure[5] (Table 33-1). Another relative contraindication is a patient with a radiculopathy into a lower extremity. Neurologic symptoms related to compression by the abnormal vertebral body or by tumor extension necessitate a cautious approach because any leakage of the PMMA could increase the compression.[5] The presence of cortical destruction or epidural or foraminal stenosis could also be of concern for leakage and compression.[5] Other relative contraindications

TABLE 33–1 Contraindications to Vertebroplasty

Absolute
Epidural involvement of the infiltrative lesion
Lack of patient consent
Coagulopathy

Relative
Extensive vertebral destruction
Significant vertebral collapse ($<\frac{1}{3}$ of original height)
Radiculopathy into the lower extremity
Disruption of the posterior vertebral wall
Lesions above T4
Patients who cannot lie prone

include disruption of the posterior vertebral wall, lesions above T4, and patients who cannot lie prone.[24]

EQUIPMENT

- 22-gauge, 3½-inch needle for deeper tissue infiltration
- 25-gauge needle for skin infiltration
- 3-mL syringe for local anesthetic infiltration
- No. 11 scalpel blade for creation of needle entry wound
- 11-gauge bone biopsy needle
- Sterile hammer
- Disposable mixing bowl and ladle
- Disposable PMMA injection syringe

DRUGS

- Codman Cranioplastic powdered polymer—13 mL
- Sterile barium sulfate powder—5 mL (6 g)
- Tobramycin powder—0.6 to 1.2 g
- Codman Cranioplastic liquid monomer—7.5 mL

PATIENT SELECTION AND PREPARATION

Patients most likely to benefit from vertebroplasty are those with a focal, intense, deep pain associated with plain film evidence of a new or progressive compression fracture.[9] This may be shown on a T2-weighted image on magnetic resonance imaging (MRI) with enhancement of the corresponding level versus a dark vertebral body that is devoid of edema.[24] Patients who seem to respond the best include those with a single level or a few levels for treatment, fractures that are present less than 2 months or a recent worsening of the fracture, and no significant sclerosis of the fractured vertebra.[24] It should also be determined if the patient is able to tolerate lying prone for 1 to 2 hours.[9]

PHYSICAL EXAMINATION

Computed tomographic (CT) imaging for the diameter of the pedicles to be entered is helpful. Recent plain radiographs should be examined.[24] Recent MRI should be available, particularly a T2-weighted sagittal image and axial views through the levels of pathology to be treated. In patients with multiple compression fractures, those vertebral bodies with enhancement demonstrate edema at that level and a greater likelihood of response.[24]

LABORATORY

- Prothrombin time, partial thromboplastin time
- Platelet function studies

PREOPERATIVE MEDICATION

Sedative analgesics in the form of fentanyl, midazolam, or propofol are administered.[9] Prior to the start of the procedure, a prophylactic antibiotic should be given intravenously. Cefazolin (Ancef) 1 g is recommended. Vancomycin may be considered as a substitute if the patient has a penicillin allergy.[24]

MONITORING

Standard monitoring includes blood pressure, heart rate, and pulse oximetry. Oxygen is supplied via a nasal canula.

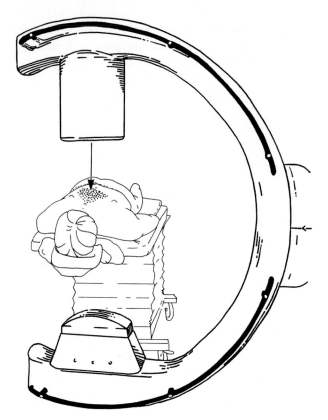

FIGURE 33–2

Drawing shows the fluoroscope positioned for a posteroanterior view of procedure side (vertebral level). The patient is prone.

PROCEDURE

POSITION OF THE PATIENT

The patient is taken to the fluoroscopy suite and placed in the prone position on the operating room table with all pressure points padded and standard monitoring applied (Fig. 33–2). Care is taken to add extra padding to the table (e.g., two egg crate mattresses) due to the osteoporotic spine and risk of rib fractures. Strict sterile technique is to be followed with full sterile drapes, masks, and gowns for all personnel in the operating room.

The level for the procedure is previously identified by physical examination and MRI. This vertebra is located in the posteroanterior fluoroscopic view.

The fluoroscope is then rotated to an oblique position to maximize the oval appearance of the pedicle (Fig. 33–3). Proper view is identified by seeing a "Scottie dog" appearance of the pedicle (Fig. 33–4). It is important to "flatten out" the end plates of the vertebral bodies; if necessary, cephalocaudad or caudocephalad fluoroscopic angle may improve the image.[24]

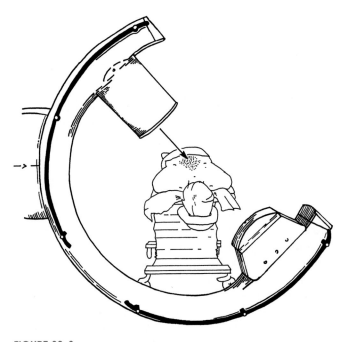

FIGURE 33–3

Drawing shows the rotation of the fluoroscope to obtain the oblique view of the vertebral level where the procedure is to be performed.

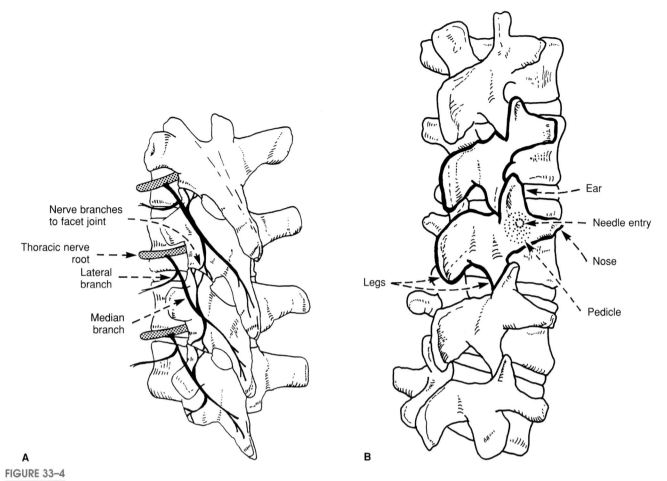

A

B

FIGURE 33-4

A, An oblique view of a thoracic vertebra shows a "Scottie dog" image. *B*, An oblique view of the lumbar vertebral bodies shows the Scottie dog image.

This will locate the pedicle well within the vertebral body in the fluoroscopic view. It is important to oblique the fluoroscopic view enough to place the facet joint in the middle of the vertebral body and the spinous processes to the contralateral side. This facilitates a central placement of the needle. The target for entry is the superior lateral quadrant of the pedicle in the fluoroscopic view.

SITE OF ENTRY

After the site of entry is identified, a skin wheal is raised over the center of the pedicle using 1 mL of 1% lidocaine and a 25-gauge needle. For patient comfort, it is advised to infiltrate to the pedicle with a 25- or 22-gauge needle with the local anesthetic.[24] A small skin incision is made with a No. 11 blade scalpel to allow insertion of a large-bore biopsy needle. An 11-gauge bone biopsy needle (Cook) is inserted through the incision. It is advanced in "gun-barrel" fashion in the oblique fluoroscopic view to monitor direction (Fig. 33-5). The oblique view will show the needle shaft end-on as a circle within the center of the pedicle.

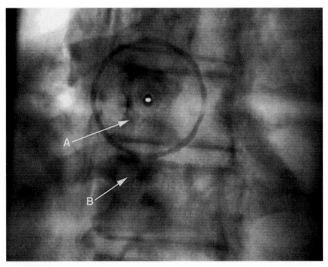

FIGURE 33-5

This radiograph shows the insertion of the needle in a gun-barrel fashion to enter the pedicle. This needle point entry needs to be done in the oblique view. *A*, Needle with wide, rounded hub inserted in the pedicles. *B*, The spine in the oblique view.

Once contact has been made with bone, insertion through the cortex of the bone may be accomplished

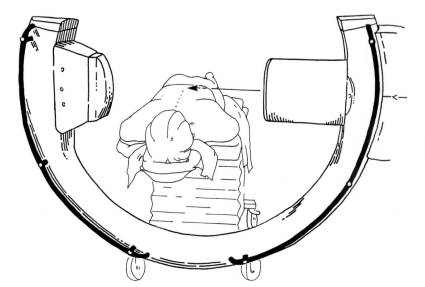

FIGURE 33–6

The position of the fluoroscope to examine the vertebral bodies in a lateral view.

with a twisting motion of the needle or gentle tapping of the needle with a sterile hammer. It is important to "set" the needle point at the exact site of entry.[24]

CONFIRMATION OF CORRECT NEEDLE POSITION

In the lateral view, the needle needs to be at the upper midpoint of the pedicle so that the needle advances in the midpoint of the pedicle (Fig. 33–6). The needle should follow a path that is parallel to the superior and inferior edges of the pedicle (Fig. 33–7). The needle is advanced to the junction of the anterior and middle third of the vertebral body (Fig. 33–8).

INJECTION OF CONTRAST MATERIAL AND ITS INTERPRETATION

After placement of the needle, the cement is prepared for injection. Codman Cranioplastic is recommended because of its radiopaque qualities. The amount to be mixed is based on the clinical observation of an average of 7 to 8 mL of cement injected in a lumbar vertebral body. Thirteen milliliters of Codman Cranioplastic polymer (powder) are mixed with 6 g of sterile barium sulfate in a container (approximately 18 mL total). Tobramycin powder (0.6 to 1.2 g) is also added. Slowly, the liquid monomer (approximately 7.5 mL) is added to the powder mixture.[24] The liquid monomer is titrated until the takes on a "toothpaste" or "cake-glaze" consistency. There are several delivery systems available that may be used to simplify the mixing and delivery in addition to decreasing fumes. If these systems are not available, 1-mL syringes may be filled and used one at a time to inject the cement into the vertebral body. The injection of the cement is followed

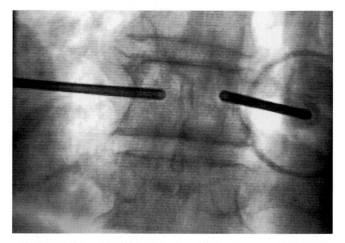

FIGURE 33–7

The radiographic image in a posteroanterior view shows the needle position on both sites of the vertebral body.

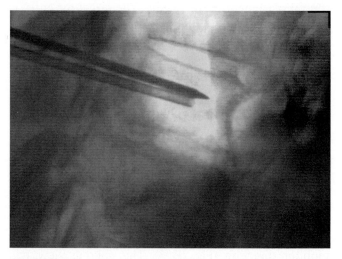

FIGURE 33–8

The radiographic image of the lateral aspect of the vertebral body shows the depth of the vertebroplasty needles inserted at the junction of posterior two thirds to the anterior one third.

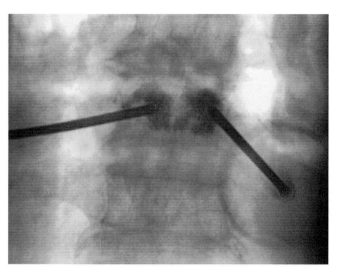

FIGURE 33–9

The radiographic image shows the cement injected through the needles and its spread in the vertebral body (posteroanterior view).

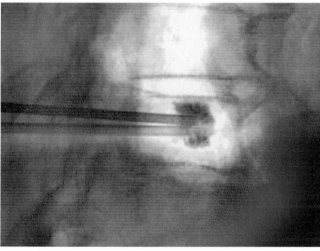

FIGURE 33–10

The radiographic image in the lateral view shows the spread of the cement in the vertebral body.

under fluoroscopic guidance in the lateral view (Fig. 33–9 and 33–10). When the spread of the cement starts to invade the posterior one third of the vertebral body, injection should be stopped. The cement is 90% fixed at 1 hour.

MONITORING OF CHANGES DUE TO PROCEDURE

After the procedure, the patient should be monitored for 3 hours in a recovery area prior to dismissal. The patient should be supine for 2 hours and then may sit.[24] A CT image through the levels (2-mm slices) is recommended for documentation purposes.[24] The patient is dismissed with routine pain medications and a graduated resumption of activity. Discharge instruction for

the patient should include advice to call the physician for the following[24]:

- New onset of back pain
- Chest pain
- Lower extremity weakness
- Fever > 100°F

COMPLICATIONS

Because of the size of the biopsy needle, there is risk of fracture of the lamina or pedicle. Preprocedural CT with pedicular diameter is helpful in assessing this risk. Owing to the vascularity of the vertebral body, there is the potential risk of pulmonary venous migration of the cement resulting in embolic phenomenon.[25]

It is important to observe the spread of the cement under direct fluoroscopy to monitor for foraminal and/or epidural extravasation. If vertebral epidural space extravasation occurs, there may be partial or complete paraplegia. Emergent operative decompression must be performed if the patient is symptomatic to minimize any damage. This risk is more common with vertebral destruction of the vertebral body from malignancy.[12]

An intradiscal leak of the PMMA may occur associated with cortical fracture or osteolysis of the vertebral end plates.[13] This does not seem to prevent pain relief. Secondary degenerative changes may develop because of this lea, but may not be deemed important due to the short life expectancy in these patients.[13]

The PMMA may leak into the adjacent paravertebral tissue because of the cortical osteolysis of the vertebral body or the hole produced by the needle after its removal.[13] This may lead to a transitory femoral neuropathy due to a leak into the psoas muscle.[13]

Aside from extravasation, the patient may complain of transient dermatomal pain due to rib fracture or mild nerve root compression.[26] Osteoporotic patients may fracture a rib with a vigorous cough. It is imperative to carefully pad the operating room table to minimize this complication.

HELPFUL HINTS

If more than one level is being performed, a Foley catheter in the bladder is inserted.

Ideally, there should be no destruction of the posterior wall of the vertebrae.

Venography may be performed at the discretion of the physician.[24] If performed, a non-ionic, water-soluble contrast dye (e.g., iohexol [Omnipaque]) is recommended. Venography may be used to assess the location of the paravertebral and epidural veins. If direct communication with a vein is observed, the needle may be advanced or the communication may be embolized with the injection of cement.

If leakage is observed into the disc space, there may be interference with visualization of the cement. It is recommended that the contrast material be washed out with saline.

A broad-spectrum antibiotic with good cerebrospinal fluid penetration for 7 days is recommended.

Follow-up after the procedure is at 1 week.

EFFICACY

Vertebroplasty is a percutaneous procedure with a low complication rate that provides immediate and long-term pain relief to patients suffering from chronic vertebral compression fracture pain. Although it remains important to provide conservative means of treatment including narcotics, adjunctive medications, and proper medical treatment of osteoporosis, vertebroplasty provides a minimally invasive procedure that may provide not only immediate relief but continued, prolonged relief that may increase the patient's daily activity level, which in turn helps provide a better quality of life. In a study performed by Jensen and coworkers,[6] 30 patients were treated with PMMA with 51 vertebral fractures. Of these patients, 90% reported immediate pain relief. Long-term pain relief (average of 255 days' follow-up) was reported in 80% of patients. In a study by Debussche-Depriester and associates,[27] PMMA was performed on 5 patients who reported the ability to ambulate in 24 to 48 hours. Weill and colleagues[28] performed 52 percutaneous vertebroplasties on 37 patients with spinal metastases. Seventy-three percent of these patients demonstrated continued improvement at 6 months.

Other peripheral nerve/myoneurals 64450; RFTC other nerve 64640.

REFERENCES

1. Follaci FM, Charnley J: A comparison of the results of femoral head prosthesis with and without cement. Clin Orthop 62:156–161, 1969.
2. Charnley J: The reaction of bone to self-curing acrylic cement: A long-term histological study in man. J Bone Joint Surg Br 52:340–353, 1970.
3. Galibert P, Deramond H, Rosat P, Le Gars D: Note preliminaire sur le traitement des angiomas vertebraux par vertebroplastic acrylic percutanee. Neurochirugie 33:166–168, 1987.
4. Bascoulergue Y, Duquesnel J, Leclercq R: Percutaneous injection of methylmethacrylate in the vertebral body for the treatment of various diseases [Abstract]. Radiology 169:372, 1988.
5. Mathis JM: Percutaneous Bone Augmentation to Treat Pain Associated with Vertebral Fracture. Presented at Vertebroplasty: A Hands-On Course, at the University of Maryland, Baltimore, MD, November 14, 1999.
6. Jensen ME, Evans AJ, Mathis JM, et al: Percutaneous polymethyl-methacrylate vertebroplasty in the treatment of osteoporotic vertebral body compression fractures: Technical aspects. AJNR Am J Neuroradiol 18:1897–1904, 1997.
7. Cotton A, Boutry N, Cortet B, et al: Percutaneous vertobroplasty: State of the art. Radiographics 18:311–322, 1998.
8. Sheperd S: Radiotherapy and the management of metastatic bone pain. Clin Radiol 39:547–550, 1988.
9. Gilbert HA, Kagam AR, Nussbaum H, et al: Evaluation of radiation therapy for bone metastases: Pain relief and quality of life. AJR Am J Roentgenol 129:1095–1096, 1977.
10. Cotton A, Dewatre F, Cortet B, et al: Percutaneous vertebroplasty for osteolytic metastases and myeloma: Effects of the percentage of lesion filling and the leakage of methylmethacrylate at clinical follow-up. Radiology 200:525–530, 1996.
11. Cotton A, Deramond H, Cortet B, et al: Preoperative percutaneous injection of methyl methacrylate and N-butyl cyanoacrylate in vertebral hemangiomas. AJNR A J Neuroradiol 17:137–142, 1996.
12. Deramond H, Galibert P, Depriester-Debussche C: Injections intra-osseus percutaneous dans le traitement palliantif des metastases occueses. Forum Metastases Os 80:36–40, 1993.
13. Deramond H, Depriester C, Toussain P: Vertebroplastie et radiology interventionnelle percutanee dans les metastases osseuses: Technique, indications, contraindications. Bull Cancer Radiother 80:277–282, 1996.
14. Deramond H, Darrasson R, Galibert P: Percutaneous vertebroplasty with acrylic cement in the treatment of aggressive spinal angiomas. Rachis 1:143–153, 1989.
15. Galibert P, Deramond H: La Vertebroplastic percutanee comme traitement des angiomas vertebraux et des affections dolorigenes et fragilisantes du rachis. Chirugie 116:326–335, 1990.
16. Deramond H, Debussche C, Pruvo JP, Galibert P: La vertebroplastie. Feuillets Radiol 30:262–268, 1990.
17. Laredo JD, Bellaiche L, Hubault A, Deramond H: Le traitement des hemangiomas vertebraux L'actualite rhumatologique (expansion scientifique) 30:332–346, 1993.
18. Kanis JA, McCloskey EV: Epidemiology of vertebral osteoporosis. Bone 13:S1–S10, 1992.
19. Rapado A: General management of vertebral fractures. Bone 18:191S–196S, 1996.
20. Melton LJ III, Kan SW, Frye MA, et al: Epidemiology of vertebral fractures in women. Am J Epidemiol 129:1000–1011, 1989.
21. Scane AC, Sutcliffe AM, Francis RM: The sequelae of vertebral compression fractures in men. Osteoporosis Int 4:89–92, 1994.
22. Young MH, Wales C: Long-term consequences of stable fractures of the thoracic and lumbar vertebral bodies. J Bone Joint Surg Br 55:295–300, 1973.
23. Heinemann DF: Osteoporosis: An overview of the National Osteoporosis Foundation clinical practice guide. Geriatrics 55:31–36, 2000.
24. Kaemmerlen P, Thiesse P, Jonas P, et al: Percutaneous injection of orthopaedic cement in metastatic vertebral lesion [Letter to the Editor]. N Engl J Med 321:121, 1989.
25. Krane SM, Holick MF: Metabolic bone disease. In Fauci AS, Braunwald E, Isselbacher KJ (eds): Harrison's Principles of Internal Medicine, 14th ed. New York, McGraw-Hill, 1998, pp 2247–2259.
26. Zoarski GH: Percutaneous Methacrylate Vertebroplasty. Presented at the 17th Annual Pain Symposium at Texas Tech University Health Sciences Center, Lubbock, TX, June 10, 2000.
27. Debussche-Depriester C, Deramond H, Fardellone P, et al: Percutaneous vertebroplasty with acrylic cement in the treatment of osteoporotic vertebral crush fracture syndrome. Neuroradiology 33(Suppl):149–152, 1991.
28. Weill A, Chiras J, Simon JM, et al: Spinal metastases: Indications for and results of percutaneous injection of acrylic surgical cement. Radiology 199:241–247, 1996.

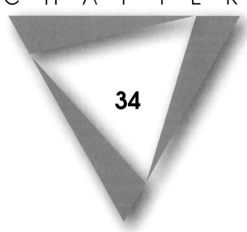

Psoas and Quadratus Lumborum Muscle Injection

HISTORY

Travell and Simons have been credited for identifying the psoas and quadratus lumborum muscles as the cause of low back pain and trigger point injections as the way of relief from their pain.[1, 2]

ANATOMY

ILIOPSOAS MUSCLE

Origins of the psoas major muscle start at the T12 vertebra and along the side of all the lumbar vertebrae. It attaches to the lesser trochanter of the femur. The iliacus muscle originates from the upper two thirds of the iliac

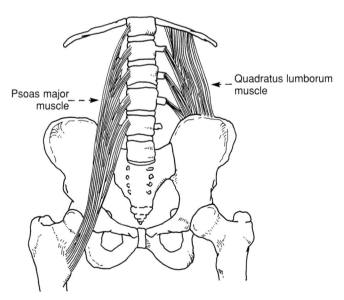

FIGURE 34–1

The drawing shows the origin and insertions of the psoas and quadratus lumborum muscles.

fossa and joins the psoas major tendon to attach directly to the femur near the lesser trochanter. The psoas muscle is active with sitting, standing, and maintaining posture. Flexion of the hip at the thigh is the primary function of the iliacus and psoas major muscle. Abduction and, possibly, some slight lateral rotation are assisted by these muscles (Fig. 34–1).

QUADRATUS LUMBORUM MUSCLE

The quadratus lumborum muscle attaches to three different structures: the ilium, the 12th rib, and the transverse processes of the upper four lumbar vertebrae. Adjacent thoracolumbar spinal nerves provide innervation. Functionally, the muscle acts as a lateral flexor and stabilizer of the lumbar spine. As a unit, the bilateral muscles can extend the lumbar spine and assist forced exhalation.

INDICATIONS

PSOAS MAJOR MUSCLE

The iliopsoas muscle, along with the quadratus lumborum muscle, is frequently responsible for failed low back postsurgical syndrome. Pain from the psoas major muscle is often referred from the ipsilateral spine in the thoracic region to the sacroiliac area. Occasionally, this pain extends to the upper buttocks.

QUADRATUS LUMBORUM MUSCLE

Symptoms of quadratus lumborum spasm are low back pain, pain with weight-bearing posture, and discomfort turning over in bed. Relief can be provided by positions or maneuvers that unload the lumbar spine of the upper body's weight. Simple coughing or sneezing can exacerbate the pain. History of irritation of pain is associated with falling, major body trauma, or any activity where one is simultaneously bending and reaching to one side to pull or lift something. Other factors that can cause persistence of this pain are leg-length discrepancies, small hemipelvis, and/or short upper arms.

CONTRAINDICATIONS

Absolute
- Local infection
- Abnormal bleeding disorders (coagulopathy)

Relative
- No radiographic imaging equipment

EQUIPMENT

- 25-gauge, 1½-inch skin infiltration needle
- 22-gauge, 5-inch needle for local anesthetic injection
- 3-mL syringe
- 10-mL three-ring syringe for contrast injection
- 20-mL syringe for local anesthetic injection
- IV T-piece extension
- Metal clamp for radiographic identification of entry site

DRUGS

- Radiographic contrast solution: iohexol (Omnipaque)

Local Anesthetics
- Lidocaine
- Bupivacaine
- Ropivacaine

Steroids
- Methylprednisolone acetate (Depo-Medrol)
- Methylprednisolone sodium succinate (Solu-Medrol)
- Dexamethasone (Decadron)
- Triamcinolone acetonide (Aristocort)

Neurolytics
- Sarapin
- 3% phenol
- 50% alcohol

Prolonged Action
- Botulinum toxin A
- Botulinum toxin B

PREPARATION OF THE PATIENT

PHYSICAL EXAMINATION

Psoas Major Muscle

Clinical examination involves tests that restrict extension of the thigh at the hip. There is increased pain with active straight-leg raise, which is decreased with passive lifting. Extension of the leg at the hip in the lateral decubitus position often increases the pain. Palpable trigger points can be performed at three locations (Fig. 34–2). Pressure at the insertion site deep in the lateral border of the femoral triangle over the trochanter elicits tenderness of the iliacus and psoas muscles. The uppermost iliacus muscle fibers can be

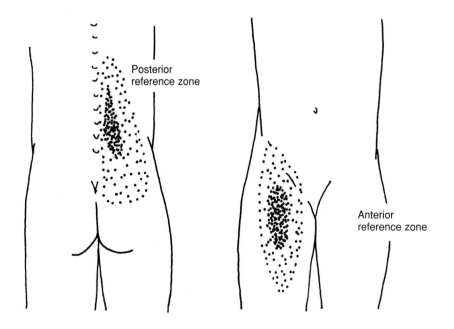

Posterior reference zone

Anterior reference zone

FIGURE 34–2

Reference zones of the psoas muscle are shown.

palpated at the ilium behind the anterior superior iliac spine. Psoas muscle tenderness is found by palpating through the abdominis muscle and compressing the psoas muscle medially against the lumbar spine (see Fig. 34–2).

Quadratus Lumborum Muscle

Physical examination shows muscular guarding and truncal rigidity with rolling over or rising into an upright posture. Trigger-point examination requires the patient to be in a prone position or any position where there is a palpable muscle area between the 12th rib and the iliac crest. There are four trigger-point locations consisting of two superficial (lateral) areas and two deep (medial) areas with a cephalad and caudal component for each pair. Palpation of the muscle just below the 12th rib and approximately 5 to 6 cm lateral to the spinous process of L1 elicits pain to the iliac crest and sometimes to the ipsilateral lower abdominal quadrant. The cephalad superficial trigger point is found at the L4 level about 1 to 2 cm above the posterior iliac crest and can refer pain to the greater trochanter. Deep or medial triggers of the quadratus lumborum muscle can be palpated at the transverse process of L3 and 2 cm above the posterior superior

iliac spine, with referred pain to the sacroiliac joint and lower buttocks, respectively (Fig. 34–3).

PREOPERATIVE MEDICATION

Standard American Society of Anesthesiologists' recommended sedation may be provided when necessary.

MONITORING

- Electrocardiogram
- Blood pressure
- Pulse oximeter
- IV access
- Nasal cannula for O_2 if necessary

PROCEDURE

POSITION OF THE PATIENT

The typical approach to the iliopsoas muscle involves fluoroscopy. The patient is placed in the prone position (Fig. 34–4).

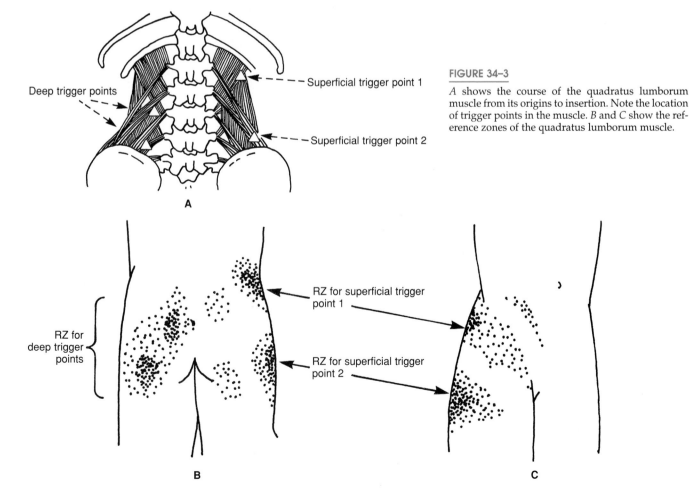

FIGURE 34–3

A shows the course of the quadratus lumborum muscle from its origins to insertion. Note the location of trigger points in the muscle. *B* and *C* show the reference zones of the quadratus lumborum muscle.

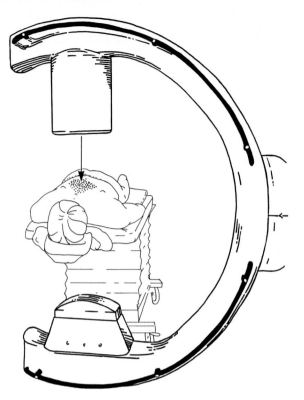

FIGURE 34–4

The patient lies in the prone position. The fluoroscope is positioned initially in the posteroanterior position to view the L3, L4, and L5 vertebrae.

SITE OF NEEDLE ENTRY

Psoas Major Muscle

Select a point approximately 5 cm lateral to the spinous process at the level of approximately the L3 level (or the top of the iliac crest). With a 22-gauge, 5-inch, B-level needle, insert the needle using a "gun-barrel" technique until the needle is approximately at the anterior one third of the vertebral body in the lateral view.

Quadratus Lumborum Muscle

Injection of the quadratus lumborum is safely done at the L3–4 level above the iliac crest. The muscle can be injected approximately 2 cm above the iliac crest and posterior superior iliac spine.

A 22-gauge, 1.5- to 2-inch B-bevel needle is inserted in a gun-barrel technique after skin infiltration with local anesthetics. The needle advancement is stopped when the needle tip is at the level of the transverse processes.

In the lateral view of the lumbar spine (Figs. 34–5 and 34–6), the tip of the needle should be behind the transverse process.

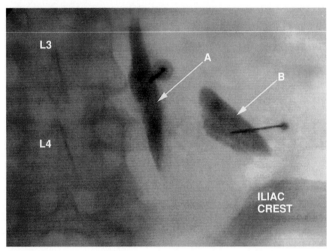

FIGURE 34–5

The fluoroscope shows the posteroanterior view of the lumbar spine. Note that *arrow A* indicates the spread of the contrast material in the psoas muscle at L3–L4. *Arrow B* shows the spread of contrast material in the quadratus lumborum muscle.

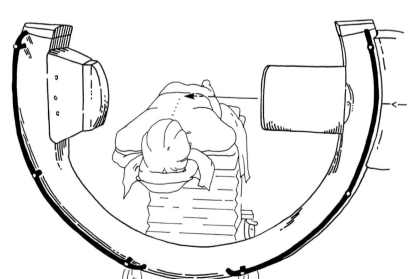

FIGURE 34–6

The position of the C-arm for viewing the lateral aspect of the lumbar spine.

CONFIRMATION OF CORRECT NEEDLE POSITION

In lateral view, psoas (Fig. 34–7, *arrow B*) major muscle spreads vertically over anterior one third of the lumbar vertebral body when contrast (iohexol) is injected. Note that it is always anterior to the foramen. The quadratus muscle, on the other hand, is seen posterior to the foramen at the level of the transverse processes (Fig. 34–7, *arrow A*). The needle should be at or below L3.

After the correct needle placement is confirmed, 8 to 10 mL of a local anesthetic–steroid mixture is injected into the psoas muscle on one side.

For the quadratus lumborum muscle, 4 to 6 mL of local anesthetic–steroid mixture should be injected. If botulinum toxin A or B is injected, one needs to follow the guidelines described in their manuals.

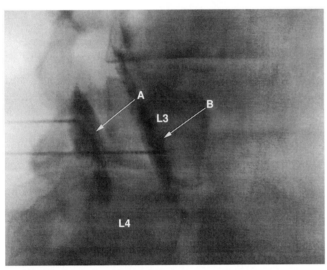

FIGURE 34–7

The fluoroscopic image shows the lateral aspect of the lumbar spine. *Arrow A* indicates the image of the contrast material in the quadratus lumborum muscle at the level and posterior to the transverse processes. *Arrow B* shows the image of contrast material in the psoas muscle at the mid and anterior one third of the vertebral bodies.

MONITORING OF CHANGES DUE TO PROCEDURE

- Relief of pain after local anesthetic injection should occur within 30 minutes.
- Botulinum toxin injection will give relief in 2 to 3 days.
- On examination, pain should be gone on flexion and extension of the hip.
- Quadratus lumborum muscle pain should be gone with flexion of the lumbosacral spine and rotation as if to tie the shoe or pick up the newspaper from the floor.

COMPLICATIONS

The complications of psoas and quadratus lumborum muscle injection include increased pain in area of injection, infection, or hematoma in the muscles.

HELPFUL HINTS

- Avoid potential damage by avoiding too long needles in the quadratus lumborum muscle injection.
- Lateral views should be used to confirm needle tip in muscular tissue.
- Psoas muscle injection should be at the lateral aspect of the transverse processes to avoid the nerve roots and the epidural space.

EFFICACY

Anecdotal reports suggest that the psoas and quadratus lumborum muscle injections are helpful. No double-blind, patient-controlled studies are available.

Other peripheral nerve/myoneurals 64450

REFERENCES

1. Travell JG, Simons DG: Myofascial Pain and Dysfunction: The Trigger Point Manual, vol 1. Baltimore, Williams & Wilkins, 1983.
2. Travell JG, Simons DG: Myofascial Pain and Dysfunction: The Trigger Point Manual, vol 2. Baltimore, Williams & Wilkins, 1992.

Sacral Nerve Root Injection

HISTORY

The origin of selective nerve root blockade (SNRB) can be traced back to 1906, when it was performed for urologic surgery. A few years later, Kappis[1] described the blockade of the brachial plexus via the cervical nerve roots. Over the ensuing century, selective root sleeve blocks have become commonplace in the diagnosis and treatment of many painful syndromes.

ANATOMY

The sacrum is a large, triangular bone composed of five fused sacral vertebrae (Fig. 35–1A). There are eight sacral foramina, each with a ventral and a dorsal opening. The dorsal sacral foramina are located just lateral to the intermediate sacral crest that represents the fused articular processes of the sacral vertebra.[2] The dorsal S1 foramen is located approximately 1 cm medial to the posterior superior iliac spine (PSIS), while the S2 foramen is 1 cm medial and 1 cm inferior to the PSIS. The S4 foramen is immediately lateral and just superior to the sacral cornu. The S3 foramen is located midway between the S2 and S4 foramina. The sacral foramina are somewhat rounded in form and diminish in size from above downward.

Nerves initially course through soft tissue spaces; the initial courses of the segmental sacral nerves are within the bony sacrum. Nerve roots divide into anterior and posterior divisions that exit the sacrum through their respective sacral foramina (S1–S4) (Fig. 35–1B and C). The fifth sacral nerve and the coccygeal nerve exit inferiorly through the sacral hiatus.

Posterior divisions supply the skin and musculature of the gluteal region. Anterior divisions, with the anterior divisions of L4 and L5, form the sacral plexus, which innervates the pelvic structures, perineum, and much of the lower extremity, mostly through its large sciatic nerve (L4–S3).

INDICATIONS

The SNRB, when combined with a careful history and physical examination, is an important tool in the diagnostic evaluation and treatment of patients with predominantly radicular symptoms.[3] It is helpful in patients with multiple level abnormalities and in patients with clearly defined clinical symptoms without significant imaging findings.[4] More specifically, an SNRB is useful in helping to (1) ascertain the specific nociceptive pathway; (2) define the mechanisms of the chronic pain state; and (3) establish the differential diagnosis of the site of the pain.[5]

SNRBs are also performed for prognostic and therapeutic purposes. Prognostically, the SNRB aids in predicting the efficacy of the neurolytic or neurosurgical treatment.[5–7]

The prognostic block also affords the patient the opportunity to experience the numbness and side effects that follow surgical resection or neurolytic block.[5] From this experience, the patient can decide whether or not to undergo the procedure. On a therapeutic basis, SNRBs are useful for treating pain not amenable to other methods of analgesia.

Clinical indications include pain secondary to nerve root compression, pain from tumor invasion of a nerve root or in the distribution of a nerve root, secondary to vertebral fractures, acute or postherpetic neuralgia, discogenic disease, or postoperative pain.[8, 9]

CONTRAINDICATIONS

- Local infection
- Coagulopathy
- Bony abnormality of the sacrum

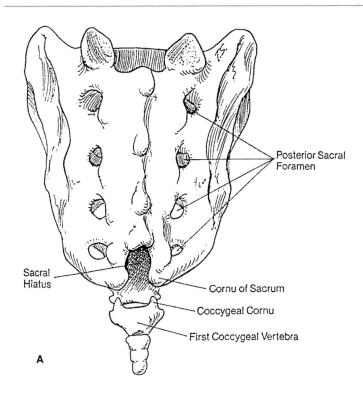

FIGURE 35–1

A, Anatomy of the sacral hiatus and dorsum of the sacrum. *B*, Anterior view of the sacrum with anterior sacral nerve root exiting. *C*, Lateral view of the sacrum that shows the sacral nerves exiting the foramen both anteriorly and posteriorly. (*A* From Raj PP [ed]: Clinical Practice of Regional Anesthesia. New York, Churchill Livingstone, 1991, p 328.)

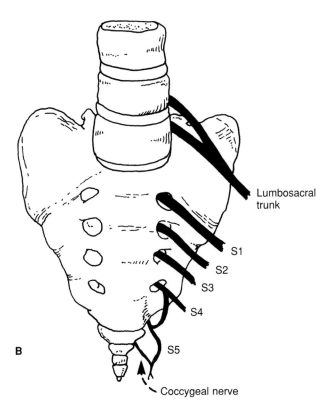

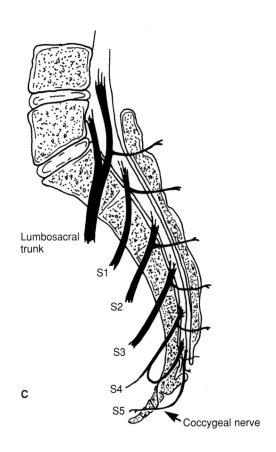

EQUIPMENT

Nerve Block
- 25-gauge needle for skin infiltration
- 20-gauge, 10-cm curved-blunt tip needle

- 16-gauge, 1½-inch angiocatheter
- 3-mL syringe
- 5-mL syringe
- 10-mL syringe
- IV T-piece extension set

Pulsed Electromagnetic Frequency or Radiofrequency Thermocoagulation—Additional Equipment

- 10-cm curved-blunt radiofrequency thermocoagulation (RFTC) needle
- RFTC electrode and connecting cables
- Grounding pad

DRUGS

- 1.5% lidocaine
- 2% lidocaine
- 0.5% bupivacaine/ropivacaine
- Steroids (optional)
- Iohexol (Omnipaque 240) radiographic contrast

PREPARATION OF THE PATIENT

One should examine for local infection and distorted anatomy that may interfere with performance of the procedure.

LABORATORY

Routine laboratory studies as indicated to rule out infection.

PREOPERATIVE MEDICATION

For preoperative medication, use the standard American Society of Anesthesiologists' recommendations for conscious sedation.

PROCEDURE

Block of the sacral nerve roots is accomplished through the posterior sacral foramen. The site of entry is visualized by adjusting the fluoroscopic beam to align the chosen posterior foramen with the anterior foramen (Fig. 35–2).[10] Insert the angiocatheter and blunt needle through the posterior foramen (Fig. 35–3) and advance the blunt needle toward the anterior foramen until the tip is just anterior to the anterior sacral plate on lateral view. Contrast material and local anesthetic can then be injected (Fig. 35–4).

A negative aspirate for blood and cerebrospinal fluid must precede any injection. All injections should be performed under fluoroscopic guidance to avoid intravascular or intrathecal spread.

A small amount (1 mL) of non-ionic, water-soluble contrast (iohexol) is injected slowly to avoid trauma to the nerve root. The spread of the contrast medium should delineate the nerve root only, with no spread into

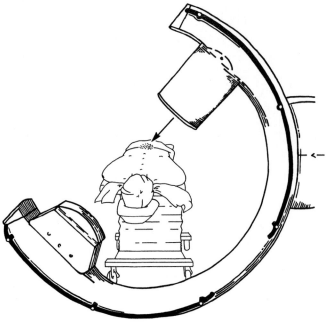

FIGURE 35–2

Line drawing of the fluoroscope C-arm and the patient position for sacral nerve root injection. The C-arm is rotated obliquely (lateral and cephalocaudal) to create a tunnel view of the posterior and anterior sacral foramen.

the epidural space or onto the peripheral plexus. If resistance is felt or vascular spread is noted, the needle must be redirected. After negative aspirate, inject 1 to 1.5 mL of local anesthetic (1% to 2% lidocaine or 0.25% to 0.5% bupivacaine) under fluoroscopic guidance. The patient should not feel any pain or paresthesia during injection. Remove the needle and place a sterile bandage.

Ganglionostomy of the sacral dorsal root ganglions (DRGs) has been done by some that requires the creation of a burr hole through the lamina or the posterior sacrum. The authors have been able to successfully place a curved-blunt tip needle through the posterior sacral foramen at the superior aspect to stimulate and lesion with RFTC or pulsed electromagnetic frequency (pEMF).

RADIOFREQUENCY OF THE SACRAL ROOTS (DRG)

The goal is to position the tip of the needle directly adjacent to the DRG of the desired nerve root. A sensory paresthesia should be felt in the desired dermatome at less the 1.0 V at 50-Hz stimulation. Ideal stimulation should be felt between 0.4 and 0.6 V. If stimulation is felt at less the 0.4 V, the tip of the needle is too close to the DRG, and if stimulation is felt at greater than 0.6 V, the tip is too far away from the DRG. Motor stimulation is then performed at 2 Hz. There should be a clear dissociation between motor

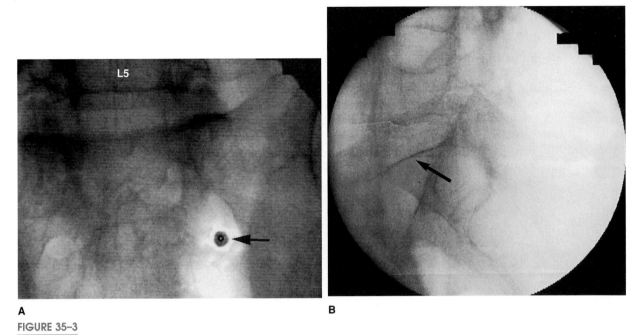

A   **B**

FIGURE 35-3

A, Oblique fluoroscopic view shows the needle over the right S1 foramen in the tunnel view. *B,* In this lateral view, the needle is shown entering from posterior to anterior SI foramen.

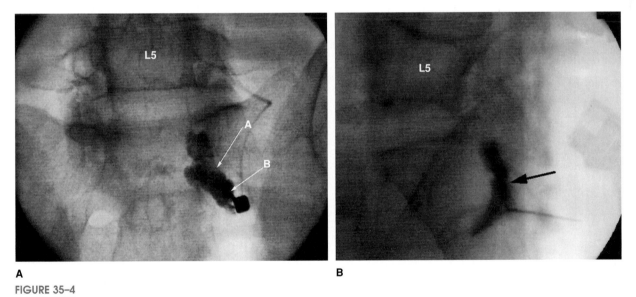

A   **B**

FIGURE 35-4

A, Anteroposterior radiographic image of a right S1 nerve root injection. *Arrow A* indicates the area where the contrast material is spreading within the bony canal and exiting with the anterior nerve root. *Arrow B* points to the needle. *B,* Lateral radiographic image with contrast material shows the spread within the bony canal and out the anterior neuroforamen *(arrow).*

and sensory stimulation; that is, the voltage required to see motor fasciculations at 2 Hz should be at least two times the voltage that produces sensory stimulation at 50 Hz.[11] Thus, if good sensory stimulation at 50 Hz is noted at 0.5 V, the motor fasciculations at 2 Hz should not be seen at voltages less than 1.0 V. The point of dissociation defines the position of the DRG. If dissociation between sensory and motor stimulation

cannot be obtained, the tip of the needle is not in alignment with the DRG, and lesioning at this point is not recommended.

Once the proper stimulation parameters have been achieved, inject 2 mL of local anesthetic with 40 mg of triamcinolone diacetate. Wait 3 to 5 minutes and then lesion at 67°C for 90 seconds with conventional radiofrequency.

PULSE ELECTRODE MAGNETIC FIELDS

For pEMF, the position of the curved tip of the needle should be similar to that placed for radiofrequency of the DRG. Once the correct site of needle is confirmed by fluoroscopy, then the sensory stimulation at 50 Hz should be done. One expects paresthesia in the distribution of that nerve root at about 0 to 3 V. PEMF is done at this site two or three times for 120 seconds and at 42°C. After pEMF, the care of the patient is similar to conventional radiofrequency.

COMPLICATIONS

One of the biggest concerns is damage to the nerve root while positioning the needle. Using a blunt-tip needle, one can reduce this complication. Neuritis after conventional radiofrequency lesioning is another concern. This is the reason for sensory and motor testing to be so important. If the proper parameters are not met, there is an increased incidence of postprocedure neuritis (30%). Injection of steroid prior to lesioning will help reduce, but not eliminate, the incidence of neuritis.

Other complications include intravascular and intrathecal injection of medication, paralysis, bowel and bladder incontinence, bruising, bleeding, increased pain, and infection.[12]

EFFICACY

No clinical data are available to evaluate the efficacy of this procedure; however, anecdotally, it has been shown to be useful.

REFERENCES

1. Kappis M: Erfahrungen mit Lokalansthesie bei Bauchoperationen. Verh Dtsch Ges Circ 43:87, 1914.
2. Blank J, Kahn C, Warfield C: Transsacral nerve root. In Hahn M, McQuillan P, Sheplock G (eds): Regional Anesthesia: An Atlas of Anatomy and Technique. St. Louis, Mosby–Year Book, 1996, pp 279–284.
3. Slosar P, White A, Wetzel F: The use of selective nerve root blocks: Diagnostic, therapeutic, or placebo? 23:2253–2256, 1998.
4. Link S, El-Khoury G, Guilford WB: Percutaneous epidural and nerve root block and percutaneous lumbar sympatholysis. Radiol Clin North Am 36:509–521, 1998.
5. Levy B: Diagnostic, prognostic, and therapeutic nerve blocks. Arch Surg 112:870–879, 1977.
6. Lamacraft G, Cousins M: Neural blockade in chronic and cancer pain. Int Anesthesiol Clin 35:131–153, 1997.
7. Guarino A, Staats P: Diagnostic neural blockade in the management of pain. Pain Digest 7:194–199, 1997.
8. Jain S: Nerve blocks. In Warfield C (ed): Principles and Practice of Pain Management. New York, McGraw-Hill, 1993, pp 379–399.
9. Pang W, Ho S, Huang M: Selective lumbar spinal nerve block: A review. Acta Anaesthesiol Sin 37:21–26, 1999.
10. Finch P, Taylor J: Functional anatomy of the spine. In Waldman S, Winnie A (eds): Interventional Pain Management. Philadelphia, WB Saunders, 1996, pp 39–64.
11. Kline M: Radiofrequency techniques in clinical practice. In Waldman S, Winnie A (eds): Interventional Pain Management. Philadelphia, WB Saunders, 1996, pp 185–218.
12. Botwin K, Gruber R, Bouchlas C, et al: Complications of fluoroscopically guided transforaminal lumbar epidural injections. Arch Phys Med Rehabil 81:1045–1050, 2000.

Hypogastric Plexus Block And Neurolysis

HISTORY

The first attempts to interrupt sympathetic pathways from the pelvis have been made by Jaboulay[1] in France and Ruggi[2] in Italy in 1899. Leriche[3] in 1921 performed a periarterial sympathectomy of the internal iliac arteries on a patient with "pelvic neuralgia," with good results. Cotte[4] presented a more systematic review in 1925. The first investigators to report superior hypogastric plexus block were Plancarte and associates.[5] Most recently, laparoscopically performed transection of the superior hypogastric plexus and stripping of the hypogastric nerves were reviewed by Chen.[6] De Leon-Casasola and colleagues[7] repeated the same study on 26 patients, but with fluoroscopy. Waldman and Wilson[8] described the use of computed tomographic scan to optimize needle placement. Kanazi and Frederick[9] have proposed an anterior approach. Other approaches to the superior hypogastric plexus have been reported, including a transvaginal approach[10] and a transdiscal technique.[11, 12]

ANATOMY

SUPERIOR HYPOGASTRIC PLEXUS

The superior hypogastric plexus is the extension of the aortic plexus in the retroperitoneal space, below the aortic bifurcation (Fig. 36–1). It receives fibers from the lumbar sympathetic nerve of L5. It is situated on the anterior aspect of L5–S1 and on the disc between L5 and S1. It lies close to sympathetic chain at this level, the common and internal iliac arteries and veins on each side. The ureter is located just lateral to these structures in close proximity to the anterolateral aspect of the L5 vertebral body. It contains almost exclusively sympathetic fibers. As it courses distally, the superior hypogastric plexus converges and forms a bilateral plexus called the *hypogastric nerve*. The hypogastric nerve follows the

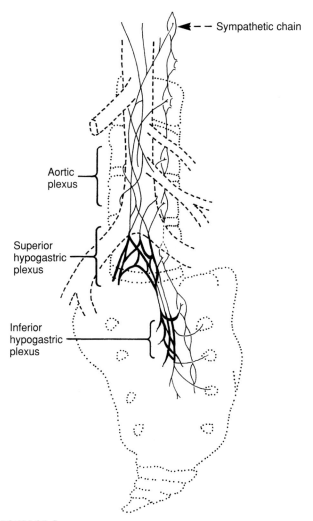

FIGURE 36–1

Anatomy of the hypogastric plexus.

internal iliac artery and vein and connects with the inferior hypogastric plexus at both sides of the pelvis. Hypogastric nerves carry sympathetic fibers only. Since the aorta is located more toward the left, the superior hypogastric plexus and the hypogastric nerves are shifted somewhat to the left as well. The anatomic location of the superior hypogastric plexus and the hypogastric nerves, the sympathetic predominance of the fibers of these plexus, and its role in transmission of most of the pain signals from the pelvic viscera should make these structures an ideal target for neural blockade.

INDICATIONS

The first group of patients consists of patients with gynecologic disorders in whom pain may or may not be dependent on the menstrual cycle. Most common causes of pain in these patients are endometriosis, adhesions, and chronic inflammation.

The second group consists of nongynecologic patients. Examples of patients in this group are those with interstitial cystitis, irritable bowel syndrome, or chronic pain after a surgical procedure such as suprapubic prostatectomy.

The third group of patients is those with neoplasms of the pelvic viscera.

CONTRAINDICATIONS

- Local infection
- Coagulopathy

EQUIPMENT

- 25-gauge, ¾-inch infiltration needle
- 20-gauge Racz-Finch radiofrequency thermocoagulation needle or curved-blunt needle
- 16-gauge, 1¾-inch angiocatheter as an introducer needle
- 22-gauge, 6-inch needle
- 18-gauge, 1½-inch needle for drawing up drugs and making skin puncture
- 3-mL syringe
- 10-mL three-ring syringe
- 10-mL syringe
- IV T-piece extension set
- Metal Markell clamp

DRUGS

- Iohexol (Omnipaque) radiopaque contrast solution
- Preservative-free normal (0.9%) saline
- 1.5% lidocaine for infiltration
- 0.5% bupivacaine or ropivacaine, preservative free
- 2% lidocaine, preservative free
- Water-soluble steroids
  Methylprednisolone
  Triamcinolone diacetate

- Triple-antibiotic ointment for skin

PREPARATION OF THE PATIENT

PHYSICAL EXAMINATION

On palpation is a usual tenderness over the ipsilateral tuberosity. This is described by Racz.[13] Other areas that can be tender are pubic bone perineum and ischial sacral fossa.

PREOPERATIVE MEDICATION

For preoperative medication, use the standard American Society of Anesthesiologists' (ASA) recommendations for conscious sedation.

MONITORING

Use the Standard ASA-recommended monitors, such as electrocardiogram, blood pressure determination, and pulse oximetry.

PROCEDURE

POSITION OF THE PATIENT

Patients are put in a prone position with fluoroscope in the posteroanterior position (Fig. 36–2).

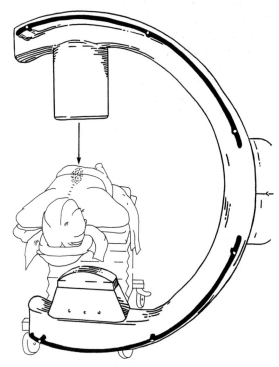

FIGURE 36–2

The patient is placed in the prone position. The beam of the C-arm fluoroscope is directed toward the L5–S1 vertebral level in the posteroanterior view.

SITE OF NEEDLE ENTRY

The L4–L5 spinous processes are identified. The skin is marked 5 to 7 cm lateral from the midline at this point (Fig. 36–3).

TECHNIQUE OF NEEDLE ENTRY

Lateral Approach

Draw a line lateral to the L4–L5 interspace and measure 7 cm. Use a 20-gauge, 15-cm needle. Direct the needle approximately 45 degrees medial and caudad to miss the transverse process of L5 and the sacral ala. In the lateral radiographic view, the needle tip needs to be at the anterior junction of L5–S1. In the anteroposterior view, the needle must be no more than 1 cm from the bony outline of L5–S1 (Figs. 36–4 and 36–5).

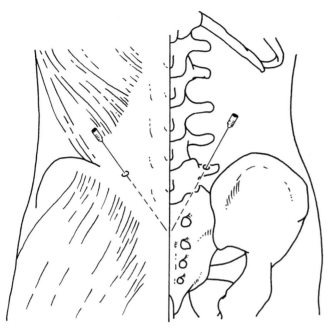

FIGURE 36–3

Lateral approach: The drawing of the landmarks in the low back region identify the needle point entry for hypogastric plexus block. Note the needle direction parallel to medial iliac border traversing toward L5–S1. (Adapted from Plancarte R, et al: Hypogastric plexus block: Retroperitoneal approach [Abstract]. Anesthesiology 71A:739, 1989.)

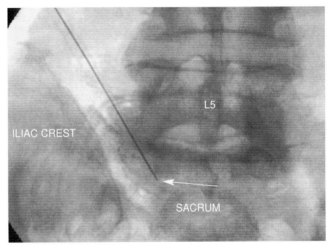

FIGURE 36–4

Posteroanterior view of a 22-gauge, 6-inch needle placed at the L5–S1 level parallel to the iliac medial border (lateral approach).

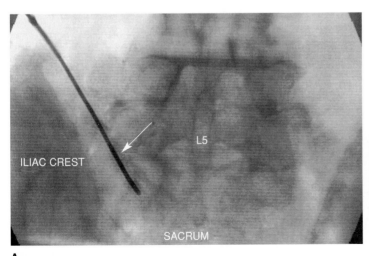

A

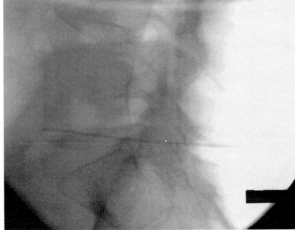

B

FIGURE 36–5

A, The posteroanterior view shows the radiofrequency needle (15 cm with 10-mm tip) in correct position for hypogastric plexus radiofrequency. B, Lateral view with the needle in position.

Medial Approach

Rotate the fluoroscopy C-arm 15 degrees caudally so that the x-ray beam looks into the pelvis (Fig. 36–6). This view enlarges the space between the L5 transverse process, sacral ala, and the posterior superior iliac spine. Under fluoroscopy using the 20-gauge, 15-cm needle, mark the most inferior and lateral part of this bone-free space. Place the needle and direct it medially and slightly caudad. Rotate the C-arm to a lateral view and observe the needle passing below this transverse process and cephalad to the superior part of the L5 neural foramen. When the anterior edge of L5 vertebral body is reached, aspirate; and if negative for blood, inject 4 to 5 mL of water-soluble contrast material. The contrast medium should be contained within the lateral bony edge, anterior to the psoas muscle, and above the sacral nerve roots (Figs. 36–7 to 36–10).

INTRADISCAL APPROACH FOR HYPOGASTRIC PLEXUS BLOCK

The procedure is performed under fluoroscopy. The patient is placed in the prone position with a pillow beneath the iliac crest to facilitate the opening of the intradiscal space. The L5–S1 intradiscal space is identified under fluoroscopy. Next, the fluoroscopy is placed in an oblique fashion and angled at 15 to 20 degrees or more for obtaining the best image of the disc to align the inferior end plates. To do so, cephalad trajectory is needed. The site of entry is point is approximately 5 to 7 cm from the midline. After local anesthetic

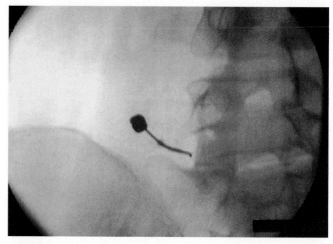

FIGURE 36–7

Medial paraspinous approach: The oblique view of the needle (curved-blunt) at the L5 level for hypogastric plexus block. The needle has traversed halfway to the site.

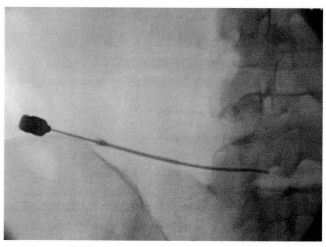

FIGURE 36–8

Medial paraspinous approach: Final position of the needle at the L5 for hypogastric plexus block (posteroanterior view).

infiltration of the skin and the tissues with 2% lidocaine, a 22-gauge block needle is introduced by tunnel vision lateral to the inferior aspect of the facet joint. The needle is introduced through the disc. While entering the disc, 1 mL of radiopaque iohexol solution is administered to verify the position of the needle within the disc. The position of the needle is controlled by lateral and anteroposterior vision.

The needle is advanced more under lateral view with a 5-mL syringe with saline until the resistance is lost. When the needle is again outside the L5–S1 intradiscal space, 2 mL of dye is administered to verify the final position of the needle. The dye is spread with a direct line image at that position. The same procedure is repeated from the opposite side. Inject the local anesthetic solution for diagnostic block or phenol for therapeutic block (Fig. 36–11).

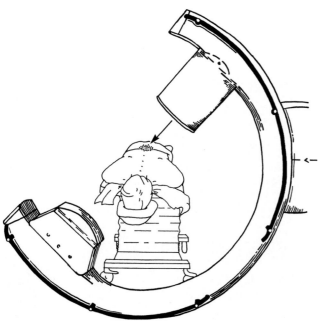

FIGURE 36–6

Position of the fluoroscope over L5–S1 for the paraspinous (medial) approach.

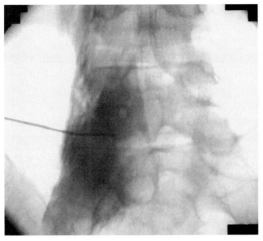

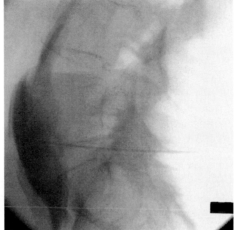

A   **B**

FIGURE 36–9

A, The posteroanterior view shows the dispersion of contrast iohexol (Omnipaque) solution to confirm the correct needle position. Note the solution spreading vertically, hugging the spine. *B,* Lateral view shows the contrast solution spreading from the L5–S1.

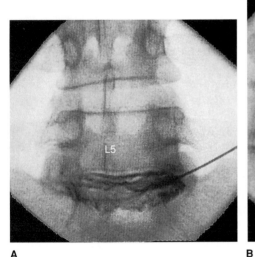

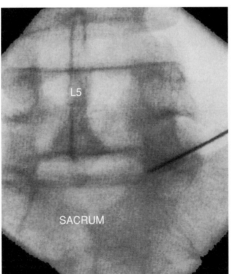

A   **B**

FIGURE 36–10

The posteroanterior view of a hypogastric plexus block through the L5–S1 disc (intradiscal technique). *A,* Step 1: needle entry in the L5–S1 disc. *B,* Step 2: contrast material in the disc confirming the needle entry in the disc.

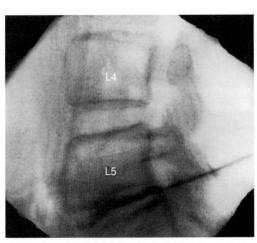

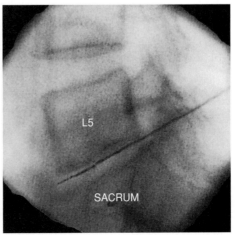

A   **B**

FIGURE 36–11

The lateral view of the needle through the L5–S1 disc while performing the hypogastric plexus block (intradiscal approach). The needle needs to be anterior to the disc. *A,* Step 3, needle in the lateral position with contrast material confirming the correct intradiscal position. *B,* Step 4, final needle position in the lateral view (intradiscal approach).

Anterior Approach

The patient is put in the supine position with the table in 15 degrees of Trendelenburg. The vertebral body of L5 can occasionally be palpated. A skin wheal is placed just 3 to 5 cm below the umbilicus. A 22-gauge, 6-cm needle is placed perpendicular to the floor and advanced until bony contact is made. At this time 20 to 30 mL of 0.25% bupivacaine is injected. Even though this technique has been performed occasionally, it is not recommended due to high risk of infection.

For diagnostic blockade, 6 to 8 mL of 0.25% bupivacaine is injected through each needle. For neurolysis, commonly 6% to 10% phenol with or without iohexol solution is injected on each side, up to 10 mL.

COMPLICATIONS

Table 36–1 lists common problems and solutions associated with hypogastric plexus block. There is a potential for intravascular injection in all approaches. A potential risk of discitis can occur with the intradiscal approach.

HELPFUL HINTS

- Measure the length of the needle required by placing the needle against the skin and taking a posteroanterior image.
- Bowel preparation prior to block is helpful to evacuate bowel content and gases.

EFFICACY

Plancarte and De Leon-Casasola[15] studied 227 patients who had chronic pelvic pain due to cancer in the largest study to date. By explicitly eliciting a history of vague, dull, poorly localized pain, the investigators attempted to select patients with predominantly visceral pain. The criteria for a successful diagnostic block were pain reduction of at least 50% lasting longer than 4 hours. Successful neurolysis was defined as a 50% pain reduction, a 40% reduction in use of opioid medication and effect lasting at least 3 weeks. It was shown that 115 (51%) of 227 patients reported good pain relief after therapeutic neurolysis of the superior hypogastric plexus; 159 of 227 patients reported good pain relief after diagnostic blockade. Limiting neurolysis to these positive responders, neurolysis was successful in 72%. A mean reduction in analgesic requirement of 43% was found in these patients. No major complications were reported. The investigators observed that effectiveness of the procedure depended mainly on the central position of the agent at L5–S1. Second neurolysis after initial failure of the procedure proved to be effective and did increase the overall success rate.

Erdine[12] presented 7 patients with chronic pelvic pain. He reported good pain relief in 5 patients, some pain relief in 1, and none in 1 patient.

In the Institute for Pain Management at the Texas Tech University Health Sciences Center (TT UHSC), superior hypogastric nerve blocks have been done for more than 10 years. The technique used at the TTUHSC is similar to the technique described by Plancarte and De Leon-Casasola.[15] A unilateral or bilateral technique is used. Because of the predominance of the plexus on the left side, the left side is always included. A blunt-curved needle is used to reduce the risk of trauma to neurovascular structures. A survey was performed on patients, who had undergone superior hypogastric plexus block for 4 years. Twenty-two patients were enrolled in this study. If these blocks were successful, most patients underwent therapeutic neurolysis with 6% phenol. Pain scores before and after treatments were obtained. A block was considered positive if more then 50% pain relief was provided for more than 4 hours. Therapeutic neurolysis was considered positive if pain relief was more than 50% and lasted longer than 1 month. Information on reduction of narcotic medication, improvement in functional status, and the occurrence of complications was obtained as well. Causes of pelvic pain were diverse and included endometriosis, adhesions, interstitial cystitis, and postprostatectomy pain. Ten (45%) of 22 patients had a positive response to diagnostic blockade (Table 36–2). Subsequently, 11 patients underwent 6% phenol injection.

▽ TABLE 36–1 Common Problems with Hypogastric Plexus Block

Problem	Solution
Touching L5 nerve root	Redirect needle
Intravascular spread of contrast material even in face of negative aspiration	Redirect; if problem not solved, abort procedure and repeat another day
Needle tip is too lateral	Withdraw and redirect

▽ TABLE 36–2 Pain Response to Hypogastric Plexus Block*

Type of Block	Pain Reduction (%)			
	0	<50	>50	100
Diagnostic	8/22	4/22	6/22	4/22
Neurolytic	3/11	4/11	3/11	1/11

*"Pain" refers to nonmalignant visceral pain. Numbers shown are the number of patients in the group with the corresponding level of pain response in relation to the total number of patients studied.

CONCLUSION

The superior hypogastric plexus, an extension of the preaortic plexus, is easily accessible to blockade by local anesthetics and neurolytic agents. Several techniques have been described. Long-lasting pain relief with this procedure has been achieved in patients with pelvic cancer pain. However, there is a discrepancy between diagnostic and therapeutic blockade in patients with non-malignant pain. Since diagnostic blockade can give significant pain relief in a large variety of patients, it is worthwhile to investigate new methods that provide lasting neural blockade of the superior hypogastric plexus and long-lasting relief of this devastating condition.

Lumbar sympathetic 64520

REFERENCES

1. Jaboulay M: Le traitement de la nevralgie pelviene par parlyse due sympathique sacre. Lyon Med 90:102, 1899.
2. Ruggi G: Della sympathectomy mia al collo ed ale abdome. Policlinoico 103, 1899.
3. Leriche R: Trans Am Surg Assoc 39:471, 1921.
4. Cotte G: Resection of the presacral nerves in the treatment of obstinate dysmenorrhea. Am J Obstet Gynecol 33:1034–1040, 1937.
5. Plancarte R, Amescua C, Patt RB, Aldrete JA: Superior hypogastric plexus block for pelvic cancer pain. Anesthesiology 73:236, 1990.
6. Chen FP: Laparoscopic presacral neurectomy for chronic pelvic pain. Chang Keng I Hsuek Tsa Chih 23:1–7, 2000.
7. De Leon-Casasola OA, Kent E, Lema MJ: Neurolytic superior hypogastric plexus block for chronic pelvic pain associated with cancer. Pain 54:145–151, 1993.
8. Waldman SD, Wilson WL: Superior hypogastric plexus block using a single needle and computed tomographic guidance: Description of a modified technique. Reg Anesth 16:286, 1991.
9. Kanazi GE, Frederick M: New technique for superior hypogastric plexus block. Reg Anesth Pain Med 24:473, 1999.
10. MacDonald JS: Management of chronic pelvic pain. Obstet Gynecol Clin North Am 20:817, 1993.
11. Ina H, Kitoh T: A new approach to superior hypogastric nerve block: Transvertebral disk L5–S1 technique. Reg Anesth 17(Suppl):123, 1992.
12. Erdine S: Transdiscal approach to the superior hypogastric plexus. Grand Rounds, Lubbock, TX, June 2000.
13. Racz GB, Noe C, Colvin J, Heavner JE: Sympathetic nerve blocks. In Raj PP (ed): Practical Management of Pain, 2nd ed. St. Louis, Mosby, 1992, pp 813–817.
14. Wechsler RJ, Maurer PM: Superior hypogastric plexus block for chronic pelvic pain in the presence of endometriosis: CT techniques and results. Radiology 196:103, 1995.
15. Plancarte R, De Leon-Casasola OA: Neurolytic superior hypogastric plexus block for chronic pelvic pain associated with cancer. Reg Anesth 22:562–568, 1997.

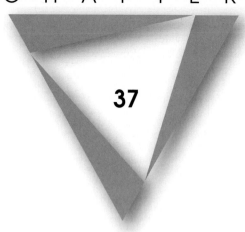

C H A P T E R

37

Ganglion Impar Block

HISTORY

The first report of interruption of the ganglion impar for relief of perineal pain appeared in 1990.[1]

ANATOMY

The ganglion impar (also known as the *ganglion of Walther* or the *sacrococcygeal ganglion*) is the most caudal ganglion of the sympathetic trunk. Thus, it marks the end of the two sympathetic chains (Fig. 37–1). Commonly, it is a single ganglion produced by the fusion of the ganglia from both sides. Because of this, it is usually located in the midline; however, it may also be lateral to the midline. Although an anatomic description of this ganglion is included in virtually every book of anatomy, one is unable to find a description of the areas that send afferent fibers to this ganglion. Clinical experience has shown that blockage at this point may be effective against some types of pain in the perineal region.

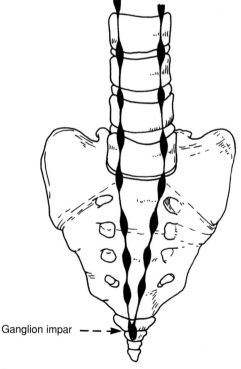

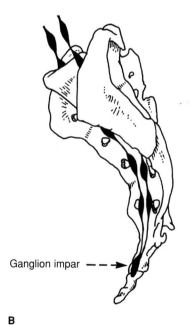

FIGURE 37–1

Anteroposterior *(A)* and lateral *(B)* illustrations of the ganglion impar, which is found in the area of sacro-coccygeal ligament anteriorly. It is composed of the terminal confluence of the left and right sympathetic chains in the midline.

Ganglion impar – – →

Ganglion impar – – →

A

B

INDICATIONS

Visceral pain or sympathetically maintained pain in the perineal area associated with malignancies of the pelvis may be effectively treated with neurolysis of the ganglion impar. Patients with a clinical picture of vague, burning, and localized perineal pain that is frequently associated with urgency may benefit from this block.

CONTRAINDICATIONS

- Local infection
- Coagulopathies
- Distorted anatomy

EQUIPMENT

- 25-gauge, ¾-inch infiltration needle
- 22-gauge, 3½-inch spinal needle, which can be shaped at one 60-degree angle or at 60 and 90-degree angles, as shown in Figure 37–2.
- IV T-piece extension

DRUGS

Local Anesthetics
- 1.5% lidocaine
- 2% lidocaine
- 0.5% bupivacaine or ropivacaine
- Iohexol (Omnipaque 240) non-ionic, water-soluble radiographic contrast

Neurolytic
- 6% phenol with contrast medium (5 to 10 mL)

PREPARATION OF THE PATIENT

PHYSICAL EXAMINATION

The perineum should be inspected for disease, infection, and ulceration. The patient must be evaluated for the ability to lie in either a prone or a lithotomy position.

PREOPERATIVE MEDICATION

For preoperative medication, use the standard American Society of Anesthesiologists' recommendations for conscious sedation.

PROCEDURE

There are multiple approaches to this block.

LATERAL TECHNIQUE

The technique for the performance of the lateral ganglion impar block is simple. As originally described,[1] the patient is placed in the lateral decubitus position with the hips flexed toward the abdomen (Fig. 37–3). The right

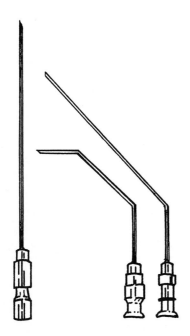

FIGURE 37–2

Drawing of the 22-gauge spinal needles used for ganglion impar blocks. Note the alternative configuration of the needles depending on the angulation of the coccyx and the approach to be used. (Adapted from Plancarte R, Velasquez R, Patt R: Neurolytic blocks of the sympathetic axis. In Patt R [ed]: Cancer Pain. Philadelphia, JB Lippincott, 1992, pp 337–427).

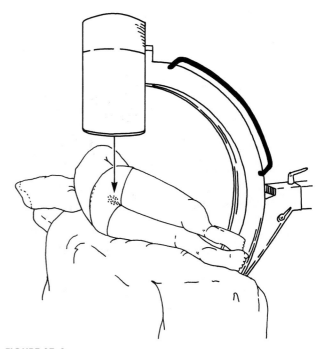

FIGURE 37–3

C-arm placed at the gluteal region in the lateral decubitus position.

lateral decubitus is used if the operator is right-handed. Local anesthesia is injected at the level of the anococcygeal ligament, which is situated midway between the anus and the tip of the coccyx (Fig. 37–4). A 22-gauge spinal needle that has been previously bent according to the curvature of the coccyx (see Fig. 37–2) is then introduced, while efforts are made to maintain the tip of the needle in the midline and outside the posterior rectal wall. Inserting the index finger in the rectum facilitates placement of the needle's tip at the level of the sacrococcygeal junction. Two milliliters of water-soluble contrast medium and biplanar fluoroscopy is used to verify adequate needle placement (Figs. 37–5 and 37–6). Neurolysis is then performed with 4 to 6 mL of 6% to 10% phenol dissolved in radiographic contrast material.

PRONE TECHNIQUE

Alternative technique approaches have been described for the prone ganglion impar block. In the trans-sacro-coccygeal approach, a 22-gauge, 3.5-inch needle is placed directly in the retroperitoneal space, in the midline at the level of sacrococcygeal junction in the prone position (Fig. 37–7).[2] An advantage of this approach is that the physician would not have to insert a finger in the rectum, which may be extremely painful in some patients, thus increasing the patient's tolerance. This is particularly important in patients with postradiation proctitis; however, fluoroscopic guidance is still needed.

LITHOTOMY TECHNIQUE

In a third alternative approach to ganglion impar block, the patient is placed in the lithotomy position (Fig. 37–8). The resulting curvature of the coccyx is decreased, allowing access to the ganglion impar with a straight 22-gauge spinal needle and facilitating needle positioning. However, placement of the finger in the rectum and fluoroscopy guidance are still

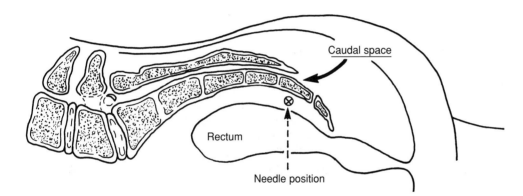

FIGURE 37–4

Lateral cross section of the sacrococcygeal area that illustrates the needle-tip position for ganglion impar block. (Adapted from Plancarte R, Velasquez R, Patt R: Neurolytic blocks of the sympathetic axis. In Patt R [ed]: Cancer Pain. Philadelphia, JB Lippincott, 1992, pp 337–427).

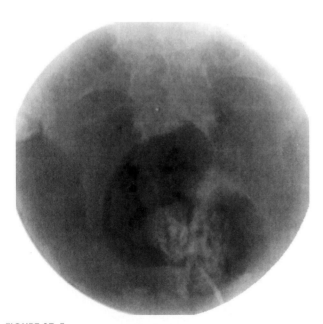

FIGURE 37–5

Anteroposterior fluoroscopic view that shows the contrast material outlining the ganglion impar.

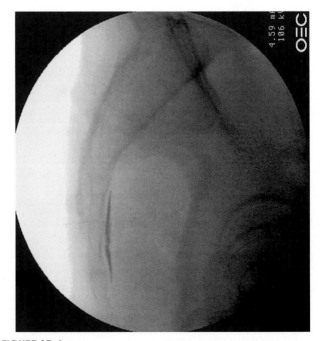

FIGURE 37–6

Lateral fluoroscopic view that shows the contrast spread anterior to the coccyx with the needle between the rectum and sacrum.

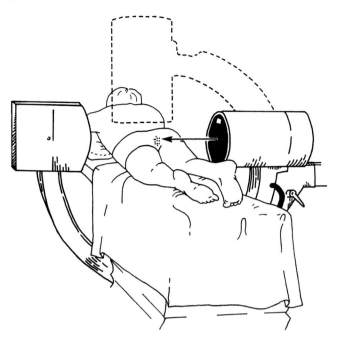

FIGURE 37-7

C-arm with the patient in the prone position for the prone technique.

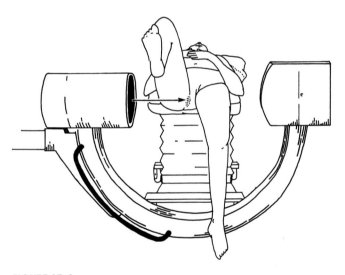

FIGURE 37-8

C-arm with the patient in the semilithotomy position for the third alternative approach.

needed. The advantages of this approach include easy needle placement and a less cumbersome fluoroscopic evaluation of the needle's tip.

A paramedial approach can be performed in the prone position for greater patient comfort. With this technique a bent 3½-inch spinal needle is used (see Fig. 37–2). The needle is inserted in the buttocks inferior and lateral to the sacral hiatus. Initially fluoroscopy in the anteroposterior position is used to confirm direction. After a change to a lateral view, the needle is advanced until bone is contacted or the needle tip is in the perirectal space parallel to the sacrococcygeal ligament. As a final anteroposterior image prior to radiographic contrast injection is obtained to ensure midline needle tip location, 1 to 2 mL of radiographic contrast medium is injected to avoid unintended spread. With confirmation of satisfactory spread, 5 mL of local anesthetic or neurolytic solution can be injected under fluoroscopy. Finger placement into the rectum is not needed for this approach.

COMPLICATIONS

- Rectum puncture
- Neurolytic injection into nerve roots and rectal cavity
- Neuritis/nerve root injection

EFFICACY

Plancarte and colleagues[1] evaluated 16 patients who experienced localized perineal pain associated with advanced cancer despite surgery, chemotherapy, radiation, and oral pharmacologic therapy. The pain was reported as burning and was associated with urgency in 8 of the patients. Complete analgesia was obtained in 8 patients, and 60% to 90% pain relief was reported for the rest of the patients. More than one block was performed in 2 of the patients with further pain improvement. Follow-up was carried out for 14 to 120 days, depending on the patient's survival. No complications have been reported to date with this block. Similarly, no further clinical studies are available documenting its efficacy.

Other peripheral nerve/myoneurals 64450; RFTC other nerve 64640

REFERENCES

1. Plancarte R, Amescua C, Patt R, Allende S: Presacral blockade of the ganglion of Walther (ganglion impar) [Abstract]. Anesthesiology 73:A751, 1990.
2. Wemm K, Saberski L: Modified approach to block the ganglion impar (ganglion of Walther) [Letter]. Reg Anesth 20:544, 1995.

C H A P T E R

38

Sacroiliac Joint Injection

HISTORY

Little history can be found for therapeutic injection of the sacroiliac joint. Much of the literature to date discusses the use of the sacroiliac joint for provocative testing.

ANATOMY

The axial spine rests on the sacrum, a triangular fusion of vertebrae arranged in a kyphotic curve and ending with the attached coccyx in the upper buttock.[1] Iliac swings (innominate bones) attach on either side, forming a bowl with a high back and a shallow front. Three joints result from this union: the pubic symphysis in the anterior midline and the left and right sacroiliac joints in the back (Fig. 38–1). Multiple ligaments and fascia attach across these joint spaces, limiting motion

and providing stability (Figs. 38–2 and 38–3).[2] The hip joints are formed by the femoral heads and the acetabular sockets deep within the innominate bones. The hips create a direct link between the lower extremities and the spine, to relay ground reaction forces from weight bearing and motion. A physiologic balance between lumbar lordosis and sacral curvature exists both at rest and in motion. Changes of pelvic tilt and lumbar lordosis occur in the anteroposterior plane, relying on attached muscles and fascia, but do not have significant effect on the sacroiliac joints owing to a self-bracing mechanism. The sacrum positioned between the innominate bones functions as a keystone in an arch, allowing

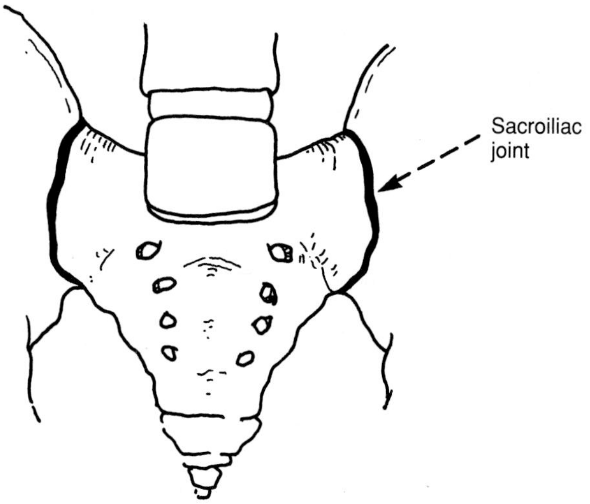

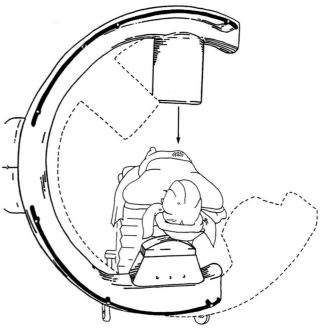

FIGURE 38–1

Line drawing of sacroiliac joint anatomy.

FIGURE 38–2

The patient lies prone. The C-arm is started in the posteroanterior view and rotated toward the oblique view until a clear view of the sacroiliac joint is obtained.

Sacroiliac joint

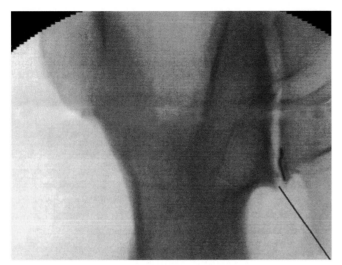

FIGURE 38–3

Sacroiliac joint enhanced fluoroscopically by oblique positioning of the C-arm.

only cephalocaudad and anteroposterior motion.[3] Innervation is varied and extensive owing to the size of this joint, which includes outflow from anterior and posterior rami of L3–L1.[4]

The S1 is a synovial (diarthrodial) joint that is more mobile in youth than later in life. The upper two thirds of the joint becomes more fibrotic in adulthood. The female pelvis is also more mobile to accommodate pregnancy and parturition. Ligament and muscle attachments help maintain stability of the pelvic ring latissimus, allowing movement within limits. Further motion is also limited by the irregular shape of the joint articulation, in which ridges and grooves increase resistance friction and add to the keystone arch structural. Prolonged loading (such as standing or sitting for long periods) and alterations of the sacral base (leg asymmetry or ligamentous injury) are associated with joint hypermobility and resultant low back pain.[3, 5, 6]

Multiple muscle attachments cross the sacroiliac joints and contribute to pelvic stability and force transfer.[3] The thoracolumbar fascia includes attachments to the 12th rib, lumbar spinous and lateral processes, and pelvic brim. Fascial and muscle attachments expand to include erector spinae, internal obliques, serratus posterior inferior, sacrotuberous ligament, dorsal S1 ligament, iliolumbar ligament, posterior iliac spine, and sacral crest. Major muscles attached to the S1 include the gluteus maximus, gluteus medius, latissimus dorsi, multifidus, biceps femoris, psoas, piriformis, obliquus, and transversus abdominis. Vleeming and coworkers[6] concluded that the purpose of these muscles is not for motion but to confer stability for loading and unloading forces produced by walking and running.

The sacroiliac joint line is densely innervated by several levels of spinal nerves (L3–S1) and may produce lumbar disc–like symptoms when stimulated.[4] Muscle insertions near the area, such as the gluteus maximus

and hamstrings, refer pain to the hip and ischial area, respectively, when stressed.

INDICATIONS

Sacroiliac pain is usually located in the gluteus and referred to the groin, hip, and thigh through its anterior plane and calf. The pain is more intense in the morning and remits during the day. Pressure on the articulation is painful.

CONTRAINDICATIONS

- Local infection

EQUIPMENT

Local Nerve Block
- 25-gauge, ¾-inch needle
- 22-gauge, 1½-inch needle
- 3-mL syringe
- IV T-piece extension

Radiofrequency Thermocoagulation
- 16-gauge, 1¼-inch angiocatheter
- 20-gauge curved Racz-Finch radiofrequency thermocoagulation needle *or*
    SMK 100-mm (active tip 0.5 cm)
    SMK 145-mm (active tip 0.5 to 1.0 cm)

DRUGS

Local Nerve Block
- 1.5% lidocaine for skin infiltration
- 0.5% bupivacaine/ropivacaine
- 2% lidocaine
- Steroids (optional)

Lubricant
- Hyaluronidase sodium (Hyalgan)

PREPARATION OF THE PATIENT

A thorough history must be taken to seek preexisting disease or injury, or new trauma, and to evaluate the patient's general health. Bladder, bowel, or sexual dysfunction or numbness often suggests an emergency that requires immediate care. The pain history should also include how long the problem has been present and treatments, including medications, injection, modalities, bracing, or manipulations and their outcomes. Provocative and palliative positions or activity can be guides to aid in treatment planning. Functional loss is significant, because it can be an indication of suffering and a measure of treatment success as the patient begins to resume activities.

PROCEDURE

The patient lies prone. The C-arm is started in the posteroanterior view and rotated toward the oblique view until a clear view of the sacroiliac joint is obtained. It is helpful first to find the L5–S1 disc space at L5–S1. Rotate cephalic 15 to 25 degrees, enough to open the disc space at L5–S1. Second, start with the oblique view, then rotate toward the anteroposterior view to visualize the widest space at the most inferior aspect of the S1 joint (see Fig. 38–2).

The scout image must shows the entire S1 joint visualized for needle entry at the most inferior aspect. The C-arm is angled in such a way that the lines of the posterior and the anterior aspects of the joint are seen to overlap (see Fig. 38–3). Injection of contrast material spreads throughout the sacroiliac joint in an inferior to superior fashion, with opacification of ventral and dorsal joint lines (Fig. 38–4).

Five to 0.5% ropivacaine with or without 40 mg of triamcinolone is injected for the diagnostic and therapeutic block. The patient is monitored for 30 minutes prior to discharge. If the local diagnostic block is successful, 2 to 5 mL of Hyalgon can be injected, twice weekly, up to 5 times.

After the radiofrequency needle is inserted in the SI joint, as described, sensory and motor testing is done.

STIMULATION PARAMETERS

- Scale: 0 to 1 V
- Sensory: 50 Hz; paresthesia of the zone must be noted above 0.5 V

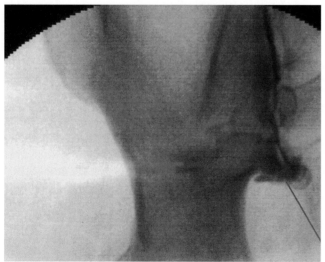

FIGURE 38–4

Sacroiliac joint with contrast material under fluoroscopy.

LESION PARAMETERS

Inject 1 mL of 2% lidocaine before the lesion radiofrequency at 80°C for 90 seconds. Multiple lesions must be completed along the entire posterior joint line. The cannula entry point must be located more medial, because the lesions are more cranial, to facilitate positioning beneath the posterior iliac crest.

COMPLICATIONS

Following sacroiliac joint radiofrequency denervation, some patients can have gluteal discomfort, hip pain, or referred posterior thigh pain that usually resolves in 10 to 15 days. Adjunct analgesic oral therapy is advisable. Patch hypoesthesia in the buttocks can be referred that resolves spontaneously within 2 to 4 weeks.

HELPFUL HINTS

The facets and root ganglia should be lesioned for the complete treatment to be performed. It is advisable to perform pulsed radiofrequency lesions in the dorsal root ganglions of S1, S2, and S3 and conventional radiofrequency in L4–L5 and L5–S1 medial branches.

The S2 segmental root contributes greatly to the innervation of the sacroiliac joint, and S2 dorsal root ganglion pulsed radiofrequency can alleviate residual symptoms after sacroiliac denervation.

EFFICACY

No randomized, controlled, prospective studies could be found. Clinical practice has found that this procedure has been efficacious. The longer durations of relief have been reported by Cavillo[7] and associates by using viscus hyaluronate.

Sacroiliac (SI) joint injection 27096

REFERENCES

1. Willard FH: The anatomy of the lumbosacral connection. Spine 9:333–955, 1995.
2. Snijders CJ, Vleeming A, Stoeckart R: Transfer of lumbosacral load to iliac bones and legs: I. Biomechanics of self-bracing of the sacroiliac joints and its significance for treatment and exercise. II. Loading of the sacroiliac joints when lifting in a stooped posture. Clin Biomech 8:285–301, 1993.
3. Soloenen KA: The sacroiliac joint in the light of anatomical, roentgenological, and clinical studies. Acta Orthop Scand 27(Suppl):27, 1957.
4. Simonian PT, Routt ML Jr, Harrington RM, et al: Biomechanical simulation of the anteroposterior compression injury of the pelvis: An understanding of instability and fixation. Clin Orthop 309:245–256, 1994.
5. Vrahas M, Hern TC, Diangelo D, et al: Ligamentous contributions to pelvic stability. Orthopedics 18:271–274, 1995.
6. Vleeming A, Pool-Goudzwaard AL, Stoeckart R, et al: The posterior layer of the thoracolumbar fascia: Its function in load transfer from spine to legs. Spine 20:753–758, 1995.
7. Calvillo O: Anatomy and pathophysiology of the sacroiliac joint. Curr Rev Pain 5:356–361, 2000.

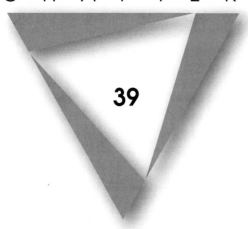

Sciatic Nerve Catheter Placement and Block

HISTORY

Labat wrote the first description of the posterior approach to the sciatic nerve in 1923.[1] The lateral approach was described by Molesworth[2] in 1944 and developed by Lchiyanagi[3] in 1959 and the anterior approach by Beck in 1963.[4] The supine sciatic approach was described by Raj and associates[5] in 1975.

ANATOMY

The sciatic nerve (L4–L5, S1–S3), the largest nerve in the body, measures 1.5 to 2 cm in width and 0.3 to 0.9 cm in diameter as it leaves the pelvis, whence it passes through a tunnel between the greater trochanter and the ischial tuberosity. At this point, the greater sciatic nerve passes posterior to the gemmules, obturator internus, and quadriceps femoris muscles and anterior to the gluteus maximus muscle (Fig. 39–1).

The posterior femoral cutaneous branch (S1–S3), which innervates the posterior aspect of the thigh, varies in proximity to the sciatic nerve and may either travel with it or separately from it cephalad. Blood vessels accompanying the sciatic nerve at this point are the sciatic artery, a branch of the inferior gluteal artery, and the inferior gluteal veins. In this region, both the artery and the veins are relatively small.

INDICATIONS

SURGERY

Sciatic nerve block is indicated together with saphenous nerve blocks for surgery and analgesia of the ankle and

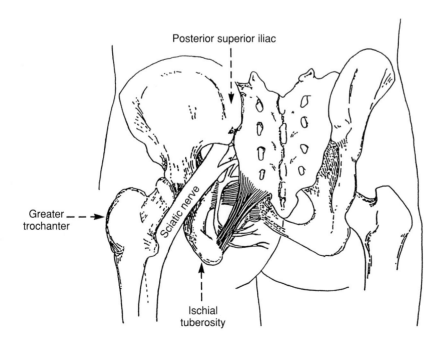

FIGURE 39–1

The drawing shows the relationship of the sciatic nerve as it transverses via the greater sciatic notch toward the lesser trochanter.

foot; for surgery and analgesia of the knee in conjunction with blocks of the femoral, obturator, and lateral femoral cutaneous nerves; and for surgery and analgesia of the leg combined with saphenous nerve blocks.

CONTINUOUS INFUSION

Patients with complex regional pain syndrome type I or II, vascular insufficiency, or unilateral leg edema (of many causes) are frequently managed with lumbar epidural catheters. There are, however, inherent risks with long-term placement of an epidural catheter. The catheter can be an alternative for such patients. It can eliminate the risk of epidural abscess, hematoma formation, and catheter erosion of the dura. The affected limb can be specifically treated without numbing or weakening the contralateral limb. Thus, ambulation is maintained. Contraindications include (1) anticoagulant therapy, (2) septicemia, (3) local infection, (4) recent injury at the site of injection to the nerve, and (5) inability of the patient to lie prone.

CONTRAINDICATIONS

Relative contraindications for this type of block include anticoagulant therapy, septicemia, local infection, recent injury at the site of injection to the nerve, inability of the patient to lie in the prone position, and distorted anatomy.

EQUIPMENT

Local Nerve Block
- 22-gauge, 6-inch B-bevel needle
- ¾-inch infiltration needle
- 3-mL syringe
- 10-mL syringe
- 20-mL syringe
- IV T-piece extension

Continuous Infusion
- B-D Longdwel catheter over 18-gauge, 6- to 8-inch needle
- 16-gauge RK epidural needle
- 24-cm Tun-L-XL epidural catheter or peripheral nerve stimulation (PN-STM) catheter

Aids to Procedure
- Nerve stimulator with appropriate clips and wires

DRUGS

- 1.5% lidocaine
- 2% lidocaine
- 0.5% bupivacaine/ ropivacaine
- Steroids

PREPARATION OF THE PATIENT

PHYSICAL EXAMINATION

Physical assessment should include a superficial examination for local infection and distorted anatomy and a neurologic examination for documentation of abnormalities or changes. Assess the patient's ability to lie prone.

PREOPERATIVE MEDICATION

For preoperative medication, use the standard American Society of Anesthesiologists' recommendations for conscious sedation.

PROCEDURE

TECHNIQUE

Block for Surgery: Posterior Approach

As discussed earlier, Labat first published his description of the posterior approach in 1923 when he placed the patient in the Sims position, then located the posterior superior iliac spine and the greater trochanter. A line was drawn between the two. A perpendicular line was dropped at the midpoint of the first line; the point of entry was at a distance of 2.5 to 3.8 cm inferior to this, located on the line drawn from the sacral hiatus to the greater trochanter. We describe a modified technique, which places the patient in the prone position (Fig. 39–2). Radiographic landmarks noted in the posterior view are described in Figure 39–3.

After skin preparation and infiltration, a 22-gauge, 9-cm needle is inserted perpendicular to the skin at the chosen landmark. After passing through the piriformis muscle, the sciatic nerve is contacted (3.8 cm deep); the latter extends at this point toward the leg from the greater sciatic notch. With the nerve stimulator, muscle stimulation of the foot is obtained as dorsiflexion or plantiflexion is noted (Fig. 39–4).

Catheter Placement[6, 7]

The patient is placed in the prone position (see Fig. 39–2). The gluteal region ipsilateral to the affected side is sterilized and draped. Landmarks are located by fluoroscopy—(1) the posterior superior iliac spine, (2) the greater trochanter, and (3) the ischial tuberosity (see Fig. 39–3). A line is drawn connecting the connecting the posterior iliac spine and the greater trochanter. The midpoint is identified and a perpendicular line drawn

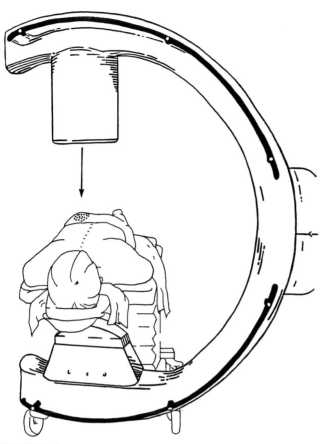

FIGURE 39-2

The patient is placed prone with the C-arm over the ipsilateral buttock for sciatic nerve block.

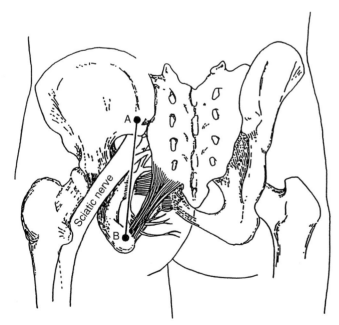

FIGURE 39-3

The drawing depicts the landmarks to be identified by fluoroscopy. The following is a key to the letters shown on the figure: A, posterior superior iliac spine; B, greater trochanter; and C, ischial tuberosity.[6,7]

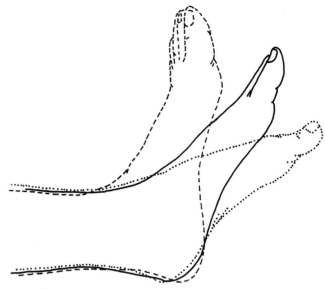

FIGURE 39-4

Plantarflexion and dorsiflexion of the foot occurring with each impulse of a nerve stimulator indicate that the needle is on the sciatic nerve.

in a caudal direction. A second line is drawn from the greater trochanter to the ischial tuberosity. This line is divided into three parts. A third line is drawn vertically from the medial third mark upward to intersect the other line. The point of entry is where the two lines meet (Fig. 39-5). A skin wheal is raised at the site with a 25-gauge needle. A larger needle (16- to 18-gauge) can pierce the skin. A 16-gauge, 7-inch blunt needle is introduced perpendicular, approximately 1 cm through the skin to reach the piriformis muscle. A 22-gauge needle is inserted subcutaneously and attached to a positive lead from the Medtronic test stimulator should be set to deliver 6 to 8 V at 1 impulse/sec. (If a peripheral nerve stimulator is used, the current should be adjusted from 3 to 0.5 mA at 1 impulse/sec.) The needle is slowly advanced anteriorly until the piriformis muscle, which is identified by contrast solution, is twitching. The needle is further advanced until the piriformis muscle stimulation stops and foot twitching (dorsiflexion) is observed in the affected limb. A stimulating catheter is then inserted through the needle. The negative lead of the stimulator is attached to the distal connect wire of the catheter. The catheter is passed to the level of the lesser trochanter for foot movement. The needle is then removed and the catheter is attached to the hub connector. Placement can be confirmed with 3 mL of contrast dye introduced via the catheter (Figs. 39-6 and 39-7). Another 3 mL of 0.2% ropivacaine may be injected, and stimulation of the sciatic nerve should cease.[6] Through an attached bacteriostatic filter, 15 to 30 mL of 2% lidocaine or 0.2% lidocaine or 0.2% ropivacaine is injected in divided doses for immediate pain relief and nerve blockade. The constant infusion of 0.1% ropivacaine

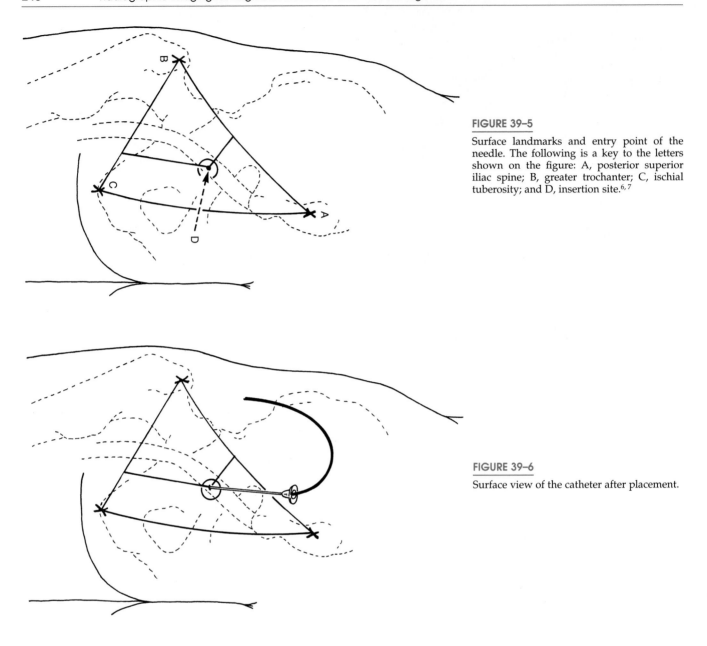

FIGURE 39–5

Surface landmarks and entry point of the needle. The following is a key to the letters shown on the figure: A, posterior superior iliac spine; B, greater trochanter; C, ischial tuberosity; and D, insertion site.[6, 7]

FIGURE 39–6

Surface view of the catheter after placement.

with fentanyl (5 µg/mL) may range from 4 to 10 mL/hr. Occasional bolus doses may be required and may be delivered by the patient through the pump with a bolus of 5 mL and a 30-minute lockout.[7] The catheter may be connected to a drug infusion balloon for outpatient care through home health services. This balloon delivers 4 mL/hr of the drug to the patient for 24 hours. (The volume of the balloon reservoir is 100 mL.)

CONFIRMATION OF BLOCK

Motor and sensory pinprick loss in the lower extremity in the area of the sciatic nerve distribution, sparing the medial aspect of the leg, indicates that block has been achieved. Sympathetic block of the leg and foot also confirms sciatic nerve block.

COMPLICATIONS

No significant complications secondary to sciatic nerve block have been documented. Residual dysesthesia may occur for as long as 3 days.

EFFICACY

Continuous regional analgesia, whether central or peripheral, is safe and efficacious. The infusions may utilize local anesthetics, opioids, or a combination of the two. These infusions are performed when prolonged analgesia is required for moderate to severe acute, chronic, or cancer pain.

Sciatic nerve 64445

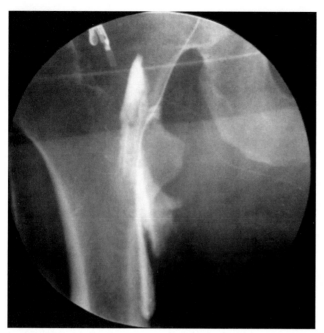

FIGURE 39-7

Fluoroscopic image of the catheter with contrast solution following the sciatic nerve sheath.[6, 7] (From Waldman SD [ed]: Interventional Pain Management, 2nd ed. Philadelphia, WB Saunders, 2001, p 431.)

REFERENCES

1. Adriani J: Labat's Regional Anesthesia: Techniques and Clinical Applications. Philadelphia, WB Saunders, 1967.
2. Molesworth HWL: Regional Anesthesia. London, Lewis, 1944.
3. Lchiyanagi K: Sciatic nerve block: Lateral approach with patient supine. Anesthesiology 20:601, 1959.
4. Beck GP: Anterior approach to sciatic nerve block. Anesthesiology 24:222, 1963.
5. Raj PP, Parks Rt, Watson TD, Jenkins MT: A new single-position supine approach to sciatic-femoral nerve block. Anesth Analg 54:489, 1975.
6. Racz G, Raj P, Lou L, et al: Posterior Sacral Approach to the Sciatic Nerve for Continuous Lidocaine Infusion: A New Technique. Presented at the 1997 meeting of the American Society of Anesthesiologists, San Diego, CA; the 1977 meeting of the PostGraduate Assembly, New York, NY; and the 1998 meeting of the International Anesthesia Research Society, Orlando, FL.
7. Racz G, Raj P, Lou L, et al: Posterior Sacral Approach to the Sciatic Nerve for Continuous Ropivacaine Infusion: A New Technique. Presented at the 1998 meeting of the PostGraduate Assembly, New York, NY.

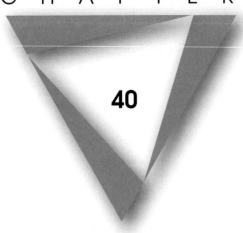

40

Piriformis Muscle Injection

HISTORY

The name of the piriformis is derived from the Latin *pirum* for "pear" and *forma* for "shape." It was coined by Adrian Spigelius, a late 16th–early 17th century Belgian anatomist. Calliet,[1] Pace,[2] and Steiner and associates[3] have recommended injection of the piriformis muscle. Pace[2] described the percutaneous spinal needle injection technique.

ANATOMY

The piriformis is a thick, bulky muscle in most individuals; it is occasionally thin and is rarely absent.[4] The piriformis muscle can be small, with only one or two sacral attachments. Conversely, it can be so broad that it joins with the capsule of the sacroiliac joint above and also with the anterior surface of the sacrotuberous and/or sacrospinous ligaments below.

This muscle is anchored *medially* to the anterior (internal) surface of the sacrum usually by three fleshy digitations between the first second, third, and fourth anterior sacral foramina.

Laterally, the muscle is secured by a rounded tendon onto the greater trochanter on the medial side of its superior surface (Fig. 40–1). This tendon often blends with the common tendon of the obturator internus and gemelli muscles.

The piriformis muscle exits the inside of the pelvis through the greater sciatic foramen. This rigid opening is formed anteriorly and superiorly by the posterior part of the ilium, posteriorly by the sacrotuberous ligament, and inferiorly by the sacrospinous ligament. When the muscle is large and fills this space, it has the potential of compressing the numerous vessels and nerves that exit the pelvis with it.

Innervation of the piriformis muscle is directly from the first and second sacral nerves. The obturator externus is supplied by the obturator nerve from spinal

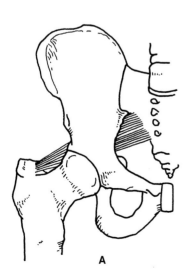
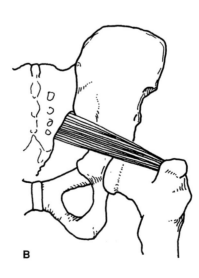

A   B

FIGURE 40–1

Anterior *(A)* and posterior *(B)* views of the piriformis muscle.

nerves L3 and L4. The remaining short lateral rotators receive innervation through motor nerves that may arise from spinal nerves L4 to S5.

Function of the piriformis in the non–weight-bearing limb is primarily lateral rotation of the thigh with the hip extended; it also acts in abduction when the hip is flexed 90 degrees. The remaining five short deep rotator muscles are primarily lateral rotators in either position. In weight-bearing activities, the piriformis restrains vigorous or excessive medial rotation of the thigh.

INDICATIONS

Pain from the piriformis muscle can be referred muscular pain or pain from entrapment of nerves and vessels. Referred pain from the muscle radiates from the sacroiliac joint to the posterior proximal two thirds of the thigh, inclusive of the buttocks and hip.

Entrapment pain associated with piriformis muscle spasm most frequently involves the sciatic nerve but can include the inferior and superior gluteal nerves and vessels; the pudendal nerve and vessels; the posterior femoral cutaneous nerve; and the nerves to the gemelli, obturator internus, and quadratus femoris muscles.

CONTRAINDICATIONS

- Local infection
- Abnormal bleeding disorders

PIRIFORMIS MUSCLE SYNDROME

The piriformis muscle syndrome frequently is characterized by such bizarre symptoms that they may seem unrelated. Pain (and paresthesias) may be reported in the low back, groin, perineum, buttock, hip, posterior, thigh and leg, foot, and during defecation, in the rectum (Fig. 40–2). Symptoms are aggravated by sitting; by a prolonged combination of hip flexion, adduction, and medial rotation; or by activity. In addition, the patient may complain of swelling in the painful limb and of sexual dysfunction dyspareunia in women and impotence in men.

It now appears that three specific conditions may contribute to the piriformis syndrome: (1) myofascial pain referred from trigger points in the piriformis muscle; (2) nerve and vascular entrapment by the piriformis muscle at the greater sciatic foramen; and (3) dysfunction of the sacroiliac joint.

Patient examination reveals a tendency for the seated patient to squirm and shift position frequently. The Pace Abduction Test is usually positive. In the supine position, the foot of the involved side is laterally rotated, and medial rotation of that limb is restricted in range as compared with the normal side. In the prone position, pelvic asymmetry may be noted. Standing examination may reveal an apparent lower limb-length inequality and a tilted sacral base. Bone scan scintigraphy may image a piriformis muscle with active trigger points. Additional evidence for entrapment of nerves passing through the greater sciatic foramen supports the diagnosis of a piriformis syndrome.

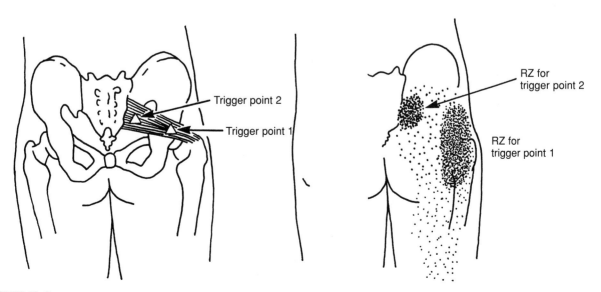

FIGURE 40–2

Trigger points and attachment of the piriformis muscle with reference zones (RZ) for trigger points 1 and 2 for the piriformis muscle.

EQUIPMENT

- 25-gauge, ¾-inch infiltration needle
- 22-gauge, 2- ,4- , or 6-inch needle
- 18-gauge, 1½-inch needle for drawing up drugs and making skin punctures
- 3-mL syringe
- 10-mL three-ring syringe
- 10-mL syringe
- IV T-piece extension set
- Metal marker/clamp
- Bandage or appropriate dressing

DRUGS

- Iohexol (Omnipaque) radiopaque contrast solution
- Preservative-free normal (0.9%) saline
- 1.5% lidocaine for infiltration
- 0.5% bupivacaine or ropivacaine, preservative free
- 2% lidocaine
- Steroids, preservative free, water soluble
      Methylprednisolone
      Triamcinolone diacetate
- Botulinum toxin

PROCEDURE

TECHNIQUE

The patient is placed prone with the C-arm directed toward the ipsilateral buttock (Fig. 40–3). Needle entry after local infiltration is just above the hip point 90 degrees to the skin midway between the greater trochanter and sacrum with a 3½-inch spinal needle.

The patient's radiographic image should confirm with a contrast solution the contrast delineating the contour of the piriformis muscle (Fig. 40–4). For diagnostic and therapeutic block, 3 mL of 0.2% ropivacaine with 40 mg of triamcinolone is injected. If the pain relief is obtained with the local anesthetic, the range of motion of the hip is evaluated at this time. For prolonged pain relief, botulinum toxin is injected (50 units) by their technique.

CONFIRMATION OF THE BLOCK

- By injecting the 2 to 5 mL of contrast solution, one can see the delineation of the part of piriformis on a muscle (see Fig. 40–4)
- By examining the patient 15 to 20 minutes after the local anesthetic injection, one can determine if the pain and function are improved.

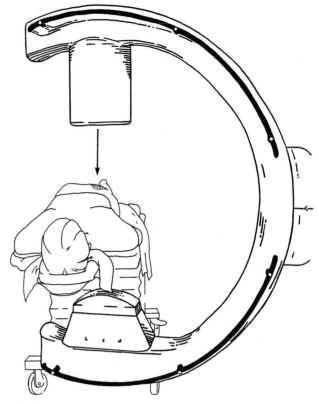

FIGURE 40–3

The C-arm position for anteroposterior viewing of the piriformis muscle injection.

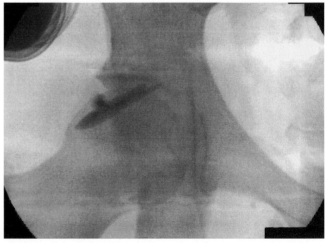

FIGURE 40–4

Radiographic image (anteroposterior view) of the piriformis muscle after contrast solution is administered.

ALTERNATIVE TECHNIQUES

Blind Technique 1: Equal distance between greater trochanter and posterior superior iliac spine, a painful trigger point is sought by the finger at the point of the site entry (Fig. 40–5)

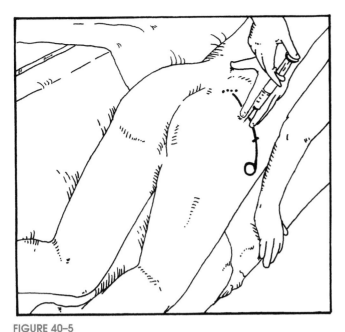

FIGURE 40–5

Identification and injection of a piriformis muscle trigger point.

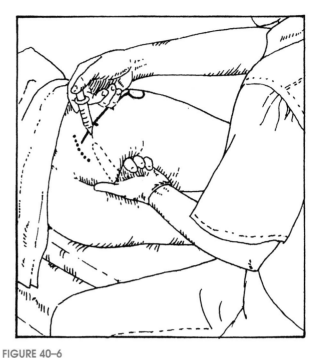

FIGURE 40–6

Identification and injection of the piriformis muscle with a finger in the rectum.

Blind Technique 2: One puts a finger in the rectum and directs the finger toward the piriformis muscle (Fig. 40–6). At a tender spot, the needle is inserted through the skin and injected.

COMPLICATIONS

- Bleeding and hematoma formation
- Injections and abscess at the site of injections
- Sciatic nerve pulse or neuropathy due to needle entry damage

HELPFUL HINTS

To avoid accidental needle penetration of the sciatic nerve, the needle should be placed in the lateral aspects of the piriformi muscle.

EFFICACY

Among the 84 patients with piriformis syndrome who received injections of 10 mL of 0.5% solution of procaine,[5] 55% of them had prompt amelioration of angiospastic signs and symptoms. The lower extremity oscillogram improved and the chilly feeling in the leg disappeared. In many patients, weak Achilles reflexes were restored, and the extent and intensity of hypalgesia were improved.

Trigger points 20552/20553

REFERENCES

1. Cailiet R (ed): Low Back Pain Syndrome, 3rd ed. Philadelphia, FA Davis, 1981.
2. Pace JB: Commonly overlooked pain syndromes responsive to simple therapy. Postgrad Med 58:107–113, 1975.
3. Steiner C, Staubs C, Ganon M, et al: Piriformis syndrome: Pathogenesis, diagnosis, and treatment. J Am Osteopath Assoc 87:318–323, 1987.
4. Travell JG, Simons DG: Myofascial Pain and Dysfunction: The Trigger Point Manual. Baltimore, Williams & Wilkins, 1983, pp 74–86, 86–87, 364–365.
5. Popelianskii II, Bobrovnikoza TI: [The syndrome of the piriformis muscle and lumbar discogenic radiculitis.] Zh Nevropatol Psikhiatr 68:656–662, 1968.

C H A P T E R

41

Decompressive Neuroplasty

HISTORY

Epidural injection for chronic pain was performed by Calthelin in 1901.[1] The initial epidurography was performed serendipitously in 1921 by Sicard and Forestier.[2] Payne and Rupp[3] in 1950 combined hyaluronidase with local anesthetic in an attempt to alter the rapidity of onset, extent, intensity, and duration of caudal anesthesia. They demonstrated maximal efficacy in a group receiving local anesthetic, hyaluronidase, and epinephrine. Hyaluronidase concentration in this study was relatively dilute at 6 U/mL, with an average volume of injection of 24 mL. In 1951 Moore[4] added 150 U of hyaluronidase in 1309 nerve blocks, including 20 caudal blocks, to enhance the spread of local anesthetic. He showed hyaluronidase to be relatively nontoxic. Lievre and coworkers reported the first use of corticosteroid injected into the epidural space for the treatment of sciatica in 1957.[5] They injected a combination of hydrocortisone and radiopaque dye in 46 patients with 31 positive results. In 1960, Goebert[6] injected procaine and hydrocortisone into the caudal epidural space. The majority of patients derived benefit from their injections of 30 mL of 1% procaine hydrochloride with 125 mg of hydrocortisone acetate. In the same year Brown injected

larger volumes, 40 to 199 mL, of normal saline followed by 80 mg of methylprednisolone in an attempt to mechanically disrupt and prevent reformation of presumably fibrotic lesions in patients with sciatica.[7] He reported complete resolution of pain for 2 months in the four patients he treated. It is notable that this investigation in 1960 laid the theoretical foundation for current therapies in which specific catheter placement is crucial to the effective treatment of epidural adhesions.

Hypertonic saline was first administered by Hitchcock[8] in 1967 for the treatment of chronic pain when he injected cold saline intrathecally. He later reported, in 1969, that it was the hypertonicity rather than the temperature of the solution that was the determining factor in its therapeutic effect.[9] Hypertonic saline was subsequently employed by Ventafridda and Spreafico[10] in 1974 for intractable cancer pain by intrathecal administration. All 21 patients in this study had pain relief at 24 hours, although only three patients reported relief at 30 days. Racz and Holubec[11] in 1989 reported the first use of epidural hypertonic saline to facilitate lysis of adhesions, and hyaluronidase was introduced as an alternative agent by Stolker and associates in 1994.[12]

The first report on this procedure was by Racz and Holubec in 1989[11] (Table 41–1). There were several vari-

▽ TABLE 41–1 Drugs Used for Decompressive Neuroplasty

	Metrizamide	Iohexol	Hyaluronidase	Lidocaine	Bupivacaine	Methylprednisolone	Triamcinolone	Hypertonic Saline
Racz and Holubec[11] (1989)	*	*	—	—	*	—	*	*
Stolker et al[12] (1994)	?	?	×	—	×	—	×	—
Arthur et al[58] (1993)	—	×	—	—	×	—	×	×
Devulder et al[59] (1995)[†]	—	*	—	*	*	*	—	*

[†] Nonspecific catheter placement.

ations in the protocol of this early study. Metrizamide was used as the contrast agent in these procedures, and hyaluronidase was not used.

In 1994 Stolker and associates added hyaluronidase to the procedure but omitted the hypertonic saline. In a study of 28 patients, they reported greater than 50% pain reduction in 64% of patients at 1 year.[12] They stressed pain patient selection criteria and suggested that the effectiveness of the procedure was based on the effect of the hyaluronidase on the adhesions and the action of the local anesthetic and steroids on the sinu-vertebral nerve.

Lysis of adhesions in the epidural space clearly is a procedure that needs to follow other simpler procedures, such as rest, nonsteroidal anti-inflammatory medications, muscle relaxants, physical therapy, activity programs, two or three single-shot epidural steroids, and transcutaneous electrical nerve stimulator unit. The more informed patients would selectively undergo procedures such as lysis of adhesions rather than surgery. The results clearly show a dramatic decline in further surgical interventions in our patient population as well as avoidance of surgical intervention in appropriately selected patients with clearly documented herniated discs and nerve root compressions. This awareness is gaining support by having the U.S. regulatory agencies, as well as courts, support the recognized effective nature of the procedure of lysis of adhesions.[11]

Scarring in the epidural space occurs frequently following surgery and causes no problems. Scarring can occur following leakage of nucleus pulposus material into the epidural space.[13] The pain associated with the scar formation originates from the nerve itself, which is irritated, swollen, and angry looking and has no space in which to move freely. In the neural foramina, nerves are normally associated with epidural veins. Epidural scarring often obstructs these epidural veins. The obstruction raises intravenous pressure, leading to additional edema formation within the epidural space.

The ideal indication for decompressive neuroplasty is radiculopathy due to epidural fibrosis and nerve root entrapment. For chemically sensitive discs, failed back surgery syndrome, and associated epidural inflammations, the placement of the catheter in the anterior epidural space has been extremely effective. In spinal stenosis the neuroplasty techniques have been helpful in some situations by decreasing edema and venous congestion with the expected effect of attenuating the compressive effects on the spinal cord and nerve roots.

In the lumbar region the caudal approach is extremely beneficial for the L5–S1 radiculopathy owing to the ease of entering the area of natural lordosis in that region. On the occasion that L4 or higher is problematic, a transforaminal approach with placement of the Racz catheter into the anterior epidural space can be done individually or in conjunction with a caudal catheter. Thoracic neuroplasty is rarely done but may be useful in situations such as acute herpes zoster or thoracic vertebral compression fractures. For the cervical region, radicular symptoms related to failed neck surgery, discogenic pain, and associated fibrosis from inflammation are the predominant indication.

DRUGS USED FOR NEUROPLASTY

Iohexol is a second-generation non-ionic, low-osmolar radiographic contrast agent. The iodine content is 46% by weight, buffered by tromethamine to a pH of 6.8 to 7.7 and preserved with 0.1 mg/mL edetate calcium disodium. The uniform coverage of the iodine atoms by the hydrophilic groups is responsible for its low toxicity.

Many concentrations (140, 210, 240, 300, 350 mgI/mL) of iohexol are available for subarachnoid, intravascular, and body cavity injections. For subarachnoid administration, the concentration should never be greater than 300 mgI/mL in adults and 210 mgI/ml in children. Because of the toxic effects of iodine, the total dose is 3.06 mg for adults and 2.94 mg for children. There is minimal protein binding in serum. Eighty-eight percent of an intrathecal dose is excreted renally in its unmetabolized form and can be found in the urine at 24 hours.[14] Chemotoxic reactions are often dose dependent and present as hypotension, dyspnea, cardiac arrest, organ failure, and/or loss of consciousness. The incidence of chemotoxic reactions with these radiographic contrasts occurs in only 1 in 100,000 patients. Intravascular injection of iohexol has been reported to have a low risk for causing renal failure.[15] There are some concerns that this risk may be increased with patients on oral hypoglycemic agents. Fortunately, these complications are infrequent with non-ionic contrast agents.

Idiosyncratic reactions consist of headaches, myalgias, nausea, vomiting, dizziness, aseptic meningitis, and other neurologic disturbances. The most common reaction is a headache, which occurs in 18% of the patients after intrathecal iohexol.[14] Aseptic meningitis and neurologic disturbances are much less common. Allergic or anaphylactoid reactions with non-ionic contrast agents are rare and less frequent than those with ionic contrast agents.[16] Ndosi and associates[17] reported that the risk of significant reaction with concentrations of 240 mgI/mL of iohexol for myelography in a placebo-controlled, double-blinded study was no greater than that related to the lumbar puncture itself. This same study reported that headaches, dizziness, nausea, vomiting, and seizures are more likely to occur with 180 and 300 mgI/mL concentrations.

HYALURONIDASE

Hyaluronidase is a lyophilized white, odorless amorphous powder that is commercially available in 150 and

1500 U. The smaller dose is supplied fully hydrated, whereas the larger amount is a solid with 1 mg of thimerosal preservative and 13.3 mg of lactose for mixing with a solute. Duran-Reynals[18] first described its spreading factor by strains of *Streptococcus* bacteria. It can be found in bee and snake venom, mammalian tissues, and sperm.[19] Its primary function is to depolymerize hyaluronic acid and to a lesser degree chondroitin-6-sulfate and chondroitin-4-sulfate. Hyaluronic acid is a large-molecule glycosaminoglycan that binds ground substance proteins that form proteoglycans. Not only are these proteoglycans found between the ground substances between cells, they are also in cheloids (dense scar tissue) and epidural adhesions.[20] Disruption of these proteoglycans is accomplished by cleaving the β-1,4 glycosidic bonds.

The breakage of the proteoglycans has been found to accelerate the diffusion of injected drugs.[21] This hypodermoclysis was subsequently found to increase the efficacy of the local anesthetic infiltrations.[22] In the epidural space, the dura is composed of collagen, elastin, and surface fibroblasts that are not affected by hyaluronidase. Intrathecal use of hyaluronidase has been documented for chronic arachnoiditis with no report of no serious adverse effects in 15 patients.[23]

Nicoll and colleagues[24] reported a 6000 retrobulbar block prospective study with the adverse effects attributed to the local anesthetic spread into the central nervous system. Because of the known homology of mammalian hyaluronidase to insect hyaluronidase, attention should be given to possible complications with patients having venom allergies.[25] Anaphylactic-like reactions have occurred in isolated cases.[26]

LOCAL ANESTHETIC

The local anesthetic used is limited to a concentration that provides only sensory blockade. With the local anesthetic immediate pain relief is possible in addition to preparation of the epidural tissues for infusion of the hypertonic saline. Hypertonic saline tends to "burn" when infused without preinjection of local anesthetics. As an additional safeguard against subdural or intrathecal injection, the local anesthetic is delivered in divided doses to monitor for nonepidural spread. For the neuroplasty technique, it also serves as a diluent for the steroids.

Bupivacaine is significant for its cardiotoxicity, which has now been attributed to the *S*-enantiomer.[27] Levobupivacaine is exclusively composed of the *S*(-) monomer of racemic bupivacaine and has proven itself to have essentially the same clinical properties and potency as racemic bupivacaine with significantly less adverse effects.[28] Ropivacaine is a third-generation *S*(-) monomer local anesthetic of the propyl-pipecoloxylidide amino-amide series with less cardiotoxicity but with potency and duration of action similar to racemic bupi-

vacaine. One significant difference of ropivacaine compared to bupivacaine is its vasoconstrictive properties and documented ability to reduce epidural blood and pial blood vessel size.[29, 30]

STEROIDS

Methylprednisolone and triamcinolone are two of the more popular choices for epidural injection. They both interact with two different receptor types: glucocorticoid and mineralocorticoid. The glucocorticoid is primarily responsible for regulation of carbohydrate metabolism and the inflammatory and immune responses, whereas the mineralocorticoid is responsible for regulation of electrolyte balance. Attempts to synthesize a steroid with anti-inflammatory properties have been difficult.

Collectively, methylprednisolone and triamcinolone are considered intermediate acting in duration with equipotent anti-inflammatory effects. Triamcinolone is a more glucocorticoid-specific agonist than methylprednisolone. Both of these drugs exhibit a lower protein binding and metabolism than endogenous corticosteroids. Unfortunately, they all are potential suppressive agents of the hypothalamic-pituitary-adrenal axis.

Triamcinolone diacetate is suspended in a solution consisting of polysorbate 80 0.20%, polyethylene glycol 3350 3%, sodium chloride 0.85%, and benzyl alcohol 0.90% as a preservative. Its pH is adjusted to approximately 6.[31] This steroid is compatible with a variety of diluents unless a preservative is present. Flocculation and clumping of triamcinolone are reported when mixed with a preserved diluent or if the steroid has been frozen and thawed. Methylprednisolone has been shown to flocculate when mixed with lidocaine.

Although systemic toxicity from epidural injection is not exactly known, suppression of the hypothalamic-pituitary-adrenal axis from triamcinolone has been shown to persist for 21 days.[32] Examples of the toxic effects are metabolic disturbances, electrolyte imbalances, fluid shifts such as edema, muscle wasting, peptic ulcers, impaired wound healing, and immunologic dysfunction[33]; allergic reactions to the steroids are rare.[34] The preservative polyethylene glycol in many commercial formulations may cause arachnoiditis when injected intrathecally.[35] Case reports of epidural abscesses, aseptic meningitis, and bacterial meningitis have also been published.[36, 37]

HYPERTONIC SALINE

Hypertonic saline was first reported as a cold saline injection into the intrathecal space for chronic back pain in 1967.[38] Hitchcock later reported that the hypertonicity of the solutions rather than the temperature was responsible for its effects.[39] Cat studies showed a selective C fiber blockade of dorsal rootlets that appeared to be related to the high chloride ion concentration.[38] Lake and Barnes's work[39] on frog spinal neurons showed that hypertonic saline decreased the spinal cord water content and depressed the lateral column evoked ventral root response by affecting the gamma aminobutyric acid (GABA) receptors. Racz and associates[43] performed a study on dogs looking at the effects of hypertonic saline in the epidural space and showed that it took 20 minutes for the cerebrospinal fluid (CSF) to equilibrate, with resultant doubling of the CSF sodium concentration.[40]

Most of the complications cited are related to intrathecal hypertonic saline. Clinical complications of intrathecal injection of hypertonic saline consist of cardiac, respiratory, and neurologic sequelae such as hypertension, tachycardia, and tachypnea with pulmonary edema.[41] The changes can occur rapidly with associated hemorrhaging.[10] As to complications directly related to epidural injection, Aldrete and colleagues[42] reported two cases of arachnoiditis from possible subdural or subarachnoid spread; no other incidences have been noted or reported.

ANATOMY

The sacrum is a large, triangular bone, situated below L5. Its apex articulates with the coccyx. Its anterior surface is concave. Anteriorly four transverse ridges cross its median part. The portions of the bone between the ridges are the bodies of the sacrum. There are four anterior sacral foramina through which the sacral nerves exit and lateral sacral arteries enter. The posterior surface of the sacrum is convex. There are rudimentary spinous processes from the first three or four sacral segments in the midline. The laminae unite to form the sacral groove. The sacral hiatus is formed by the failure of the laminae of S5 to unite posteriorly. The tubercles that represent remnants of the inferior articular processes are known as the *sacral cornua*; they are connected inferiorly to the coccygeal cornua. Laterally one can identify four dorsal sacral foramina. They transmit the posterior divisions of the sacral nerves. The sacrum may have many variations. The bodies of the S1 and S2 may fail to unite or the sacral canal may remain open throughout its length (Fig. 41–1).

RADIOLOGIC LANDMARKS OF THE CAUDAL CANAL

In a lateral view (Fig. 41–2), the caudal canal appears as a slight step off on the most posterior part of the sacrum. The median sacral crest is seen as an opaque line posterior to the caudal canal. While still in the lateral view, the sacral hiatus is usually visible as a translucent opening at the base of the caudal canal. To aid identification of the sacral hiatus, the coccyx can be seen articulating with the inferior surface of the sacrum.

On the anteroposterior view, the intermediate sacral crests are seen as opaque vertical lines on either side of the midline (Fig. 41–3). The sacral foramina are seen as translucent near-circular areas lateral to the intermediate sacral crests. Note that the presence of bowel gas can make recognition of these structures difficult.

INDICATIONS

- Failed back surgery syndrome
- Epidural fibrosis
- Lumbar radiculopathy
- Spinal stenosis

CONTRAINDICATIONS

- Local infection
- Coagulopathies
- Unstable lumbar spine
- Inability to lie in prone position

EQUIPMENT

- 25 gauge, ¾-inch infiltration needle
- 18-gauge, 1½-inch needle
- 16-gauge Epimed RK epidural needle
- Epimed Tun-L or Tun-L-XL epidural catheter, 24 cm
- Loss-of-resistance syringe
- 3-mL syringe
- 2 10-mL syringes
- Needle driver
- 3-0 nylon on cutting needle
- Scissors

DRUGS

- 1.5% lidocaine for skin infiltration
- 2% preservative-free lidocaine
- 0.5% preservative-free levobupivacaine or ropivacaine
- 0.9% preservative-free normal saline
- 10% preservative-free hypertonic saline
- 1500 U of hyaluronidase

PREPARATION OF THE PATIENT

PHYSICAL EXAMINATION

- Straight leg raise: positive radicular signs at less than 60 degrees

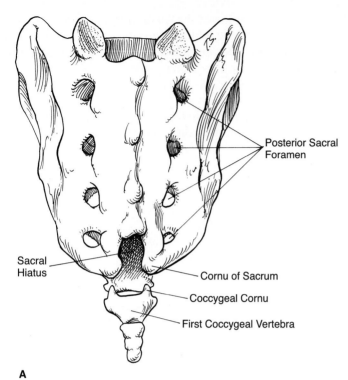

A

FIGURE 41–1

A, Anatomy of the sacral hiatus and dorsum of the sacrum. Also shown is the course of sacral nerve roots in anteroposterior *(B)* and lateral *(C)* views. (*A* From Raj PP [ed]: Clinical Practice of Regional Anesthesia. New York, Churchill Livingstone, 1991, p 328.)

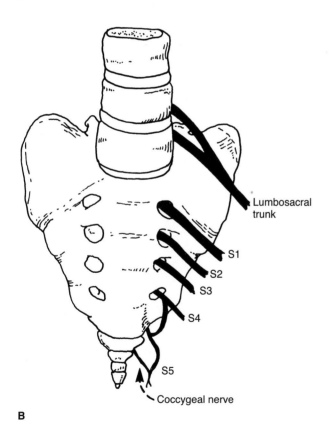

B

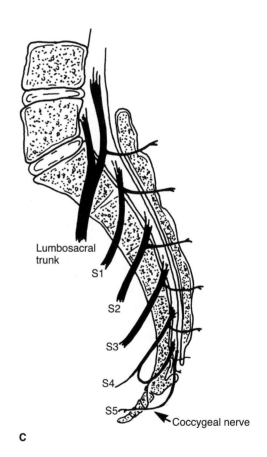

C

- Identification of pain to nerve root levels
- Functional evaluation
- Confirm stable vital signs
- Ability to lie prone for 60 minutes

LABORATORY

Indicated laboratory and radiologic studies should be obtained. Prothrombin time, partial thromboplastin time, bleeding time, white blood cell count with differential, urine analysis, and magnetic resonance imaging of the affected area are usually reviewed.

PREOPERATIVE MEDICATION

It may be necessary to sedate the patient with 1 to 2 mg midazolam and 25 to 50 µg of fentanyl.

■ Ceftriaxone (Rocephin) 1 g preoperative intravenously.

MONITORING PROCEDURES

Usual monitoring includes an automated blood pressure cuff, electrocardiogram, and pulse oximeter; the patient should have a patent intravenous catheter. Fluoroscopy is essential to the performance of safe adhesiolysis. To minimize radiation exposure, it is preferable to use a fluoroscope with memory capabilities and efficient computed image processing. For documentation purposes, videotaping the fluoroscopy screen during the procedure or printouts for subsequent review is recommended. For personal safety, the physician should use appropriate protective measures such as leaded gloves, apron, thyroid shield, and leaded glasses. An addition of a leaded skirt around the fluoroscopy table can further decrease radiation exposure. Lastly, fluoroscopy is important in obtaining the maximum benefit from this procedure, that is, for verification of needle placement, visualization of dye spread, and proper catheter placement.

TECHNIQUE

On the fluoroscopy table the patient is placed prone with a pillow under the abdomen to straighten the lumbar spine. Monitors are applied, including an electrocardiogram, pulse oximeter, and a blood pressure monitoring device, preferably an automated one. The sacral area is then sterilely prepared and draped from the top of the iliac crest to the bottom of the buttocks. Abduction of the legs and internal rotation of the feet facilitates entry into the sacral hiatus. The sacral cornua and the sacral hiatus are palpated with the index finger of the nondominant hand rolled laterally over the sacral hiatus. For entry through the skin, a spot approximately 1 to 2 cm lateral and 2 to 3 cm inferior to the sacral hiatus in the contralateral gluteal region on the affected side for treatment is accessed (Fig. 41–4). This point of entry inherently allows the needle, as well as the catheter, to be directed toward the affected side. The entry point is infiltrated with a local anesthetic, such as 1% lidocaine. A 16-gauge epidural needle, preferably an Epimed RK epidural needle, is passed through the described entry point, into the sacral hiatus and through the sacrococcygeal ligament. Using the sacral cornua as

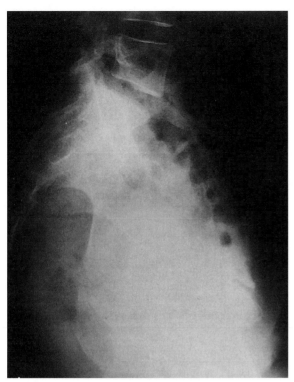

FIGURE 41–2

Lateral radiograph of caudal space. (From Waldman SD [ed]: Interventional Pain Management, 2nd ed. Philadelphia, WB Saunders, 2001, p 435.)

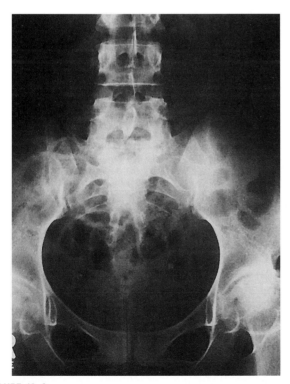

FIGURE 41–3

Anteroposterior view of the lumbosacral region. (From Waldman SD [ed]: Interventional Pain Management, 2nd ed. Philadelphia, WB Saunders, 2001, p 435.)

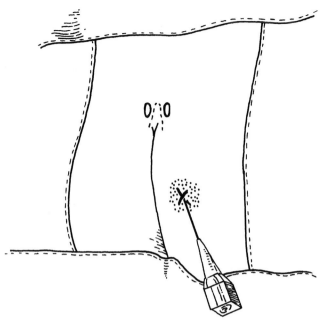

FIGURE 41-4

Drawing of the site of entry in the gluteal fold for caudal neuroplasty.

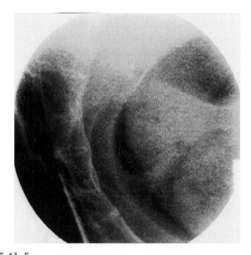

FIGURE 41-5

Lateral radiographic image of the caudal canal that shows the needle entering into the space.

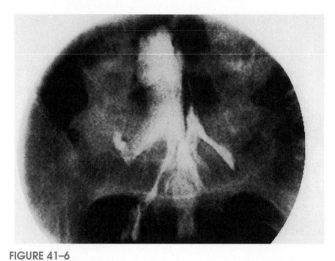

FIGURE 41-6

Radiographic image of the caudal canal after contrast material (iohexol) has been injected during neuroplasty. One can discern a "Christmas tree" appearance of the contrast solution.

▼ TABLE 41-2 Solutions Used in Caudal Neuroplasty

When Used	Solution	Volume(mL)
Day of operation	Iohexol 240 mgI/mL	20
	Hyaluronidase in PFNS, 150 U/mL	10
	Bupivacaine, 0.25% triamcinolone diacetate, 4 mg/mL	10
	NaCl, 10%	10
	prn bupivacaine, 0.25%	2
	PFNS	2
Postoperative day 1	Bupivacaine, 0.25%	10
	NaCl, 10%	10
	prn bupivacaine, 0.25%	2
	PFNS	2
Postoperative day 2	Bupivacaine, 0.25%	10
	NaCl, 10%	10
	prn bupivacaine, 0.25%	2
	PFNS	2

PFNS, preservative-free normal saline,

landmarks to locate the hiatus, the needle is advanced to a level no higher than the S3 foramen to avoid damaging the sacral nerve roots. Placement is confirmed by a lateral fluoroscopic view prior to any injections to determine that the needle is within the bony canal (Fig. 41–5). This is important because anatomic variations of the sacrum could lead to incorrect needle placement, which may "feel" correct. Next, an anteroposterior view should verify needle tip placement toward the affected side. To facilitate the passage of the catheter to the anterior epidural space, the epidural needle is turned with the bevel facing either the 7 o'clock position for the left or the 5 o'clock position for the right.

After negative aspiration for blood and CSF, 10 mL of iohexol (Omnipaque 240) or metrizamide (Amipaque) is injected under fluoroscopy for an epidurogram (Fig. 41–6 and Table 41–2). If venous runoff is noted, the needle tip is moved during injection until contrast media is seen spreading within the epidural space. As contrast media is injected into the epidural space, a "Christmas tree" shape will be noted as the dye spreads into the perineural structures inside the bony canal and along the nerves as they exit the vertebral column. Epidural adhesions will prevent dye spread, such that there will be a marked absence of dye outlining the involved nerve roots. A lateral view will also show a lack of dye outlining the scarred nerve roots.

If the needle tip is subarachnoid, dye spread will be noted centrally and cephalad many levels above L5. If the needle tip is subdural, dye spread will also be central and cephalad but will not be as wide as that of a subarachnoid injection. The contrast will enhance the view of the outline of the nerve roots and the dura from the circumferential spread within the less resistant subdural space. Injection of local anesthetic into the subarachnoid or subdural space will result in a motor block that is notably more profound, with a more rapid onset of the block than that seen after injection into the epidural space. A subdural block is often typified by a segmental motor block with a diffuse sensory block to the level expected from a subarachnoid injection of local anesthetic.

If CSF is aspirated, it is best to abort the procedure and repeat it another day. If blood is aspirated, the needle is first retracted caudally in the sacral canal until no blood can be aspirated. If this is unsuccessful, an attempt can be made to proceed with catheter placement into the proper location. Aspiration of this catheter should be negative for blood, and lack of venous runoff should be confirmed through the injection of contrast agent.

The ideal epidural catheter for use is a stainless-steel, fluoropolymer-coated, spiral-tipped Racz Tun-L-Kath.[43,44] A Racz catheter is passed through the needle into the scar tissue (Fig. 41–7). The bevel of the needle should be facing the ventrolateral aspect of the caudal canal of the affected side. This turning of the needle facilitates passage of the catheter to the desired side and decreases the chance of shearing the catheter. Because scar formation is usually uneven, multiple passes may be necessary to place the catheter into the scarred area. For this reason, it is best to use a 16-gauge RK epidural needle, which has been specially designed to allow multiple passes of the catheter.[45] To facilitate steering of the catheter into the desired location, a 15-degree bend is placed at the distal end of the catheter. After final placement of the catheter and negative aspiration, another 3 to 5 mL of contrast medium (maximum of a total of 20 mL) is injected through the catheter. This additional dye should be seen spreading into the area of the previous filling defect with outlining of the targeted nerve root. Next, 1500 U of hyaluronidase (Wydase) in solution with 10 mL of preservative-free normal saline is injected rapidly. Afterward 10 mL of 0.2% ropivacaine and 40 mg of triamcinolone are injected through the catheter in divided doses after negative aspiration. This additional volume is helpful in further lysis of adhesions because the catheter tip is in the scar tissue. The area of scarring and subsequent scar dissection should be noted and recorded. The steroids cannot be injected through the 22-μm bacteriostatic filter, so the steroid must be injected prior to placement of the in-line filter.

If contrast media is not used because of an allergic history, the procedure is the same except for the absence of dye. Aspiration should be negative for CSF and blood prior to any injection. Additionally, a test dose of local anesthetic should be given to verify that the needle and subsequently the catheter are not subarachnoid or sub-

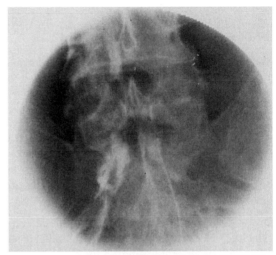

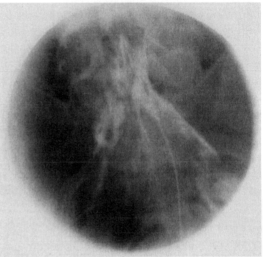

FIGURE 41–7

A, The Racz Tun-L-Kath epidural catheter is threaded to the right side of the epidural space into the area scarred. *B*, Injection of 5 mL of contrast medium shows spread into the area scarred previously. This was followed by injection of 9 mL of 0.2% ropivacaine with 40 mg (1 mL) of triamcinolone and, 30 minutes later, by 10 mL 10% saline. The patient had complete pain relief after the procedure. (From Waldman SD [ed]: Interventional Pain Management, 2nd ed. Philadelphia, WB Saunders, 2001, p 437.)

dural. When properly placed, the patient often reports pain with injection in the dermatomal distribution of the scarred area.

When the procedure is completed, the catheter should be secured to the skin with 3-0 nylon on a cutting needle. Caution must be taken to not puncture the catheter with the needle as well as not cutting the catheter coating while wrapping it. Triple-antibiotic ointment, such as polymyxin, and two 2 × 2-inch split gauze pads are used to cover the catheter exit site. The surrounding skin is sprayed or covered with tincture of benzoin and, with a single loop of the catheter toward midline, all of the above is covered with a 4 × 6-inch size sterile transparent surgical dressing. On top of the transparent dressing, we place two 4 × 4-inch gauze pads over the puncture site and apply four pieces of

6-inch long Hypafix tape over the area . This Hypafix tape has the unique ability of being elastic yet porous, so that the patient does not "sweat it off" during the 3 days that the catheter is kept in place. Prior to undraping the sterile field, the catheter is connected to an adapter and a 22-μm bacteriostatic filter that are not removed during the duration of the three daily injections. The filter is capped, and the catheter is taped to the flank of the patient. In the preoperative area and during hospitalization, the patient is given intravenous antibiotics in the form of cephalosporins, such as ceftriaxone (Rocephin), 1 g daily intravenously. Prophylactic antibiotics are given to prevent bacterial colonization, which is especially hazardous in view of the epidurally administered steroid. It is also our practice to send a patient home on an oral antibiotic for 5 additional days as epidural abscess prophylaxis.

Once the patient is taken to the recovery room and vital signs are obtained, 10 mL of the 10% hypertonic saline is infused over 20 to 30 minutes. Occasionally, the patient may complain of severe burning pain during the infusion. The burning is usually from the introduction of hypertonic saline to unanesthetized epidural tissue. Should this occur, the infusion must be stopped and a 3- to 5-mL bolus of additional local anesthetic is injected. After 5 minutes the hypertonic saline infusion can be restarted without incident. Following completion of the hypertonic saline infusion, 1.5 mL of preservative-free normal saline is used to flush the catheter. Once this task is completed, the cap is replaced on the filter.

The hypertonic saline has a mild, reversible local anesthetic effect and also reduces edema of previously scarred or inflamed nerve roots.[46,47] Injection of hypertonic solutions into the normal epidural space is quite painful unless preceded by local anesthetic. If the hypertonic saline spread is greater than the coverage area of the local anesthetic, the patient may have severe pain. The pain caused by the hypertonic saline in the epidural space rarely persists more than 5 minutes.

The catheter is left in place for 3 days. On the second and third days, the catheter is injected once a day with 10 mL of 0.2% ropivacaine after negative aspiration from the catheter. Fifteen minutes later, 9 mL of 10% saline is infused over 20 minutes for patient comfort. As with all hypertonic saline infusion series, the catheter must be flushed with 1.5 mL of preservative-free normal saline. On the third day the catheter is removed 10 minutes after the last injection. A triple-antibiotic ointment is placed on the wound and is covered by a bandage or other appropriate dressing.

HELPFUL HINTS

We inject only one dose of steroid and do so in the operating room under total sterile conditions. After the bac-

teriostatic filter is placed, it is not removed during the series of reinjections. We have demonstrated in our laboratory that when methylprednisolone (Depo-Medrol) plus local anesthetic or triamcinolone (Aristocort) and local anesthetic are injected through a bacteriostatic filter, the filter screens out virtually all of the steroid.[48]

During the time the catheter is indwelling, the patient should keep the insertion site dry. We also recommend that the patient keep the area dry for 48 hours after removal to decrease the chance of infection. Showering is permitted after this period, but immersion of the wound such as in a bath or pool therapy should be avoided for a minimum of 7 to 10 days.

This procedure is usually followed by significant improvement in pain and motor function. With improvement of pain, it is important to initiate aggressive physical therapy to improve muscle strength and tone, which is usually decreased from lack of use secondary to pain. Often it is not possible to completely lyse existing epidural adhesions because of the extensive amount of scar tissue. If necessary, we repeat the procedure. Because of the steroids used, a 3-month delay between procedures is necessary, during which time the patient should be encouraged to continue intense physical therapy. This therapy should begin immediately, when possible. Initiation of neural flossing techniques, especially while the local anesthetic is still active, provides a prime opportunity to maximize the adhesiolysis process with the least discomfort to the patient. One month of aquatic therapy followed by aggressive, graded physical therapy and work hardening is also recommended.

After negative aspiration is noted, all solutions should be injected slowly. Observation of the fluoroscopies often initially reveals massive epidural scar formation, as seen in the series of radiographs shown in Figure 41–8. In Figure 41–8A, after injection of 10 mL of Omnipaque 240, one can see the dye preferentially spreading toward the right-hand side, opening up the right L4–5 and S1–2 nerve roots, whereas there is a complete filling defect of the left L4 and S1 and partial filling of the L5 nerve root. In Figure 41–8B a Racz Tun-L-XL catheter is threaded into the L5 neural foramen area, and through this, an injection of an additional 10 mL of Omnipaque is seen to open up the L5, S1 nerve root (Fig. 41–8C), as well as to spread cephalad as evidenced by the disappearance of the L4–5 disc space because this space is masked by the spreading contrast (Fig. 41–8D). This is followed by the injection of 10 mL of preservative-free saline, 1500 U of hyaluronidase spreading to L4 and L5, and finally the 10 mL of 0.2% ropivacaine and 40 mL of triamcinolone (Fig. 41–8E). The contrast is spreading up to L4, L5, and then to S1, evenly, almost like a Christmas tree appearance. The foot drop dramatically improved the following day as a result of the decompression of the L4–5, S1 nerve

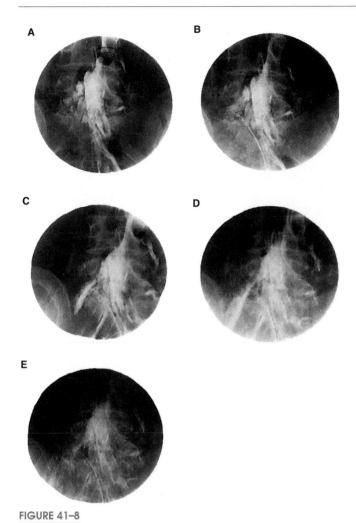

FIGURE 41–8

Radiographs from a patient with left lower extremity pain and foot drop. *A,* After 10 mL of iohexol (Omnipaque) 240. Note complete filling defect on the left at L4 and S1 and partial filling of the L5 spinal nerve. *B,* Racz Tun-L-Kath-SL threaded into the L5 neural foramen. *C,* After injection of another 10 mL of iohexol, note the opening of the L5–S1 nerve root and cephalad spread of contrast medium. *D* and *E,* Further opening of filling defect and cephalad spread of contrast medium. (From Waldman SD [ed]: Interventional Pain Management, 2nd ed. Philadelphia, WB Saunders, 2001, p 441.)

roots by dissection of the perineural space with the injected material.

COMPLICATIONS

Injection of local anesthetic into the subarachnoid or subdural space (Fig. 41–9) results in a motor block that is notably more profound and of more rapid onset than that subsequent to injection into the epidural space. A subdural block is often typified by a segmental motor block with a diffuse sensory block to the level expected from a subarachnoid injection of local anesthetic.

If CSF is aspirated, it is best to abort the procedure and repeat it another day. If blood is aspirated, the needle is first retracted caudad in the sacral canal until

no blood can be aspirated. If this is unsuccessful, an attempt can be made to proceed with catheter placement into the proper site. Aspiration through this catheter should be negative for blood, and lack of venous runoff should be confirmed with injection of contrast medium. The adverse effects include bruising, transient hypotension, transient breathing difficulty, numbness of the extremities, bowel or bladder dysfunction, paralysis, infection, sexual dysfunction, and the possibility that the catheter might shear.

The most common idiosyncratic reaction occurring after intrathecal iohexol is headache, which occurs in approximately 18% of patients.[14] Myalgias, nausea, vomiting, and dizziness may also occur. Aseptic meningitis and neurologic disturbances have been reported as infrequent complications. In addition, allergic or anaphylactoid reactions may occur rarely with non-ionic agents, but far less frequently than with their ionic predecessors.[16]

The exact complication rate of iohexol epidurography is unknown; however, a number of studies on the complications of iohexol myelography have provided some indications regarding the safety margin of epidurography. Ndosi and colleagues[17] determined in a double-blinded, placebo-controlled trial that myelography with appropriate concentrations of iohexol (240 mgI/mL) carried no more risk of significant reaction than a diagnostic lumbar puncture. The same study demonstrated that iohexol concentrations of 180 and 300 mgI/mL were more likely to result in headache, dizziness, nausea, vomiting, and seizures.

Insect hyaluronidase is an allergen in stinging insect venoms and has a known homology to mammalian hyaluronidase.[25] Anaphylactic-like reactions have occurred in isolated cases.[26] Heightened awareness of this complication should be considered when treating patients with a history of venom allergy.

The significant toxicity of bupivacaine is cardiotoxicity. This usually results from accidental intravascular administration of large doses of bupivacaine. Bupivacaine disassociates from sodium channels more slowly than lidocaine during cardiac diastole; therefore, its effect is more pronounced and cumulative. This leads to severe cardiac arrhythmias and myocardial depression.

Systemic toxicity of triamcinolone diacetate depends on the dose and duration of treatment and the rapidity with which it is absorbed from the epidural space. These kinetics have not yet been elucidated; however, after epidural administration, suppression of the hypothalamic-pituitary-adrenal axis has been shown to persist for 21 days.[32] The potential systemic toxic effects, though rare, are related to its glucocorticoid activity and include fluid, electrolyte, and metabolic disturbances; muscle wasting; peptic ulcer; and impaired would healing and immunologic function.[33] Allergic reactions have been reported in rare instances.[34] Intrathecal corticosteroid administration may be a serious complication of epidural corticosteroid injections since depot formulations commonly contain

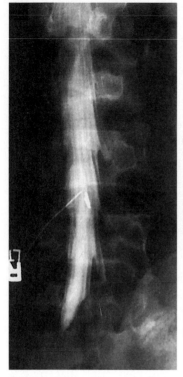

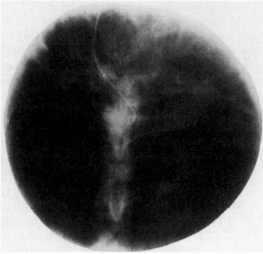

B

A

FIGURE 41-9

A, Subarachnoid spread of contrast medium. B, Subdural spread of contrast medium. Observe the contrast medium spreading centrally, without a "Christmas tree" configuration. The catheter is in the central part of the canal. (From Waldman SD [ed]: Interventional Pain Management, 2nd ed. Philadelphia, WB Saunders, 2001, p 437.)

polyethylene glycol, which may cause arachnoiditis when administered intrathecally. Cases of aseptic and bacterial meningitis, as well as epidural abscess, have been reported rarely.[36,37]

Clinical complications of intrathecal hypertonic saline have been well described in multiple investigations. They include cardiac, respiratory, or neurologic sequelae in approximately 10% of patients.[8] In addition, the discomfort associated with intrathecal administration requires general anesthesia. Serious complications can occur when osmotic effects of hypertonic saline cause elevated CSF pressure, which in turn results in hypertension, tachycardia, and tachypnea with pulmonary edema. These changes can occur precipitously and with hemorrhagic consequences.[9]

Conversely, such complications from hypertonic saline injected epidurally are not observed, although two cases of arachnoiditis were reported by Aldrete and others.[42] It was suggested the solutions may have been injected into the subarachnoid space in these cases. These researchers' results were based on a survey of 72 patients who were randomly selected from a pool of approximately 200 patients who had the procedure performed, as well as follow-up with these patients, which occurred between 6 months to 1 year later. They found that 25.0% of the patients did not decrease their use of pain medication, 43.0% decreased their dosage and frequency of their medication use, 16.7% discontinued pain medication, and only 1.4% increased their use of pain medication. Although 72.2% of the patients reported pain relief on discharge, 25.0% reported no

TABLE 41-3 Outcomes

	Total Volume on Day 1 (mL)	Number of Patients	Outcomes
Racz and Holubec[11] (1989)	50	72	Initial pain relief: 72.2% Return to work/daily function: 30.6%
Stolker et al[12] (1994)	?	28	50% pain relief at 12 months: 64%
Arthur et al[58] (1993)	40–50	50	Initial pain relief: 65% Persistent relief: 14%
Devulder et al[59] (1995)*	40	34	Pain relief at 1 month: 33.3% Pain relief at 12 months: 0%

* Nonspecific catheter placement

relief and 2.8% reported worse pain on discharge; 37.5% of the patients reported less than 1 month's relief, 30.5% reported 1 to 3 months' relief, and 12.5% reported 3 to 6 months' relief. In total, 30.6% of the patients returned to work or returned to daily functions.

Arthur and colleagues[54] described a study at the 7th World Congress on Pain in which the technique was identical to the present technique except that hyaluronidase was injected in only 50 of the 100 patients. The results showed 81.6% of the hyaluronidase group had relief of pain, with 12.3% having persistent relief; 68.0% of the no-hyaluronidase group had relief of pain, with 14.0% having persistent relief[49] (Table 41–3).

A study by Devulder and coworkers[50] in 1995 was based on 34 patients in whom epidural adhesions were suspected based on either magnetic resonance imaging or their history of back surgery. In their protocol, in which hyaluronidase was not employed, an epidural catheter was placed via the sacral hiatus under fluoroscopy but without direction toward the affected site. The catheter was simply advanced 10 cm into the epidural space and 10 mL of contrast agent (10 hexol 240 mgI/mL) was injected. Defects that corresponded to the patient's pain were demonstrated in 30 of the 34 patients' resulting epidurograms. Injection of 20 mL of 2% lidocaine with 80 mg of methylprednisolone added was followed by 10 mL of 10% hypertonic saline. The procedures were repeated on the second and third day via the indwelling catheter. The researchers noted a regression of adhesions in 14 of the 30 patients who had had defects. Seven of these patients reported marked improvement of their pain, defined as a visual analog scale score of less than 4 at 1 month. Only two of these patients reported this level of improvement at 3 months, and at 1 year this entire group of patients had undergone a different treatment because of return of their pain. Only four of the patients without any improvement of contrast spread reported marked pain relief at 1 month, two at 3 months; and one remained pain free at 1 year. Chi-square analysis of these data showed no statistically significant correlation between enhanced contrast spread after the injections and a better outcome. This procedure has been criticized for the lack of guidance of the catheter tip into the lesion and demonstrates the importance of directing the catheter tip into the lesion.

TRANSFORAMINAL NEUROPLASTY

HISTORY

Lumbar transforaminal injections were first developed as a method to inject the dorsal root ganglion.

ANATOMY

The lumbar spine consists of five lumbar vertebrae. The borders of the lumbar foramen consist of the vertebral body and disc anteriorly, the pedicles superiorly and inferiorly, and the facet articular processes posteriorly. Within the foramen the nerve root exits in an anterocaudal direction. Anterior to the nerve root, radicular vessels can be found to follow the nerve root into the epidural space. Posterior to the nerve root is the dorsal root ganglion.

INDICATIONS

Transforaminal neuroplasty may be indicated on those occasions when the nerve roots are difficult to "open" or when access to the anterior space is needed.

CONTRAINDICATIONS

The main contraindications to transforaminal neuroplasty are local infection and coagulopathies.

DRUGS AND EQUIPMENT

See sections on caudal neuroplasty and caudal neuroplasty for drugs and equipment.

PATIENT POSITION

The patient is in the prone position with enough table clearance to provide full range of rotation of the fluoroscopy.

TECHNIQUE

After consent, the patient is placed in the prone position. Using sterile preparation and technique, the back is cleansed with a sterilizing solution from just below the scapula to the lower margin of the buttocks. Preparation of the lumbar region is appropriate only if the upper lumbar region is the source of the problem, without sciatic involvement. Using fluoroscopy the desired lumbar level and side are identified. The fluoroscope is then oblique to the ipsilateral side of the desired foramina to 15 to 20 degrees. Once a "Scottie dog" image is obtained, the fluoroscope is then rotated in a caudal-cephalad direction for 15 to 20 degrees. A caudal-cephalad rotation elongates the superior articular process ("ear of the Scottie dog"). The tip of the ear or superior articular process in a "gun barrel" technique is marked on the skin. This spot is the skin entry site, and local anesthetic is injected for skin infiltration. An 18-gauge needle is used to make a puncture wound. Through this wound a 16-gauge Epimed RK epidural needle is advanced anteriorly, until bone is contacted (Fig. 41–10). Next, a lateral fluoroscopic view is obtained prior to further introduction of the needle. To facilitate passage of the needle past the articular process, the epidural needle is turned laterally to slide past the bone and stopped just after a "pop" is felt. The needle tip on a lateral view should be in the posterior aspect of the foramen. An Epimed Tun-L-XL epidural catheter is then inserted through the epidural needle. Occasionally, the epidural needle must be tilted at the hub laterally to aid entry of the epidural catheter into the anterior epidural space. The catheter is advanced medial to the pedicle (Fig. 41–10C). After catheter placement is confirmed to be in the anterior epidural space under lateral view (Fig. 41–10D), the stylet is removed from the catheter and a connector is placed on the proximal end of the epidural catheter. Aspiration should be negative before 3 mL of iohexol (Omnipaque 240) radiographic contrast is injected. The contrast injection

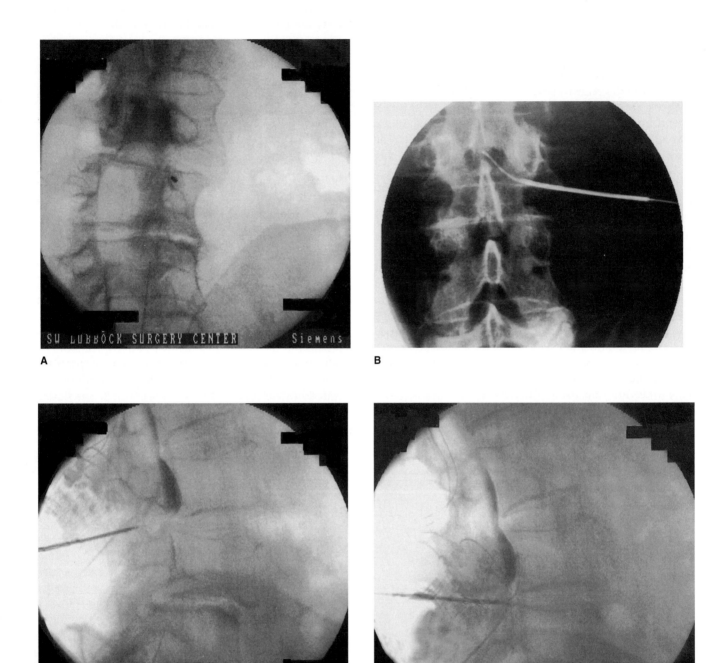

FIGURE 41–10

A, Oblique view of the lumbar spine showing the needle entry point for the transforaminal technique. *B*, Anteroposterior view of the transforaminal technique with the catheter entering the epidural space. *C*, Lateral view of the transforaminal technique with the catheter entering the epidural space. *D*, Lateral radiographic imaging of the lumbosacral region in the transforaminal technique showing the passage of the catheter anteriorly with contrast spread from the tip.

should show opening of the entered neuroforamen with contrast agent exiting along the path of the nerve root. When satisfactory contrast spread is seen, 8 mL of 1500 U of hyaluronidase and preservative-free normal saline is injected to further the opening of other adhesions. Lastly, 8 mL of 0.2% ropivacaine or 0.25% bupivacaine with 20 to 40 mg of triamcinolone diacetate is injected. The catheter is then secured into place with 2-0 nylon on a cutting needle. The dressing consists of triple-antibiotic ointment over the wound site, a 2×2-slotted gauge pad over the ointment, small loop inferior loop of the catheter, and a cover with a transparent surgical dressing. For added security, the dressing is further covered by Micropore tape.

After the patient is transported to the recovery room and negative aspiration of the catheter is confirmed, 7 mL of 10% hypertonic saline is infused over 20 minutes. Once the infusion is completed, the epidural catheter is cleared with 1 to 2 mL of preservative-free normal saline. The epidural catheter is then left in place for reinjections 2 and 3. For reinjections 2 and 3, the catheter is checked for negative aspiration. The local anesthetic is given in divided doses (2 mL and 4 to 6 mL) at 5-minute intervals. As with the first injection, the hypertonic saline (7 mL) is infused over 20 minutes and flushed with 1 to 2 mL of normal saline.

Subdural or intravascular injection should be monitored. Removal of the catheter is performed after the third infusion. Care must be taken to remove the epidural catheter intact.

EFFICACY

While there are no controlled studies on the clinical effectiveness of transforaminal epidural injections, many clinical reports have been supportive.

CERVICAL NEUROPLASTY

HISTORY

Cervical epidural blockade was first reported by Dogliotti in 1933.[51] Cervical neuroplasty is a derivative of caudal neuroplasty. It was conceived by Racz in 1989 as a method to address the epidural fibrosis associated with failed neck surgery syndrome, disc bulges, and inflammation not responsive to single-shot epidural steroid injection. Because of the narrowness and potential for profound spinal cord injury, fluoroscopy was introduced as safety tool for the pain physician. Naturally, the use of non-ionic water-soluble radiographic contrast was soon added to monitor vascular runoff. The technique has been modified to include selective nerve root stimulation for localization of the painful nerve root. This modification is called *neural mapping*.

ANATOMY

The cervical spine consists of seven vertebrae and eight nerve roots. C1 and C2 nerve roots exit the central neuraxis posteriorly through the intralaminar space to innervate the posterior upper neck and scalp of the occipital region. Cervical nerve roots C3–C8 exit from neuroforamina. These differences are important for nerve-specific epidural catheter placement and adhesiolysis.

For the placement of the epidural needle, several key points need to be mentioned. The posterior wall of the bony canal is composed of the spinous process and lamina. Knowledge of these landmarks is important for radiographic identification. Just after the bone of the vertebrae is the ligamentum flavum. The interspinous ligament covers the interspinous spaces.

PATIENT POSITIONING

The standard used by our team is a left lateral decubitus position. In lateral decubitus, the potential of the patient moving into your needle is greatly diminished. By providing an outlet direction for movement, the patient tends to move away from the epidural needle. If the prone or sitting position is used, caution must be used to ensure that the patient does not move. Securing the patient may require extensive strapping and taping of the head and torso.

TECHNIQUE

Because of the potential for dural puncture and spinal cord injury, the upper thoracic approach (T1–T2) is used. After sterile preparation and maintaining sterile technique, the skin entry point is marked 1 to 1½ vertebral levels lower. Using the spinous process as midline, the site for skin entry is anesthestized with 1.5% lidocaine using a 25-gauge infiltration about 1 cm paramedial on the contralateral side. The entry of the epidural needle is facilitated with a puncture wound from an 18-gauge needle. Using fluoroscopy in the anteroposterior view (Fig. 41–11*A*), a 16-gauge, 3½-inch Epimed RK epidural needle is inserted toward the T1–T2 interspace with the tip of the needle directed to midline. At the skin the needle will appear to be progressing in a 70- to 80-degree angle owing to the lordosis of the spine at that level. Once the direction of the needle is considered satisfactory and before the needle crosses into the interlaminar zone, the fluoroscope is changed to a lateral view to visualize the "straight line" of the anterior spinous process (Fig. 41–11*B*). Just before this line is breached, the fluoroscope is returned into the anteroposterior view to confirm the proper direction of the needle (Fig. 41–11*C*). The final 2 to 3 mm of needle

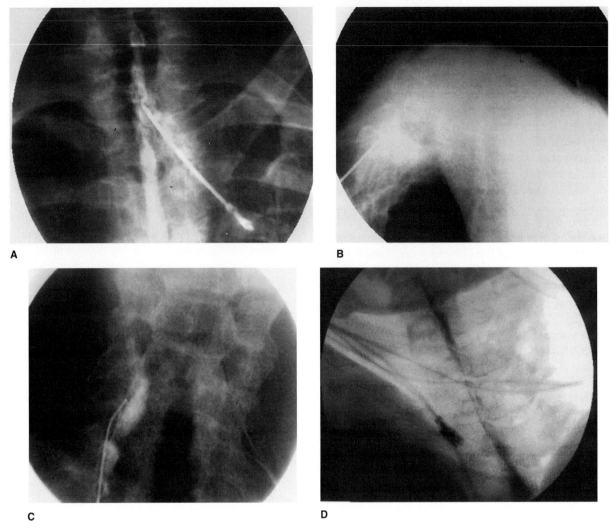

FIGURE 41-11

A, Entry of the RK needle in the anteroposterior view with contrast spread during cervical neuroplasty. *B,* Lateral view of needle during cervical neuroplasty. The RK needle is in the epidural space. *C,* Anteroposterior view of a cervical catheter in place with early spread of a small amount of contrast solution. *D,* Spread of contrast solution in the cervical region during cervical neuroplasty.

advancement is done with the loss-of-resistance technique. Our practice is to use 2 mL of preservative-free normal saline and 2 mL of air.

After the needle is in place, 3 to 5 mL of Omnipaque 240 contrast material is injected to create an epidurogram. Once a scarred area is delineated, a styleted, saline-flushed Epimed Tun-L-XL catheter is prepared for introduction through the epidural needle. A 10-degree bend is placed at the distal 2.5 to 3 cm of the epidural catheter. The bend facilitates steering of the catheter. By using purposeful twisting of the epidural catheter, the tip is guided through the scarred area and specifically placed at that nerve root.

If a clearly scarred nerve root cannot be found, the Racz Tun-L-XL epidural lends itself to electrostimulation. The distal tip is metallic and the stylet can be withdrawn 1 to 2 cm for clamping with alligator clip cables. The negative (black) electrode is placed on the catheter

stylet and the positive (red) alligator clamp is placed on the epidural needle or a 22-gauge needle placed into the skin as a ground. In these situations the catheter tip is placed at the lowest suspected nerve root and progressively manipulated over each successive superior nerve root and vice versa. The Medtronic trial screener is the pulse generator used. (Standard pulse generator settings are 0 negative, 3 positive, and 1 and 2 off; rate = 50; pulse width = 450.) Commonly, the patient vocalizes reproduction of pain or paresthesia in the affected painful area with electrostimulation.

When final placement is determined, the epidural catheter is often reinjected with 1 to 2 mL of radiographic contrast to evaluate the "opening" of the nerve root (Fig. 41-11*D*). Once this is confirmed, the catheter is thereafter injected with 6 mL of 1500 U of hyaluronidase in preservative-free 0.9% saline. Radiographic imaging during injection of these agents is recommended to rule out intravascular and intrathecal injection. As an added precaution the catheter should always be aspirated prior to injection of any drugs. Lastly, 6 mL total of 0.2% ropivacaine or 0.25% bupivacaine and 40 mg of triamcinolone diacetate is injected in 2- and 4-mL boluses. It is extremely important to wait 5 minutes between boluses of local anesthetics to guard against inadvertent spread or injection. Active monitoring of the patient during local anesthetic injections should be maintained.

The catheter is now ready for securing. To prevent accidental displacement of the epidural catheter, the epidural needle is removed under fluoroscopic assistance. The catheter tip is watched. After the epidural needle is removed, the catheter is sewn into place with 2-0 nylon on a cutting needle. The permanent connector and 22-μm bacteriostatic filter are attached to the catheter. Once triple-antibiotic ointment is placed at the wound site, a slotted 2 × 2 gauze is placed over the catheter exit site. A small loop of the catheter is then held into place and covered, along with the gauze dressing, by a transparent surgical dressing.

Infusion of the 5 mL of preservative-free hypertonic (10%) saline is delivered over 20 minutes in the recovery room. Should the patient complain of pain, burning, or other noxious stimuli during the infusion of hypertonic saline, the infusion must be stopped and re-evaluated. Occasionally, 1 to 3 mL of additional 0.2% ropivacaine needs to be injected to anesthetize the newly exposed neural tissue. After 5 minutes, the hypertonic saline infusion can be restarted without further complaints. When the hypertonic saline infusion is complete, the epidural catheter is flushed with 1 to 2 mL of preservative-free normal saline. The epidural catheter is then recapped.

For neuroplasty stages 2 and 3, the epidural catheter is reaccessed. Aspiration of the catheter should be negative. Once again, 6 mL of local anesthetic (0.2% ropivacaine) is injected in divided doses, with attention given to possible intrathecal, subdural, or intravascular injection. The patient is then asked to lie in the lateral decubitus position with the painful side down to allow for gravitational spread to the affected nerve root. Similar to the previous hypertonic saline infusion, 5 mL is delivered over 20 minutes. Once the infusions are completed, 1 to 2 mL of preservative-free normal saline is used to flush the catheter. After the third infusion the suture is cut and the intact epidural catheter is carefully removed. Another application of triple-antibiotic ointment is applied over the wound and covered by a bandage.

INDICATIONS

- Failed neck surgery syndrome
- Epidural fibrosis
- Cervical radiculopathy
- Spinal stenosis
- Cervical disc bulges

CONTRAINDICATIONS

- Local infection
- Coagulopathies
- Unstable cervical spine
- Inability to lie in prone or in lateral decubitus position

EQUIPMENT

- 25-gauge, ¾-inch infiltration needle
- 18-gauge, 1½-inch needle
- 16-gauge Epimed RK epidural needle
- Epimed Tun-L or Tun-L-XL epidural catheter, 24 cm
- Loss-of-resistance syringe
- 3-mL syringe
- 2 10-mL syringes
- Needle driver
- 3-0 nylon on cutting needle
- Scissors

DRUGS

- 1.5% lidocaine for skin infiltration
- 2% preservative-free lidocaine
- 0.5% preservative-free levobupivacaine or ropivacaine
- 0.9% preservative-free normal saline
- 10% preservative-free hypertonic saline
- 1500 U of hyaluronidase

HELPFUL HINTS

The initial placement of the epidural needle is facilitated by perfectly aligned anteroposterior and lateral fluoroscopic images. Slight oblique images can cause inaccurate placement of the epidural needle. Good midline needle entry is important if C1 and C2 are to be targeted. Paramedial epidural needle entry allows for easy coverage of C3–C8 nerve roots but difficult catheter steering in the posterior midline for C1 and C2 coverage.

Another common situation is with the infusion of hypertonic saline. Frequently, the patient complains of pain at the initiation of infusion. Often this can be treated not by injecting more local anesthetic but by time: A rapidly moving environment, the local anesthetic and steroid injected in the operating theater has not fully reached peak effect—an additional 5 to 10 minutes prevents the need for more local anesthetics.

Choosing cervical neuroplasty is dependent on many factors. The most important factor is the safety of the initial approach. While single-shot posterior approach cervical epidural steroid procedures can and have been used frequently and safely, in the more stenotic and scarred epidural spaces the placement of the epidural needle can be extremely hazardous. In skilled hands, the "hanging-drop" and "loss-of-resistance" techniques facilitate safe entry into the epidural space in most situations. Unfortunately, severe and sometimes fatal consequences of complications in this region may occur with the use of the "old" standard methods of epidural access.

For this reason the "three-D" technique applied to cervical epidural entry is especially pertinent. The first D is *direction*, followed by *depth*, and lastly, *direction* again. Fluoroscopy is an important key to this technique. With the ability to see the relationship of the epidural needle to the vertebra, the needle can be advanced in a safe fashion.

Neural mapping is very useful in complex pain complaints. Frequently, the patient may complain of a pain that involves multiple dermatomes. If the pain is centrally mediated, the ability to determine the actual nerve roots that are painful allows for directed treatment.

Percutaneous lysis of epidural adhesion 62263; epidurography 72275–26; fluoroscopic guidance 76005–26

REFERENCES

1. Burn JMB: Treatment of chronic lumbosciatic pain. Proc R Soc Med 66:544, 1973.
2. Sicard JA, Forestier J: Methode radiographique d/exploration de la cavite epidurale par le Lipiodol. Rev Neurol 28:1264–1266, 1921.
3. Payne JN, Rupp NH: The use of hyaluronidase in caudal block anesthesia. Anesthesiology 12:164–172, 1951.
4. Moore DC: The use of hyaluronidase in local and nerve block analgesia other than spinal block—1520 cases. Anesthesiology 12:644–626, 1951.
5. Lievre JA, Block-Michel H, Atali P: L'injection trans-sacree: Etude clinique et radiologique. Bull Sac Med Paris 73:110–118, 1957.
6. Goebert HW, Jallo SJ, Gardner WJ, et al: Sciatica: Treatment with epidural injections of procaine and hydrocortisone. Cleve Clin Q 27:191–197, 1960.
7. Brown JH: Pressure caudal anesthesia and back manipulation. NW Med 59:905–909, 1960.
8. Hitchcock E: Hypothermic subarachnoid irrigation for intractable pain. Lancet 1:1133–1135, 1967.
9. Hitchcock E: Osmolytic neurolysis for intractable facial pain. Lancet 1:434–436, 1969.
10. Ventafridda V, Spreafico R: Subarachnoid saline perfusion. Adv Neurol 4:477–484, 1974.
11. Racz GB, Holubec JT: Lysis of adhesions in the epidural space. In Raj P (ed): Techniques of Neurolysis. Boston, Kluwer, 1989, pp 57–72.
12. Stolker RJ, Vervest ACM, Gerbrand JG: The management of chronic spinal pain by blockades: A review. Pain 58:1–19, 1994.
13. McCarron RF, Wimpee MW, Hudkins PG, Laros GS: The inflammatory effect of the nucleus pulposus: A possible element in the pathogenesis of low back pain. Spine 12:760–764, 1987.
14. Omnipaque product insert. Princeton, NJ, Nycomed, 1996.
15. Lasser EC, Lyon SG, Berry CB: Reports on contrast media reactions: Analysis of data from reports to the U.S. Food and Drug Administration. Radiology 203:605–610, 1997.
16. Halpin SF, Guest PJ, Byrne JV: Theory and practice: How much contrast for myelography? Neuroradiology 33:411–413, 1991.
17. Ndosi BN, Ndosi NK, Kazema RR: Myelography with Omnipaque (iohexol) using basic radiographic facilities: The main adverse effects. Cent Afr J Med 42:192–195, 1996.
18. Duran-Reynals F: Tissue permeability and the spreading factors in infection. Bact Rev 6:197, 1942.
19. Lewandowski EW: The efficacy of solutions used in caudal neuroplasty. Pain Digest 7:323–330, 1997.
20. Benoist M, Ficat C, Baraf P: Postoperative lumbar epiduro-arachnoiditis: Diagnostic and therapeutic aspects. Spine 5:432–436, 1980.
21. Hechter O, Dopkeen SK, Yudell MH: Clinical use of hyaluronidase in hypodermoclysis. J Pediatr 30:645–656, 1947.
22. Kirby CK, Eickenhoff JE, Looby JP: Use of hyaluronidase with local anesthetic agents in nerve block and infiltration anesthesia. Surgery 25:101, 1949.
23. Gourie-Devi M, Satish P: Intrathecal hyaluronidase treatment of chronic spinal arachnoiditis of noninfective etiology. Surg Neurol 22:231–233, 1984.
24. Nicoll JMV, Acharya PA, Ahlen K, et al: Central nervous system complications after 6000 retrobulbar blocks. Anesth Analg 66:1298–1302, 1987.
25. King TP, Lu G, Gonzalez M: Yellow jacket venom allergens, hyaluronidase, and phospholipase: Sequence similarity and antigenic cross-reactivity with their hornet and wasp homologs and possible implications for clinical allergy. J Allergy Clin Immunol 98:588–600, 1996.
26. Wydase product insert. Philadelphia, Wyeth Laboratories, 1994.
27. Graf BM, Martin E, Bosnjak ZJ, Stowe DF: Stereospecific effect of bupivacaine isomers on atrioventricular conduction in the isolated perfused guinea pig heart. Anesthesiology 86:410–419, 1996.
28. Lyons G, Columb M, Wilson RC, Johnson RV: Epidural pain relief in labour: Potencies of levobupivacaine and racemic bupivacaine. Br J Anaesth 81:899–901, 1998.
29. de Jong RH: Ropivacaine. Anesth Clin North Am 2:109–130, 1998.
30. Iida H, Watanabe Y, Dohi S, Ishiyama T: Direct effects of ropivacaine and bupivacaine on spinal pial vessels in canines. Anesthesiology 87:75–81, 1997.
31. Aristocort Forte product insert. Deerfield, IL, Fujisawa USA, 1994.
32. Jacobs S, Pullan PT, Potter JM, et al: Adrenal suppression following extradural steroids. Anaesthesia 38:953–956, 1983.
33. Abram SE, O'Connor TC: Complications associated with epidural steroid injections. Reg Anesth 21:149–162, 1996.
34. Simon DL, Kunz RD, German JD, et al: Allergic or pseudoallergic reaction following epidural steroid deposition and skin testing. Reg Anesth 14:253–255, 1989.
35. Nelson DA, Vates TS, Thomas RB: Complications from intrathecal steroid therapy in patients with multiple sclerosis. Acta Neurol Scand 49:176–188, 1973.
36. Dougherty JH, Fraser RAR: Complications following intraspinal injections of steroids. J Neurosurg 48:1023–1025, 1978.
37. Shealy CN: Dangers of spinal injections without proper diagnosis. JAMA 197:156–158, 1966.
38. King JS, Jewett DL, Sundberg HR: Differential blockade of cat dorsal root C fibers by various chloride solutions. J Neurosurg 36:569–583, 1972.
39. Lake DA, Barnes CD: Effects of changes in osmolality on spinal cord activity. Exp Neurol 68:555–567, 1980.
40. Racz GB, Heavner JE, Singleton W, Carline M: Hypertonic saline and corticosteroid injected epidurally for pain control. In Racz GB (ed): Techniques of Neurolysis. Boston, Kluwer, 1988, pp 73–86.
41. Lucas JT, Ducker TB, Perot PL: Adverse reactions to intrathecal saline injection for control of pain. J Neurosurg 42:557, 1975.
42. Aldrete JA, Zapata JC, Ghaly R: Arachnoiditis following epidural adhesiolysis with hypertonic saline: Report of two cases. Pain Digest 6:368–370, 1996.
43. Racz GB, Sabonghy M, Gintautas J, Kline WM: Intractable pain therapy using a new epidural catheter. JAMA 248:579–581, 1982.
44. Racz GB, Haynsworth RF, Lipton S: Experiences with an improved epidural catheter. Pain Clin 1:21–27, 1986.
45. Racz GB, Kline WN: New epidural adapter and epidural needle. In Racz GB (ed): Techniques of Neurolysis. Boston, Kluwer, 1988.
46. Katz J (ed): Atlas of Regional Anesthesia. Norwalk, CT, Appleton-Century-Crofts, 1985, p 124.
47. MacNab I: The mechanism of spondylogenic pain. In Hirsch C, Zotterman Y (eds): Cervical Pain. Oxford, Pergamon, 1972, pp 89–94.

48. Racz GB, Heavner JE: Aristocort and Depo-Medrol passage through a 0.2-micron filter [Abstract]. Reg Anesth 15(Suppl):25, 1991.

49. Arthur J, Racz G, Heinrich R, et al: Epidural space: Identification of filling defects and lysis of adhesions in the treatment of chronic painful conditions. Abstracts of the 7th World Congress on Pain. Paris, IASP Publications, 1993.

50. Devulder J, Bogaert L, Castille F, et al: Relevance of epidurography and epidural adhesiolysis in chronic failed back surgery patients. Clin J Pain 11:147–150, 1995.

51. Dogliotti AM: Segmental peridural anesthesia. Am J Surg 20:107, 1933.

42 Epiduroscopy

HISTORY

In 1931, Michael Burman[1] removed 11 vertebral columns from cadavers and examined the anatomy with arthroscopic equipment. Elias Stern described a spinascope and trocar for in vivo examination of the spinal canal in 1936.[2, 3]

The first in vivo examination of the spinal canal was performed by J. Lawrence Pool in 1937.[2, 4] The first examination was complicated by hemorrhage. However, prior to the loss of visualization, a glimpse was gained of the lumbosacral nerves. Subsequently, Poole examined seven more patients without complication and observed the cauda equina. He also noted the flow of blood through the epidural blood vessels.[2, 4] By 1942, Pool was able to report on 400 cases he had performed. The technique was used for diagnostic preparation for surgery.[2, 5, 6] Pool was able to identify neuritis, herniated nucleus pulposus, hypertrophied ligamentum flavum, neoplasms, and arachnoid adhesions.[5, 6]

Ooi and Morisaki in Japan developed an endoscope in the 1960s.[2, 7-9] With the advent of the fiberoptic light source in the 1970s, the scope was more amenable to percutaneous placement, which simplified the procedure.[2] From 1967 to 1977, Ooi and colleagues[10, 11] performed 208 myeloscopies using various types of equipment.

Rune Blomberg[12] of Sweden was the next to describe a method of epiduroscopy and spinaloscopy. Using the technique, Blomberg noted the epidural space contents varied in regard to fat and connective tissue. He also noted that adhesions between the dura mater and ligamentum flavum could restrict the opening of the epidural space despite flushing with normal saline.[2, 12] Blomberg was also able to visualize the entry of Tuohy needles through the ligamentum flavum into the epidural space. Dural tenting was seen when an epidural catheter was threaded through the Tuohy needle into the epidural space.[2, 12]

In 1991, Shimoji and associates[13] visualized the epidural space after withdrawing the endoscope from the subarachnoid space. By visualizing the epidural space in this manner, they confirmed it as a potential space.[2] They were the first group to publish their endoscopic experience using both a fiberoptic light source and a flexible fiberoptic catheter instead of the traditional rigid metal endoscopes.[2, 13] The investigators identified the spinal level by using a concomitant radiograph. They were able to observe aseptic adhesive arachnoiditis where nerve roots were matted or clumped by filamentous tissue.[2, 13]

ANATOMY AND PHYSIOLOGY

The epidural space is largely a potential space, its average depth being probably no greater than 3 mm. In vivo, the actual depth of the space is highly dependent on the relationship of epidural pressure to cerebrospinal fluid (CSF) pressure. Determination of epidural space morphology in cadavers has yielded variable results, depending on whether attempts were made to approximate physiologic CSF volumes in the specimens.[14] Distention of the epidural space with irrigation solutions occurs only when the pressure within the epidural space exceeds CSF pressure, thereby displacing CSF. Distention of the epidural space is nonuniform, with the dorsomedial portion being the most distensible. The dorsolateral epidural space distends only minimally, and the ventral epidural space distends little, if at all. At its point of maximum distention, the depth of the epidural space is 9 mm (Fig. 42–1).[14]

These anatomic characteristics limit the ability to fully examine epidural structures. It is usually

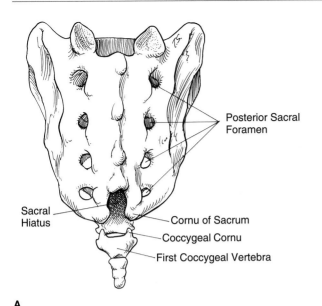

A

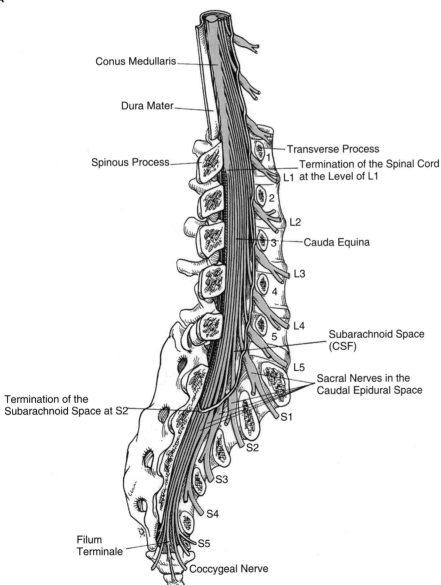

B

FIGURE 42–1

A, This figure shows the sacral hiatus and its anatomic relationships. This is the site where the epiduroscope is inserted. *B*, The longitudinal section of the lumbosacral vertebral spine demonstrates the neural contents as they traverse toward their foramina. CSF, cerebrospinal fluid. (*A* and *B*, From Raj PP [ed]: Clinical Practice of Regional Anesthesia. New York, Churchill Livingstone, 1991, pp 328, 329.)

possible to obtain tangential views of the dura and proximal nerve root sleeves and to identify the junctions of the sleeves with the thecal sac. It is difficult to visualize the lateral recesses or to view the lateral portions of the sleeves. It is not possible to examine the anterior epidural space. Because distention of the epidural space involves displacement of CSF, injection of irrigation solution during epiduroscopy causes a transitory, but substantial, rise in lumbar CSF pressures. Concurrent lumbar CSF pressure monitoring undergoing epiduroscopy has shown an increase in lumbar CSF pressure to 60 mm Hg with 30 mL of irrigant injected over a 60-second period.

INDICATIONS

DIAGNOSIS

Examination of the epidural space in patients with chronic radicular pain symptoms without radiographic or magnetic resonance imaging (MRI) evidence of disc injury has shown the presence of inflammation involving the nerve root corresponding to the symptomatic area.[15] These findings suggest that factors other than direct mechanical compression may cause radicular symptoms. Myeloscopy may therefore be useful in confirming a physiologic basis for radicular pain when other diagnostic studies are negative. With epiduroscopy, direct clinical observation is possible for adhesions and fibrosis, tissue changes after epidural blocks, structural changes with aging, neuritis, herniated nucleus pulposus, and hypertrophied ligamentum flavum.

EPIDURAL STEROID INJECTION IN PATIENTS WITH PREVIOUS SPINAL SURGERY

Recently, Fredman and colleagues[16] have shown using fluoroscopy that in patients with previous back surgery, epidurally injected depot steroid solution will spread to reach the level of pathology in only 26% of cases. Myeloscopy allows more accurate placement of drugs within the epidural space, which may improve the efficacy of epidural steroids in "failed back surgery syndrome." Additional studies are needed to evaluate this assertion.

LYSIS OF PERINEURAL ADHESIONS

Perineural epidural scarring has been postulated as a cause of chronic pain following laminectomy. During endoscopy, these adhesions may be lysed by manipulation of the fiberscope tip, by pressure of the irrigating solution, or by a probe introduced through a second portal.

PUNCTURE AND ASPIRATION OF EPIDURAL CYSTS

Some investigators have successfully fenestrated both synovial cysts and CSF inclusion cysts using the tip of the endoscope.

CONTRAINDICATIONS

Injection of large volumes of fluids and epiduroscopy should be avoided in patients with a coagulopathy, local infection, cerebrovascular disease, and central nervous system space-occupying lesions. Patients with sacral nerve injury may be at further risk for bladder and bowel dysfunction during or after administration of large volumes of epidural saline.[17]

EQUIPMENT (Fig. 42–2)

- 9- and 10-French Arrow central access catheter with dilators
- Guidewire (Fig. 42–3)
- 0.8- to 1.0-mm fiberoptic scope
- 25-gauge, ¾-inch infiltration needle
- 18-gauge needle
- No. 11 blade scalpel
- 4- to 10-mL syringe
- IV T-piece extension
- 16-gauge Epimed RK epidural needle
- Needle driver
- 2-0 nylon suture on CT needle—Epimed
- 36-cm epidural (Tun-L) catheter
- Epidural catheter connector
- 2 2 × 2 split IV sponges
- 3-mL syringe
- Transparent surgical dressing
- Nerve stimulators (optional)

DRUGS

- 5% lidocaine for skin infiltration
- 0.25% bupivacaine or 0.2% ropivacaine
- Preservative-free normal saline
- 1500 units hyaluronidase (Wydase)
- 10% hypertonic saline
- Steroids
- Iohexol (Omnipaque 240) radiographic contrast

PREPARATION OF THE PATIENT

PHYSICAL EXAMINATION

Examine the entry site for local infection and distorted anatomy. There should be a positive "straight-leg raise" test for documentation of radiculopathy.

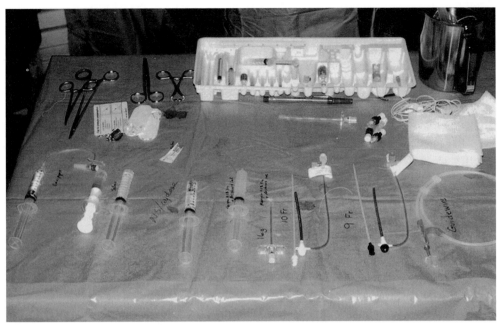

FIGURE 42-2

Illustration of how a sterile table has to be set up for flexible epiduroscopy.

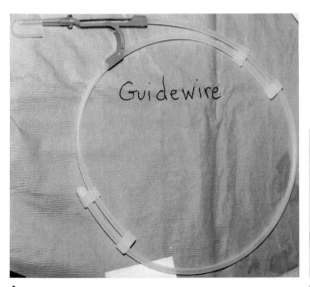

A

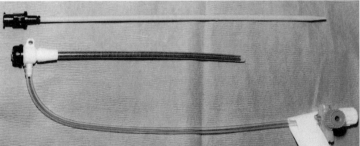

B

FIGURE 42-3

The guidewire *(A)* and a dilator *(B)* are shown here.

LABORATORY

- Complete blood count with platelets
- Prothrombin time, partial thromboplastin time
- Platelet function studies and bleeding time
- Urinalysis

PREOPERATIVE MEDICATION

For preoperative medication, use the standard American Society of Anesthesiologists' recommendations for conscious sedation.

PROCEDURE

POSITION OF THE PATIENT

The patient is in the prone position.

TECHNIQUE

There are currently at least three steerable catheters available for use within the spinal canal. Catheter outer diameters range from 2.4 to 2.4 mm. The fiberscopes are 0.8 to 1.0 mm, providing up to 10,000 pixels. The current technique for epiduroscopy involves the introduction of the catheter through the sacral hiatus. This is performed at Texas Tech University Health Science Center in the operating room suite. After adequate preoperative work-up that includes lumbosacral MRI, urology evaluation (if necessary), and laboratory studies (normal values in complete blood count, prothrombin and partial thromboplastin times, and platelet function), the patient is placed in the prone position on a fluoroscopy table. The procedure is performed under local anesthetic and monitored anesthesia care. The patient is given 1 g of ceftriaxone (Rocephin) intravenously prior to the start of the case. (Ciprofloxin [Cipro], 400 mg, for 1 hour before the case may be substituted if there is concern about allergy.) A pillow may be placed under the lower abdomen to decrease the lordosis of the lumbar spine. The patient is prepared and draped in a sterile manner (Figs. 42–4 and 42–5).

A skin wheal is raised over the sacral hiatus using 1 to 2 mL of 1% lidocaine and a 25-gauge needle (Fig. 42–6A). An 18-gauge needle is used to penetrate the skin. A 16-gauge RK epidural needle is then inserted through the puncture site and into the sacral hiatus (Fig. 42–6B). This may be verified in both the anteroposterior (AP) and lateral fluoroscopic views (Fig. 42–7A). An epidurogram is then performed with 10 mL of water-soluble non-ionic dye (Fig. 42–7B). After the epidurogram, a guidewire is inserted through the needle and advanced to approximately the L5 or S1 level. A small incision is made with a No. 10 × 1-blade scalpel to the level of the sacral ligament to decrease the "drag" of the skin and subcutaneous tissues on the introducer/sheaths. A 9-French introducer is then inserted over the guidewire into the sacral space. This is then removed

and the introducer with sheath is placed over the guidewire into the space (Fig. 42–8). It is important to check the guidewire for freedom of movement because the physician does not want to kink it. The 9-French introducer and sheath is then removed and a 10-French introducer is placed over the guidewire in the sacral space. If there is ease of movement, the 10-French introducer with sheath is then placed into the sacral space. This method is used to slowly dilate the space because there are anatomic differences in size. The 10-French introducer and the guidewire are then removed, leaving the sheath in place.

The steerable fiberscope is inserted through the introducer sheaths (Fig. 42–9). Fluoroscopy is necessary to verify the proper intraspinal placement. During the epiduroscopy procedure, care must be taken to use the minimal amount of saline for irrigation and local distention. Injection rates should not exceed 30 mL/minute. The total *infused* volume should not exceed 100 mL. (There is often considerable retrograde flow of irrigation fluid out of the catheter or introducer, which should not be counted with the amount actually infused). Continuous CSF pressure monitoring through a lumbar subarachnoid needle should be considered during prolonged cases with larger irrigation volumes. In addition to monitoring the volume infused, it is strongly suggested that the time in the epidural space with the steerable catheter also be monitored. In clinical practice at our institution, that time should not be more than 30 minutes.

The steerable fiberscope allows for three-dimensional direct clinical observation. The operator may observe normal peridural fat in the sacral canal. Dense granuloma tissue may be noted. Swollen, angry nerve roots may be identified by the surrounding

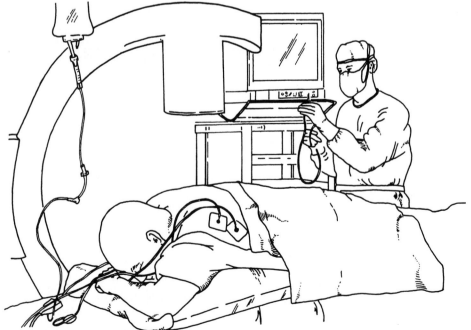

FIGURE 42–4

The patient is draped in a sterile manner in the prone position with all other connections in place.

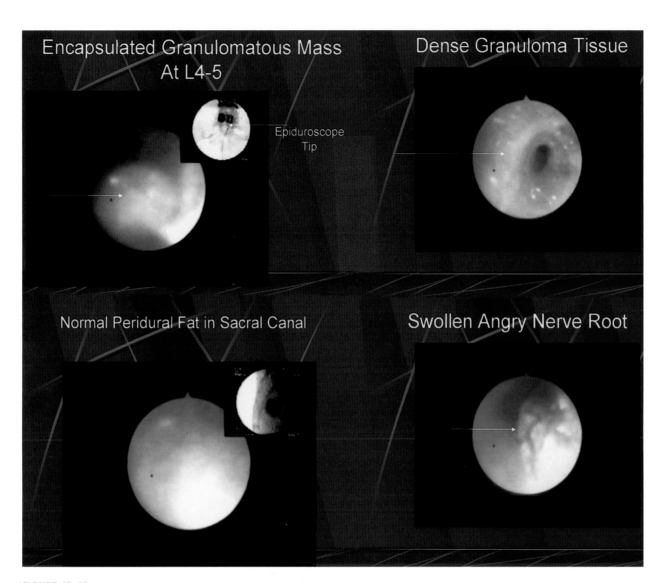

FIGURE 42–10

Fiberscopic views of normal peridural fat *(lower left)*, encapsulated granulomatous mass at L4–5 *(upper left)*, dense granuloma tissue *(arrow) (upper right)*, and swollen nerve root *(arrow) (lower right)*.

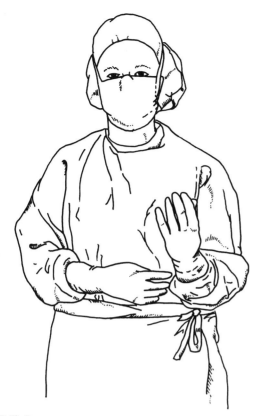

FIGURE 42–5

The drawing shows the physician appropriately draped and gloved.

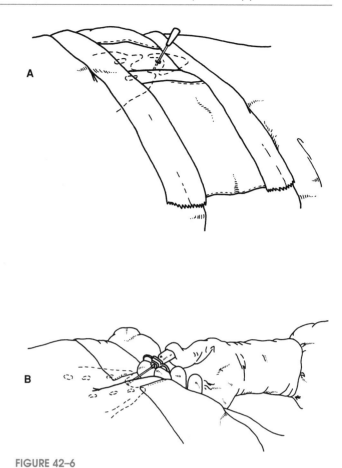

FIGURE 42–6

A, Introduction of infiltration needle in the caudal region. *B*, Insertion of epidural needle in the caudal space.

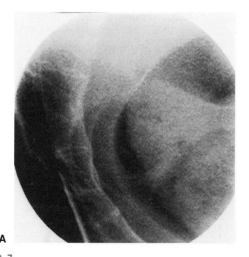

FIGURE 42–7

A, Lateral view of the RK needle *(arrow B)* in the caudal canal *(arrow A)*. *B*, The radiographic dye spread in the caudal canal confirms the correct position of the needle.

granulomatous tissue and distended vasculature that follows the root. There may also be incidental findings such as an encapsulated granulomatous mass (Fig. 42–10, see Color Plate).

At Texas Tech University Health Sciences Center, epiduroscopy is combined with caudal epidural neurolysis technique. After performing the epiduroscopy, while the steerable scope is in place, an Epimed Tun-

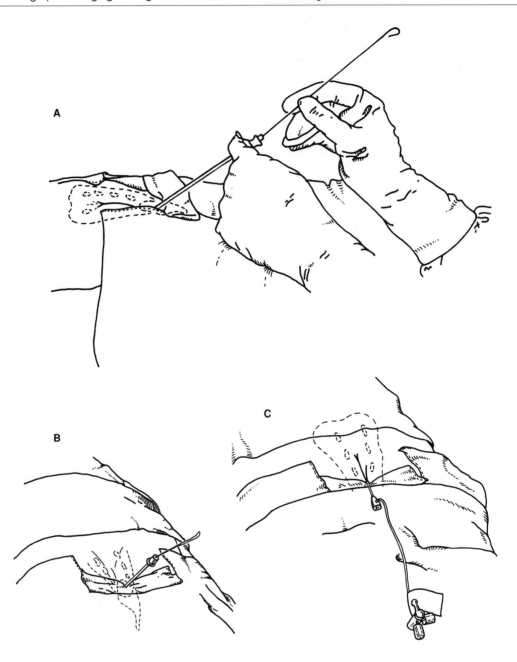

FIGURE 42–8

A, This drawing shows the guidewire being inserted through the RK needle. *B,* Then the RK needle is then removed and a 9- or 10-French dilator catheter is inserted over the guidewire. *C,* After the dilation, the guidewire is recovered and the introduction sheath is in place for the fiberscope to be introduced.

L-XL catheter is placed through the working channel and advanced to the desired site of position. The fluoroscopic view allows determination of the level of the placement. It also allows for determination of ventral or dorsal epidural placement. The epiduroscope view ensures visualization of the placement of the catheter, which will be used for further therapy. The epiduroscope is then threaded off the catheter, with attention emphasized on the retainment of the position of the catheter tip. Once the epiduroscope is removed from the space, a skin wheal is made approximately 1 cm lateral and 2 cm caudal to the sacral space. The skin is punctured with an 18-gauge

needle (Fig. 42–11). The RK epidural needle is then inserted throughout the puncture site and tunneled subcutaneously to exit at the sacral hiatus site. The epidural catheter is threaded through the needle and out the lateral incision. The needle is then carefully removed. The sacral hiatus incision should be closed with a single, interrupted stitch with 2-0 silk or nylon. An anchor stitch should be placed to hold the catheter in place with the 2-0 silk or nylon. The site is then covered with antibiotic ointment, two 2 × 2 sponges, transparent dressing, folded 4 × 4, and tape. The protocol for caudal epidural neurolysis is then followed with testing the catheter, treatment

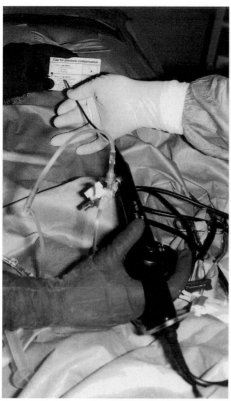
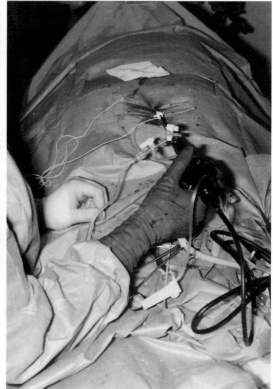

A   **B**

FIGURE 42–9

A, The figure shows the fiber-scope focused for clear vision prior to introduction. *B,* The fiberscope introduced in the sheath for direct vision of the caudal space.

with local anesthetic and steroid, injection of hyaluronidase, and hypertonic saline infusion.

COMPLICATIONS

To date, there have been no complications reported in the literature. There is one instance of epidural abscess. Some investigators use routine prophylactic antibiotic with no subsequent infections. There are three known cases of macular hemorrhage with visual impairment following the procedure. These may be related to increased CSF pressure from infusion of irrigation fluid.[18] Spinal endoscopy is associated with postdural puncture headache and fever. Dysesthesia during the procedure has also been reported.[13]

HELPFUL HINTS

For epiduroscopy to be performed, the epidural space needs to be distended by repeated injections of saline. If the procedure takes a long time, the excessive saline volumes may generate significant epidural pressures and affect local perfusion. Sustained pressure epidurally could potentially compromise perfusion or cause barotraumas at locations remote from injection.[2, 19] The amount of the fluid injected must therefore be accurately monitored. Epiduroscopy should not be performed in anesthetized patients.

Identification of the correct spinal level is almost impossible without simultaneous fluoroscopy. Furthermore, due to the presence of abundant epidural adipose tissue and the limited field of vision of superfine fiberscopes, it may be difficult to distinguish normal discs. Perioperative epiduroscopy could identify the herniating disc in only one of five patients.[20]

- The epidural space is only a potential space that opens on introduction of an epiduroscope or epidural and spinal needles and catheters.
- During epiduroscopy, the epidural space can be visualized only if it is kept distended by repeated injections of saline (or air).
- The endoscopic view is much clearer and more distinct as the scope is being withdrawn.
- Easily recognized structures include dura mater, ligamentum flavum, epidural fat, fibrous connective tissue, and blood vessels. Spinal nerve roots can be difficult to identify. The presence of a dorsomedian connective tissue band, which divides the epidural space into compartments, has been demonstrated in some[21] but not in other[22, 23] studies.
- In direct observation of epidural pathology, the following have been demonstrated:
  1. Presence of adhesions and fibrosis in the epidural space after spinal surgery[24]
  2. Tissue changes after regular epidural blocks[25]
  3. Structural changes in the epidural space with increasing age.[26]

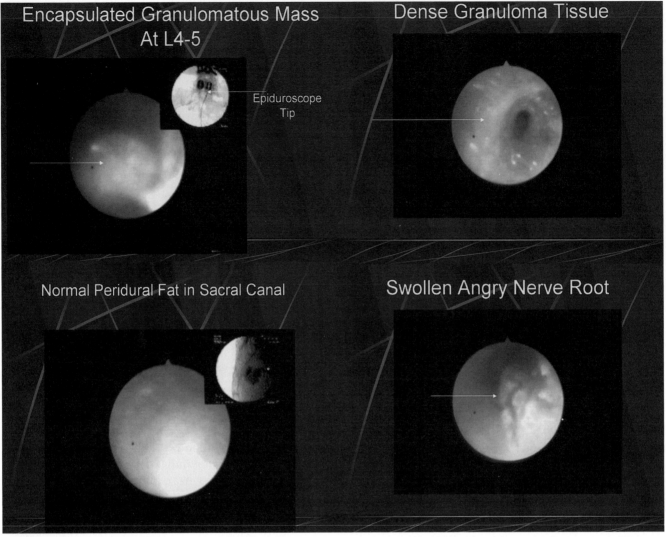

FIGURE 42–10

Fiberscopic views of normal peridural fat *(lower left)*, encapsulated granulomatous mass at L4–5 *(upper left)*, dense granuloma tissue *(arrow) (upper right)*, and swollen nerve root *(arrow) (lower right)*. (See color plate.)

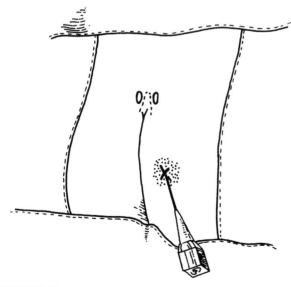

FIGURE 42–11

After the caudal neuroplasty (see Chapter 41), the catheter is tunneled to the buttock fold. The site for skin infiltration is marked with an X.

■ Spinaloscopy studies in patients have demonstrated the presence of neuritis, herniated nucleus pulposus, hypertrophied ligamentum flavum,[5] and adhesive arachnoiditis.[13] Technical aspects of epidural, spinal, and combined spinal epidural (CSE) techniques have been described. Spinal endoscopic studies have evaluated the risk of epidural catheter migration into the subarachnoid space,[27] technical and mechanical problems with spinal catheter placement,[28] and the risk of catheter migration during performance of the CSE block.[22] The risk due to rotation of the epidural needle in the epidural space and the possibility of looping of the epidural catheters have also been demonstrated.[22]

EFFICACY

The initial study was designed to assess the outcome and safety of epidural steroid injection made with fiberoptic assistance (improved targeting) on patients with persistent lumbar radiculopathy who did not respond to physical therapy after two or three caudal injections. It was the premise of the initial study that an epidural injection might fail because medication was not delivered to the proper area, owing to scar, fat, or other morphologic anomalies adjacent to the nerve roots in question. Unfortunately, despite widespread acceptance of spinal canal endoscopy for delivery of targeted injections, outcome data have been hard to come by. Clinical data have been collected from tens of thousands of procedures worldwide. Case reports and retrospectives have started to be published, and findings have been presented at various symposia. There have been no controlled studies, to date, comparing the outcomes of early spinal canal endoscopy and discectomy. In one study, preprocedural and postprocedural survey data from 77 patients demonstrated a decreased need for medication and improved functional capacity as long as 6 months after spinal endoscopy.

REFERENCES

1. Burman MS: Myeloscopy or the direct visualization of the spinal cord. J Bone Joint Surg 13:695–696, 1931.
2. Saberski LR: Spinal endoscopy: Current concepts. In Waldman SD (ed): Interventional Pain Management, 2nd ed. Philadelphia, WB Saunders, 2001, pp 143–161.
3. Stern EL: The spinascope: A new instrument for visualizing the spinal canal and its contents. Med Rec (NY) 143:31–32, 1936.
4. Pool JL: Direct visualization of dorsal nerve roots of the cauda equina by means of a myeloscope. Arch Neurol Psychiatry 39:1308–1312, 1938.
5. Pool JL: Myeloscopy: Intraspinal endoscopy. Surgery 11:169–182, 1942.
6. Pool JL: Myeloscopy: Diagnostic inspection of the cauda equina by means of an endoscope. Bull Neurol Inst NY 7:178–189, 1938.
7. Ooi Y, Morisaki N: Intrathecal lumbar endoscope. Clin Orthop Surg (Jpn) 4:295–297, 1969.
8. Ooi Y, Satoh Y, Morisaki N: Myeloscopy. Igakuno Ayumi (Jpn) 81:209–212, 1972.
9. Ooi Y, Satoh Y, Morisaki N: Myeloscopy. Orthop Surg (Jpn) 24:181–186, 1973.
10. Ooi Y, Satoh Y, Inoue K, et al: Myeloscopy. Acta Orthop Belg 44:881, 1978.
11. Satoh Y, Hirose K, Ooi Y, Mikanagi K: Myeloscopy in the diagnosis of low back pain syndrome. Presented at the Third Congress of International Rehabilitation Medicine Association, Basel, Switzerland, July 2–9, 1978.
12. Blomberg R: A method for spinal canal endoscopy and spinaloscopy: Presentation of preliminary results. Acta Anaesthesiol Scand 21:113–116, 1985.
13. Shimoji K, Fujioka H, Onodera M, et al: Observation of spinal canal and cisternae with the newly developed small-diameter, flexible fiberscopes. Anesthesiology 75:341–344, 1991.
14. Harrison GR, Parkin IG, Shah JL: Resin injection studies of the lumbar extradural space. Br J Anaesth 57:333–336, 1985.
15. Rizor RF: Epiduroscopy: Technique for examination of the lumbar epidural space. Presented at the 19th meeting of the American Society of Regional Anesthesia, Chicago, 1994.
16. Fredman B, Ben Nun B, Zohar E, et al: Epidural steroids for treating "failed back surgery syndrome": Is fluoroscopy really necessary? Anesth Analg 88:3667–3672, 1999.
17. Blomberg R: Technical advantages of the paramedian approach for lumbar epidural puncture and catheter introduction. Anesthesiology 43:837–843, 1988.
18. Saberski LR: Personal communication.
19. Serpell MG, Coombs DW, Colburn RW, et al: Intrathecal Pressure Recordings Due to Saline Instillation In The Epidural Space (Abstract 1535). In Abstracts of the Seventh World Congress on Pain, Paris, Raven Press, August 1993.
20. Rosenberg PH: Fiberoptic epiduroscopy: Current research [Abstract]. Int Pain Clin 7:124, 1996.
21. Blomberg R: The dorsomedian connective tissue band in the lumbar epidural space of humans: An anatomical study using epiduroscopy in autopsy cases. Anesth Analg 65:747–752, 1986.
22. Holmstrom B, Rawal N, Axelsson K, et al: Risk of catheter migration during combined spinal epidural block: Percutaneous epiduroscopy study. Anesth Analg 80:747–753, 1995.
23. Igarashi T, Hirabayaski Y, Saitoh Fukuda H: Thoracic and lumbar extradural structure examined by extraduroscope. Br J Anaesth 81:121–125, 1998.
24. Schutze G, Kurtze H: Direct observation of the epidural space with a catheter-secured epiduroscopic unit. Reg Anesth 19:85–89, 1994.
25. Kitamura A, Sakamoto A, Aoki S, et al: Epiduroscopic changes in patients undergoing single and repeated epidural injections. Anesth Analg 82:88–90, 1996.
26. Igarashi T, Hirabayashi Y, Shimizu R, et al: The lumbar extradural structure changes with increasing age. Br J Anaesth 78:149–152, 1997.
27. Blomberg RG: The lumbar subdural extra-arachnoid space of humans: An anatomical study using spinaloscopy in autopsy cases. Anesth Analg 66:177–180, 1987.
28. Mollmann M, Holst D, Lubbesmeyer H, et al: Continuous spinal anesthesia: Mechanical and technical problems of catheter placement. Reg Anesth 18:469–472, 1993.

Augmentation Techniques

43

HISTORY

Spinal cord stimulation (SCS) for control of pain was first introduced in 1967 by Shealy and colleagues.[1] They proposed that via peripheral nociceptors information from the periphery is transmitted to the spinal cord in small-diameter, unmyelinated C fibers and lightly myelinated A delta fibers. These fibers terminate at the substantia gelatinosa of the dorsal horn, are then transmitted cephalad via the spinal cord. Other sensory input, such as touch or vibration, is transmitted via large myelinated A beta fibers. The basic premise of this theory is that reception of large-fiber information such as touch or vibration would turn off or close the gate to reception of small-fiber information. The effect of this gate closure, these authors theorized, would be analgesia.

Because these authors believed that electrical stimulation is effective only at the dorsal horns of the spinal cord, they called this stimulation modality *dorsal column stimulation* (DCS). Since it is now known that inhibition of nociception can occur with electrical stimulation almost anywhere in the spinal cord, DCS has been supplanted in the literature by the more general, but accurate, term *SCS*.

Studies supporting segmental antidromic inhibition of spinothalamic projection cells by electrically stimulating the dorsal columns soon appeared.[2] Foreman and coworkers investigated the effects of DSC on spinothalamic tract cells in anesthetized monkeys.[2] Dorsal column stimuli were applied to mid-thoracic or cervical levels of the spinal cord while responses of spinothalamic cells to von Frey hair activation of the sural nerves were examined. These authors found that DSC depressed the activity of spinothalamic tract cells for about 150 milliseconds and that the best points for stimulation producing inhibition were over the ipsilateral dorsal columns. Responses to electrical stimulation of periph-

eral nerves and mechanical stimulation of cutaneous nociceptors were similarly depressed by DCS. Lesioning the dorsal columns eliminated this depression of activity by DCS stimulation below the lesion. Lesioning the lateral columns in this model had no effects. Likewise, Handwerker and associates[3] and Feldman[4], in studies from single dorsal horn neurons in anesthetized cats, found that the discharges of class 2 cells in the dorsal horn that respond to both noxious radiant heat stimulation and input from low-threshold cutaneous mechanoreceptors, were suppressed by electrical stimulation of cutaneous, myelinated, afferent nerve fibers. The mechanism of SCS is summarized in Table 43–1.

In this chapter, the techniques of placement of suboccipital, cervical, thoracicolumbar and sacral electrodes are described in the section on specific augmentation procedures.

▽ TABLE 43–1 SPINAL CORD STIMULATION: MECHANISMS OF ACTION[5]

Segmental, antidromic activation restricted to A beta afferents. With a diameter of ≥ 10.7 µm (gate control theory)

Blocking of transmission in the spinothalamic tract

Supraspinal pain inhibition

Activation of central inhibitory mechanisms influencing sympathetic efferent neurons

Activation of putative neurotransmitters or neuromodulators

A maximum of four to five fibers (≥ 10.7 µm) may be recruited in each dermatome near the discomfort threshold

Paresthesia and pain relief in a dermatome may be affected by the stimulation of a single large A beta fiber

The depth of stimulation may be increased twofold to threefold when stimulation is applied optimally (a narrow bi/triple or a transverse tripole).

The A beta fibers (12 µm) recruited when stimulation is applied in the dorsal epidural space

Anodal exaltation and propagation are unlikely to occur with spinal cord stimulation

INDICATIONS

- Failed back surgery syndrome
- Peripheral vascular disease and associated ischemic pain
- Complex regional pain syndrome
- Other painful conditions
   Phantom limb pain
   Postherpetic neuralgia
   Deafferentation pain
- Axial pain
- Vascular pain
   Thoracoabdominal aortic aneurysm
   Cardiovascular (angina) pain
- Motor disorders
   Cerebral palsy
   Multiple sclerosis

CONTRAINDICATIONS

Absolute
- Sepsis
- Coagulopathy
- Previous surgery or trauma that obliterates the spinal canal
- Local infection at implantation site

Relative
- Physical and/or cognitive disability that interferes with proper usage of and understanding of the device
- Spinal bifida

EQUIPMENT

Trial of Spinal Cord Stimulation Procedures
- Epimed Stim-Cath or Medtronic trial screening electrode
- 16-gauge RK epidural needle or 15-gauge Medtronic epidural needle
- 25-gauge infiltration needle
- 18-gauge needle
- 3-mL syringe
- 10-mL syringe
- Loss-of-resistance syringe
- Metal marker
- 2-0 nylon suture on CT needle
- Needle driver
- Connecting cables to stimulator box
- Medtronic trial screener pulse generator

Permanent Percutaneous Placement of Electrodes and Batteries (Pulse Generator or Receiver)
- Medtronics electrodes Pisces Quad or Quad-Plus electrodes or percutaneous Advanced Neuro-modulation Systems electrodes (e.g., Cervitrode, Quattrode, Octrode)

- Implantation accessories such as anchors, guide-wires, stylet for electrodes, and protective sheaths
- Connecting stimulation extension wire
- Implanted pulse generator or receiver
- 2-0 nylon on CT needle
- 2-0 silk suture or rounded needle for pursestring closure
- Needle driver
- Forceps
- 3-0 Vicryl
- 4-0 Monocryl
- No. 10 blade scalpel
- Surgical kit for implantation or suturing

DRUGS

- 1% lidocaine with 1:200,000 or 1:400,000 epine-phrine for skin infiltration
- Preservative-free normal saline
- Sterile water
- Triple-antibiotics to soak the implant
- Triple-antibiotic ointment for surface dressing

SPECIFIC AUGMENTATION PROCEDURES

OCCIPITAL NERVE STIMULATION

History

Initial reports of occipital nerve stimulation date back to the late 1970s when the electrode was actually applied to surgically exposed C2 and C3 nerves (i.e., greater and lesser occipital nerves).[6]

Anatomy

The technique of occipital placement of electrodes is primarily subcutaneous at the C1–C2 level. Innervation of the region is by the medial branch of the C2 and C3 posterior primary rami; the lesser occipital nerve is supplied by the C3 posterior primary ramus. The greater occipital nerve exits the spinal canal between the posterior arches of C1 and C2 and then transverses the paraspinal (semispinalis and trapezius) muscles near the nuchal ridge of the occipital bone (Fig. 43–1).

Indications

- Greater occipital neuralgia (common cause of headaches)
- Tension-type headaches in the occipital region
- Whiplash injuries causing irritation or compression of suboccipital nerves
- Migraine headaches
- Damage of the greater occipital nerve after halo pin placement for cervical spine or intracranial procedures[7]

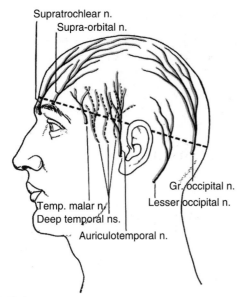

FIGURE 43–1

Innervation of the scalp and cranium. (From Raj PP [ed]: Clinical Practice of Regional Anesthesia. New York, Churchill Livingstone, 1991, p 198.)

Contraindications

- Local infection
- Coagulopathies
- Cognitive deficit in a patient

Equipment

- 25-gauge ¾-inch infiltration needle
- 18-gauge 1¼-inch needle
- 15-gauge, 3½-inch Tuohy epidural needle
- 1 or 2 Medtronic pies Quad, Quad Plus, or custom electrode or ANS Octrode

Electrode Placement for Trial Stimulation

- Medtronic verify electrode
- Medtronic trial screener

Electrode Placement for Permanent Implantation

- Connecting wires
- Tunneling equipment
- Itrel 3 or Synergy implantable pulse generator battery
- No. 10 blade scalpel
- Tenotomy scissors

Drugs

- 1.5% lidocaine or equivalent for infiltration

Preparation of the Patient

All patients should have previously had diagnostic and therapeutic local anesthetic blocks into the region of the affected occipital nerve with initial benefit. Others might also have had some type of ablative treatment of

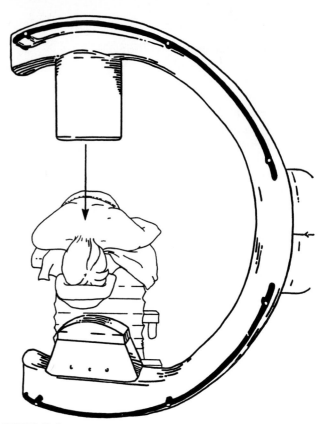

FIGURE 43–2

Position of the patient in the prone position with the C-arm for radiographic imaging during occipital stimulation.

the occipital nerve such as cryoprobe freezing or alcohol injections prior to referral for trial stimulation.

LABORATORY

- Complete blood count with platelets
- Prothrombin time, partial thromboplastin time
- Bleeding time or platelet function studies

PREOPERATIVE MEDICATION AND MONITORING

Follow the standard American Society of Anesthesiologists' recommendations for preoperative medication and monitoring.

Procedure

The prone position is commonly used, with the head in a horseshoe frame or other suitable device (Fig. 43–2). However, other patients are positioned laterally to allow for electrode or extender wire tunneling medial to the scapula for flank, abdominal, or buttock receiver-generator pocketing (Fig. 43–3). The supine position with the head turned to the opposite side allows for anterior tunneling to the subclavicular or abdominal regions. However, care must be taken to avoid proximity of the extender wire connector to the carotid artery. This is easily solved with a longer wire electrode-connector array.

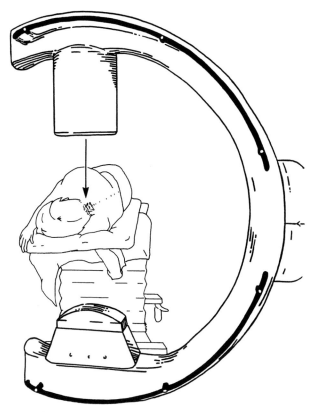

FIGURE 43–3

Position of the patient in a lateral position with the C-arm for radiographic imaging during occipital stimulation.

TECHNIQUE OF NEEDLE ENTRY AND PLACEMENT OF ELECTRODES

Using local anesthesia, a 2-cm vertical skin incision is made at the level of C1 lamina either medial and inferior to the mastoid process or in the midline posteriorly: The subcutaneous tissues immediately lateral to the incision are undermined with sharp scissors to accept a loop of wire electrode created after placement and tunneling to prevent electrode migration. A Tuohy needle is gently curved to conform to transverse cervical curvature (bevel inward) and without further dissection is passed transversely in the subcutaneous space at the level of C1. (Fig. 43–4A). Single or dual quadripolar or octapolar electrodes may be passed from a midline incision to either affected side or alternatively placed to traverse the entire cervical curvature bilaterally from a single side. Rapid needle insertion usually obviates the need for even a short-acting general anesthetic. Following placement of the electrode through the Tuohy needle (Fig. 43–4B), the needle is withdrawn and the electrode connected to an extender cable for intraoperative testing (Fig. 43–4C). Stimulation is then applied using a temporary radiofrequency (RF) transmitter to various selected electrode combinations, enabling the patient to report stimulation location, intensity, overall sensation, and effect.

STIMULATION

Most of the patients have reported immediate stimulation in the selected occipital nerve distribution with voltage settings usually below 2 V. A report of burning pain or muscle pulling should alert the interventionist that the electrode is probably placed either too close to the fascia or too far above or below the C1 level, and it should be repositioned more superficially in the subcutaneous space. Repeated needle passage for electrode placement should be avoided to reduce the risk of subcutaneous edema and/or hematoma formation, which can result in loss of stimulation.

The electrode is then sutured to the underlying fascia with the silicone fastener and 2-0 silk suture. A loop of electrode is also sutured in place to reduce the risk of electrode migration (Fig. 43–4D). A short-acting general anesthetic is used to tunnel the electrodes or extender wire to the distal site for connection and implantation of the receiver-generator. Typical stimulator parameters include pulse widths of 90 to 180 μs, frequency of 60 to 130 Hz, and power of 0.5 to 2 V. Higher rates of up to 400 Hz with RF systems have also been beneficial. An example of dual suboccipital subcutaneous electrode placement is shown in Figure 43–5.

Complications

- Electrode fracture and/or displacement
- Infection
- Subcutaneous tension causing dehiscence

Helpful Hints

- Infection can be decreased by careful through cleansing of the whole neck. The risk of infection is due to bacterial population in the hairline.
- Bending the tunneling epidural needle to the contour of the neck facilitates placement of the electrode.
- To prevent migration, the distal top of the electrode can be sutured into place.

Efficacy

Although still relatively new, the follow-up success appears to be relatively high with this technique.[8] In one study, 12 of 17 patients had greater than 50% reduction in pain at last follow-up. This is the only study known at this time. Further studies are needed.

CERVICAL SPINAL CORD STIMULATION

Anatomy

Anatomy of the epidural space is described elsewhere (see Chapter 16) and is not discussed here.

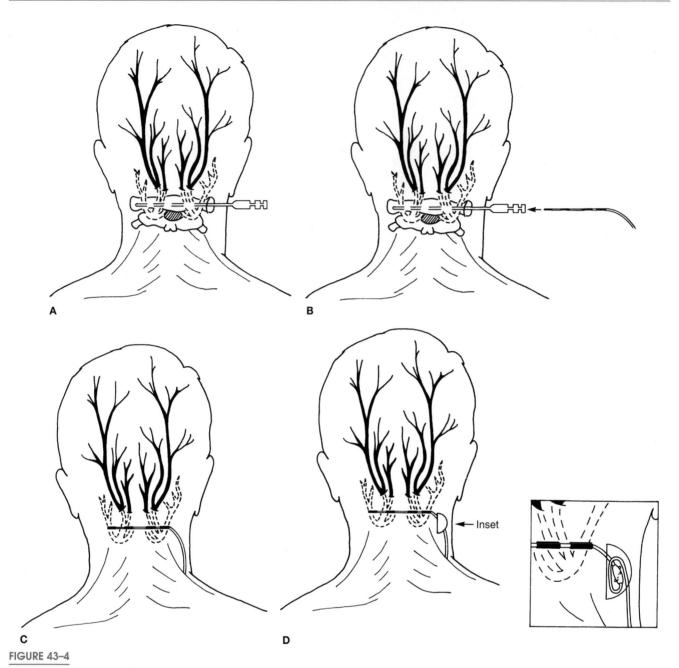

FIGURE 43-4

A, Therapy placement at the C1 level during the procedure for occipital stimulation. *B,* Electrode placement through the Tuohy needle. *C,* Removal of Tuohy needle with the occipital electrode in place. *D,* Lead anchored to fascia with an electrode loop to prevent migration.

Cervical placement of the SCS is indicated for painful conditions of the neck, upper extremities, and upper torso for which cervical SCS is indicated.

Typical diagnoses include the following:

- Complex regional pain syndrome
- Peripheral neuropathy of the upper extremity
- Brachial plexus injuries, including
     Stretch injury
     Radiation burns
     Traumatic injuries
- Somatic skeletal injuries (e.g., whiplash)
- Carpal tunnel syndrome

- Postherpetic neuralgia
- Scleroderma
- Failed surgical procedures in the neck

Contraindications

- Sepsis
- Coagulopathy

Preparation of the Patient

SELECTION OF THE PATIENT

To be considered for SCS procedure, the patient must meet the following general criteria:

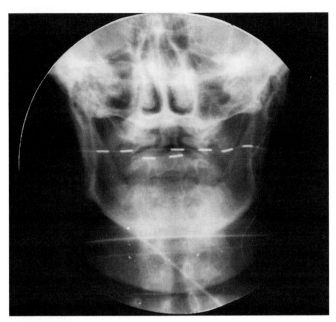

FIGURE 43–5

Two occipital electrodes in place for the patient with headaches.

- There is a demonstrable pathology and an objective basis for the pain complaint.
- Conservative therapies have failed.
- Further major surgical intervention is not indicated.
- No serious drug habituation problems exist.
- Psychiatric or psychological clearance has been obtained.
- The patient has primarily radiating extremity pain.
- Trial stimulation has been successful or will be done prior to permanent placement.

LABORATORY

- Complete blood count with platelets
- Prothrombin time, partial thromboplastin time
- Platelet function studies or bleeding times
- Urinalysis, electrocardiogram, and chest radiograph when appropriate

PREOPERATIVE MEDICATION AND MONITORING

For preoperative medication and for monitoring, use the standard American Society of Anesthesiologists' recommendations.

Procedure

- Prone (Fig. 43–6) *or*
- Lateral decubitus (see Fig. 43–3)

SCREENING TRIAL: TECHNIQUE FOR PLACEMENT OF A PERCUTANEOUS CERVICAL SPINAL CORD STIMULATION ELECTRODE

As with all trial placements of SCS electrodes, an alert and communicative patient is essential to correct lead

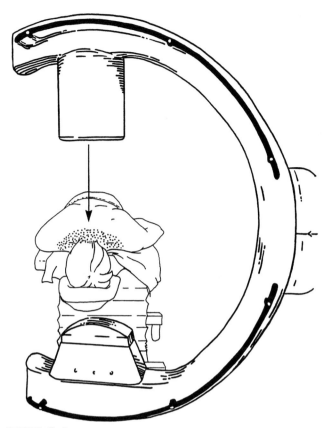

FIGURE 43–6

Position of the patient and the C-arm for cervical electrode placement.

positioning. The patient should be made comfortable with local anesthesia infiltration at the insertion site.

The patient should lie in the left lateral position. With the fluoroscopic C-arm in the anteroposterior (AP) view at the T1–2 level, the spinous process and the patient's chest should be perfectly vertical and not tilting forward. The target for needle entry should be the T1–2 interspace on the side opposite of the pain. For bilateral pain, a paramedian needle entry approach is still appropriate, with electrode placement at the midline. The direction of the shaft of the needle and the curved tip of the guidewire influence where the electrode travels.

Using a paramedian approach with a shallow angle ½ inch off midline, the physician aims the needle at the target, moving toward the painful side. The use of an angled paramedian approach for the needle, as opposed to a midline approach, is a recent improvement in technique, which speeds lead placement considerably in the upper cervical area (Fig. 43–7*A*).

The C-arm is then rotated to the lateral view to look down on the patient. The needle is advanced with the stylet in place to the ligamentum flavum area. Then, by rotating the C-arm back to the AP view, any necessary corrections can be made to get the needle to the target area (Fig. 43–7*B*). The stylet is then removed and a syringe is attached to the needle, which is then advanced into the epidural space using the "loss of

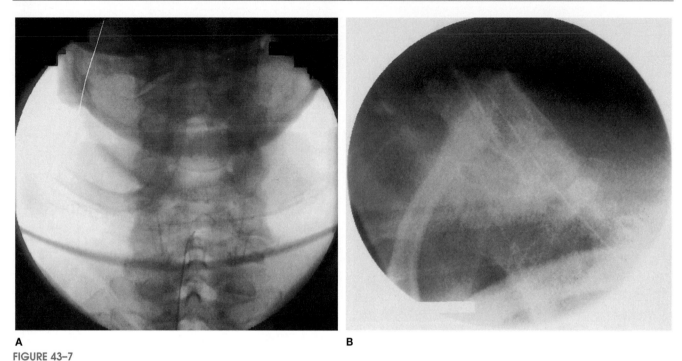

A   **B**

FIGURE 43–7

Anteroposterior *(A)* and lateral *(B)* views of cervical trial electrocatheter in place ready to be stimulated.

bounce" technique. With the syringe filled with 4 mL of preservative-free saline and 2 mL of air, the physician bounces the plunger constantly with the right hand while advancing the needle with the left hand until there is a loss of bounce. The physician then attempts to pass the electrode. If the electrode will not pass easily, it is probable that an insufficient portion of the needle has entered the epidural space. The needle should be advanced further or should be repositioned to allow the electrode to pass easily. The target area for the "0" electrode (most distal) should be just off midline to the painful side, with placement depending on the pain pattern. If there is specific nerve root involvement, such as in cases of postherpetic neuralgia or intercostal neuritis, the electrode may be placed on the nerve root itself lateral to the spinal cord for entry zone stimulation.

TESTING THE STIMULATION (TRIAL)

One can use a trial screening lead during the screening trial. Once the screening lead is positioned, it is connected to a temporary, external power source (screener). If the patient does not experience satisfactory paresthesia, one should reposition the lead and try again. When both the patient and physician are satisfied that the stimulation coverage is satisfactory, then complete the circuits using an external ground patch on the patient's abdomen and tape the screener to the patient's body. To verify the electrode position, AP and lateral radiographs should be obtained (Fig. 43–8).

For the next 24 hours following lead placement, the patient wears a soft cervical collar and is instructed to remain flat while sleeping to reduce the chance of

lead migration. After an overnight stay at the hospital, patients are sent home to test the stimulation with the screener for 4 or 5 days as they go about their normal activities. After that time, regardless of their decision about permanent stimulation, we cut the sutures and remove the screener and the lead.

Those who elect to have a permanent cervical SCS system implanted are scheduled for surgery 1 month later. This wait between the screening and the permanent SCS system implantation allows everyone to carefully consider the decision of whether or not to implant. At the same time, this is enough time for trial site of entry to be completely healed.

PERMANENT IMPLANTATION OF THE CERVICAL SPINAL CORD STIMULATION ELECTRODE

Surgical Technique

For additional information, see Figures 43–14 to 43–18 in the thoracolumbar SCS implantation technique.

Following a successful screening and month-long consideration period, if the patient elects to have a permanent SCS system implanted, one can use either a Medtronic Pisces Quad lead or Pisces Quad Plus lead as described in the screening section earlier. Equivalent cervical electrodes from other companies are also available. Two recent advances in the Pisces Quad Plus lead have made lead placement easier: a new radiopaque tip that allows the lead to be visualized on fluoroscopy and an 18-degree bend in the stylet tip that provides improved steerability. Directional control of the lead tip is also enhanced by a special ball-and-socket insertion mechanism in the lead tip, which allows one to snap the

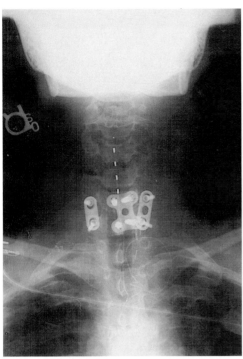 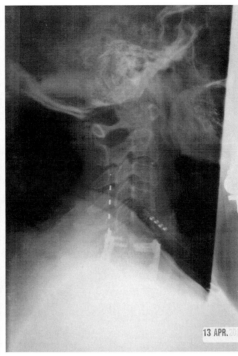

A   **B**

FIGURE 43–8

Anteroposterior *(A)* and lateral *(B)* views of quadripolar electrode in place in the cervical region.

ball-tipped stylet into the lead tip. This mechanism provides a one-to-one torque capability for excellent turning response.

When the electrode is in place, it is connected to the screener and paresthesia patterns are tested. When excellent stimulation coverage is achieved, the lead is anchored using both silicone anchors in the Medtronic lead kit. One is then ready for implantation of the pulse generator.

OPTIMAL ELECTRODE PLACEMENT FOR VARIOUS PAIN SITES

Typically, good stimulation can be achieved using the following upper cervical placements for specific nerve involvement:

- C2–3—for upper neck
- C4–5—for radial nerve
- Just below C5—for median nerve
- C6–7—for ulnar nerve

A percutaneous lead with a broad area of coverage can provide good stimulation for these areas with a single quadripolar lead. When pain is bilateral, the lead should be placed at the midline.

ANCHORING AND TUNNELING

Ideally, dissection of subcutaneous tissue using combined blunt and sharp dissection with Metzenbaum scissors is targeted at exposing the supraspinous ligament, which is shiny and striated, in contrast to the fat and subcutaneous tissue. A dry sponge is helpful in removing fatty tissue and exposing this target to fix the lead anchors. Failure to suture the anchors securely to the ligament and the lead

to the anchor is the most common cause of lead migration. Traditional soft anchors have either a butterfly or a lead-through configuration. Medtronic has introduced a new rigid snap-close anchor that eliminates lead motion at the anchor. This anchor still needs to be carefully attached to the ligament for long-term stabilization. Tunneling rods of various configurations are supplied in the SCS system surgical kits. Depending on the type, they have different end pieces for tunneling and pulling through leads or extensions. With the patient in the prone position, many surgeons are placing Itrel generators in the posterosuperior aspect of the buttock. RF receivers can be placed in the midaxillary line, over the lower rib margin. Placement in the buttock region, with the patient in the prone position, is also becoming popular.

POCKET FORMATION

Preparing the pocket for either an RF receiver or an implanted pulse generator is a relatively straightforward and simple procedure. After infiltration of the proposed incision with local anesthetic, an incision of appropriate length is made, the goal being to produce a pocket that is the right size for the device and for any extra lead or extension that may be coiled behind it.

RF receivers must be no more than 1 cm (<1 inch) from the skin surface and implanted generators. Formation of these pockets can be accomplished mainly with blunt finger dissection, when necessary, by instrument dissection. General principles of tissue handling and hemostasis with electrocautery are standard. Pockets are best closed in two layers to prevent stress on the suture line from the implant. Integrity of the system should always by tested before the patient leaves the operating room to detect easily correctable errors.

IMPLANTATION OF THE PULSE GENERATOR

There are two common placements for the pulse generator when the lead is placed in the upper cervical spine: The anterior chest wall, lower quadrant, same side as the pain, or just below the iliac crest away from the sacroiliac joint in the buttock. A pocket is made for the pulse generator. A tunnel is made for the lead, and the lead and pulse generator are connected using an extension. One can keep the patient in the same position so that redraping is not necessary. It is important to use nonabsorbable sutures when suturing the pulse generator to the deep fascia to help prevent lead migration.

POSTIMPLANT PROCEDURE

Patients need to wear a soft cervical collar for the first 24 hours following surgery and are instructed to remain flat while sleeping to reduce the possibility of lead migration. Patients typically remain in the hospital 2 or 3 days following implantation. During that time, staff assesses them frequently to make any necessary adjustments in the stimulation. The patients are then discharged home with appropriate instructions for home care and a return visit in the outpatient clinic for wound inspection and, if necessary, for future removal and/or reprogramming of the SCS.

THORACOLUMBAR SPINAL CORD STIMULATION

Anatomy

Anatomy of the epidural space is described in Chapter 24 and is not duplicated here.

Indications

In the United States, the primary indications for SCS are failed back surgery syndrome, sympathetically mediated pain, and sympathetically independent pain of complex regional pain syndrome.[9-13] In Europe, interest in SCS has been greatest in connection with treatment of chronic, intractable angina and pain and disability due to peripheral vascular disease.[13-22]

Contraindications

The complications of thoracolumbar spinal cord stimulation are similar to other implantation procedures.

Procedures

- Once the trial for SCS is scheduled, the patient is seen in the clinic the day before surgery, at which time a thorough history and physical examination are performed and appropriate laboratory studies are obtained.

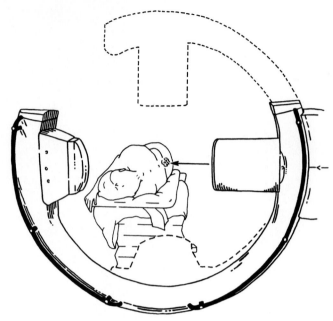

FIGURE 43–9

A drawing of the patient in the lateral position with the C-arm in anteroposterior and lateral positions for entry of Tuohy needle.

- All patients should have undergone a thorough psychological assessment and clearance.
- On the morning of the procedure, the patient is admitted to outpatient surgery for the trial stimulation procedure and 24-hour observation.
- The patient is placed in the lateral position for electrode placement (Fig. 43–9). The lateral position minimizes the risk of spinal cord damage caused by the patient moving back onto the needle suddenly.
- Minimal intravenous sedation is given, because it is important to be able to communicate with the patient while positioning the stimulating electrode.
- The initial dose of antibiotics is given prophylactically at this time.
- The patient is then prepared and draped in a sterile fashion, and local anesthetic is infiltrated at the site of entry.
- A 16-gauge RK needle (Epimed) is placed paramedially to the epidural space at a point roughly two or three segments below the target site using the three-dimensional technique: direction, depth, direction (Fig. 43–10).
- A Lectrocath (Epimed) is placed through the needle to the epidural space and threaded to the appropriate level. A 15-degree bend in the catheter roughly 2 cm from the end facilitates steering of the catheter to a specific site. A trial-stimulating unit is connected to the proximal end of the catheter via alligator chips with the negative lead connected to the catheter wired to the positive electrode grounded to the patient. The

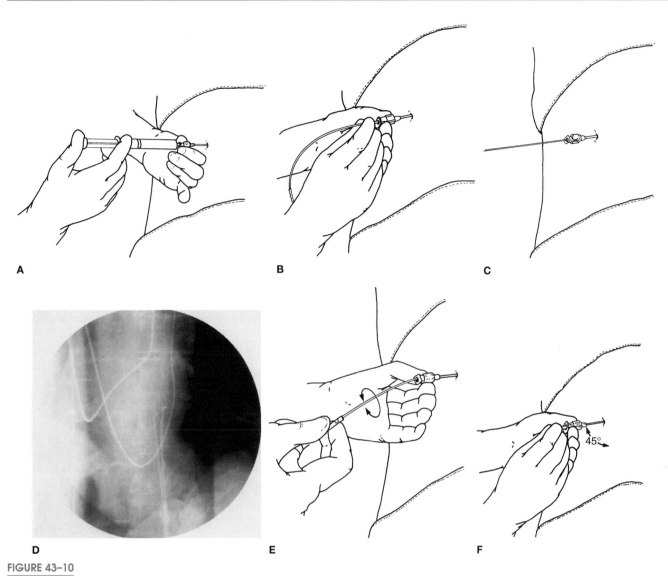

FIGURE 43–10

A, Insertion of a Tuohy needle with the beveled edge facing cephalad. *B,* Trial screening electrode inserted through the Tuohy needle. *C,* If there is difficulty, a guidewire is inserted to facilitate the track. *D,* Racz's electrocatheter in place in the thoracolumbar region for stimulation trial. *E,* the verification screening electrode is now connected to the stimulator screening box to test stimulation. *F,* Once the electrode is in good position, the Tuohy needle is cautiously removed without pushing the electrode any further.

primary goal during the testing period in the operating room is to evaluate the stimulation pattern obtained (Fig. 43–11). Once adequate stimulation over the site of the patient's pain is achieved, the needle is removed under fluoroscopic visualization with care being taken to maintain the position of the catheter tip. The catheter is then sutured to the skin. The distal end of the catheter electrode is permanently anchored with skin suture and dressing (Fig. 43–12). AP and lateral radiographs are taken in the postanesthesia department to document catheter position (Fig. 43–13). The patient is instructed to lie flat overnight to minimize the risk of electrode migration.

PERMANENT PLACEMENT OF THORACOLUMBAR ELECTRODES AND PULSE GENERATOR

Once the type of electrode and style of system are chosen, the surgical technique for all implantation is similar. The practitioner must become familiar with the specific issues of each manufacturer's equipment and of the different models. ANS lead systems are available as one-piece units that must be connected in the generator pocket, although extensions are available and are used mainly for cervical implantation. All Medtronic lead systems use a lead extension, and the lead-lead extension connection is made at the spinal incision. For an RF receiver system, a pocket of the correct depth is paramount. An RF receiver system must be implanted no deeper than 1 cm, whereas an Itrel implantable pulse

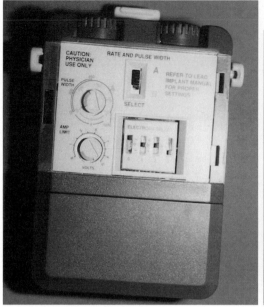

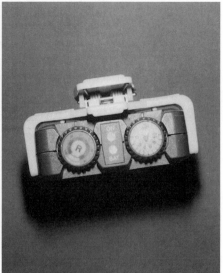

FIGURE 43–11

A, The trial stimulator is used by the patient to evaluate the effect of stimulation for next 5 days. *B,* View from the top of the same screener.

A   **B**

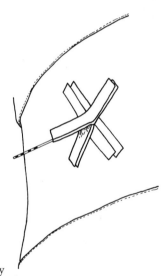

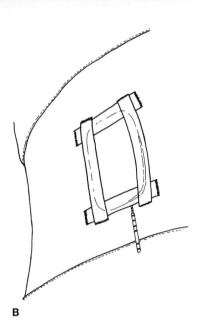

FIGURE 43–12

A and *B,* The distal end of the catheter electrode is permanently anchored with skin suture and dressing.   **A**   **B**

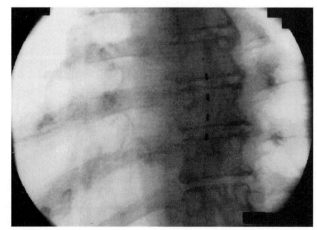

FIGURE 43–13

Medtronic single lead in place with four sites of stimulation.

generator is generally placed deeper, but no deeper than 1 inch.

THORACOLUMBAR ELECTRODE PLACEMENT

For lead placement, the patient can lie in the lateral decubitus position, but increasingly the prone position is being used and a bolster placed under the costal margin to promote adequate flexion of the spine and facilitate epidural lead placement. The patient is prepared and draped in the usual manner for surgery, with a strict aseptic technique. The site of entry of the epidural needle for patients with lower extremity, hip, or back pain is L1–L2 (Fig. 43–14). Fluoroscopy is used to guide and confirm the needle of entry into the epidural space. Care must be taken to drape the fluoroscopy unit and to provide an extra side drape, to

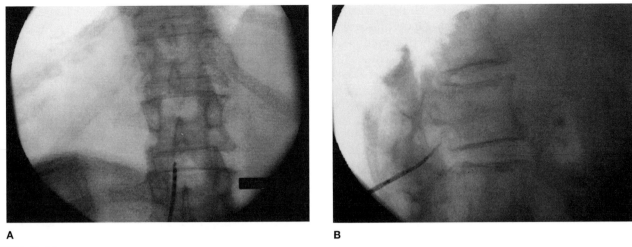

FIGURE 43–14

A, Step 1. In the anteroposterior view, the site of entry of the Tuohy needle between L1–L2 interspace just lateral to the spinous process. *B,* In the lateral view, the needle is confirmed to be in the epidural space after a positive "loss of bounce" technique.

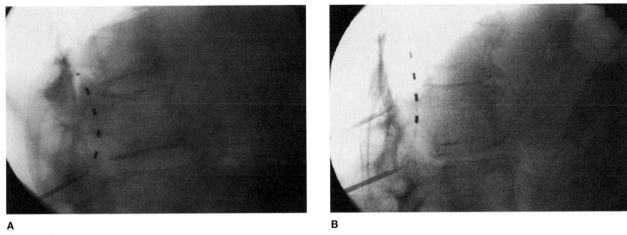

FIGURE 43–15

A, When the electrode is inserted, the lateral view is important. The electrode has to remain posterior. In this radiograph the electrode has gone anteriorly and the tip is bounced back posteriorly. *B,* In this radiograph the electrode is more posterior than in *A.*

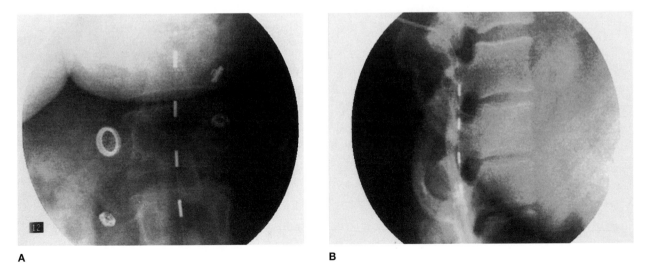

FIGURE 43–16

Anteroposterior *(A)* and lateral *(B)* views of correct quadripolar electrode placement.

prevent contamination of the surgical field during cross-table views. Fluoroscopy helps guide placement of two leads, if needed, for bilateral pain distribution. A combination of 1% lidocaine and 0.5% bupivacaine with epinephrine is a useful mixture for both preoperative and postoperative analgesia. Once the needle is confirmed to be in the epidural space, a lateral view is taken to confirm that the electrode enters cephalad dorsally (Figs. 43–15 and 43–16).

Two-stage initial lead placement or definitive placement of an SCS system after a successful trial proceeds with a midline or slightly paramedian skin incision after

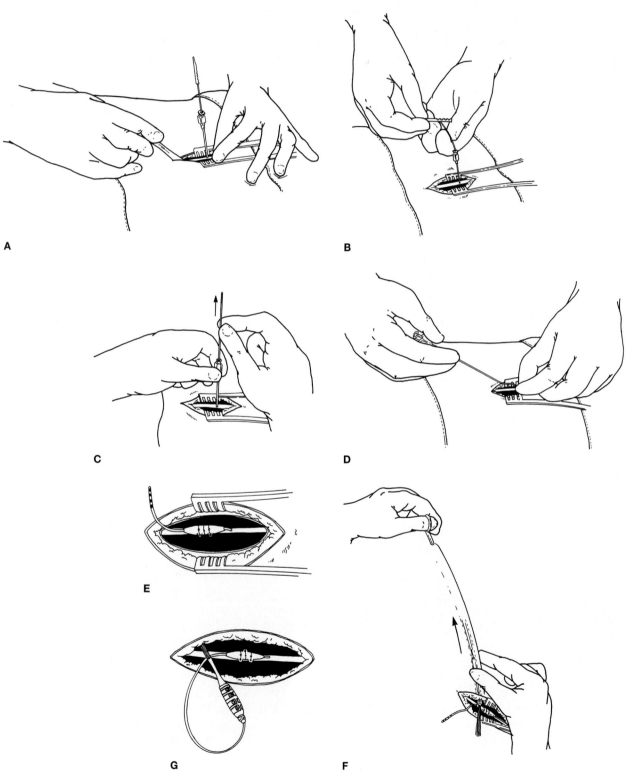

A

B

C

D

E

G

F

FIGURE 43–17

See legend on facing page.

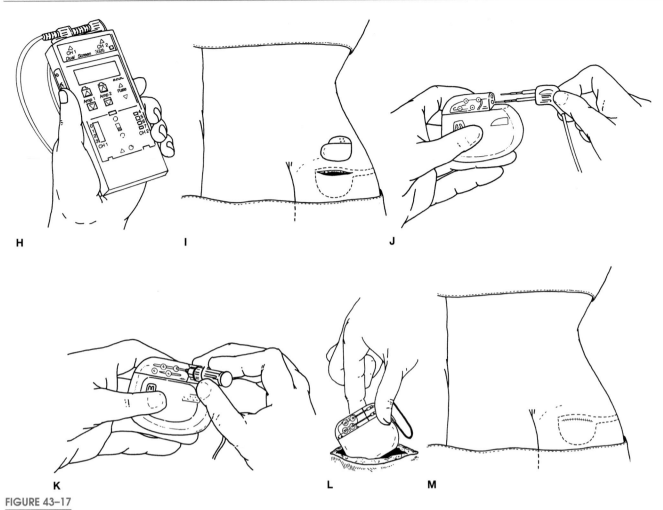

FIGURE 43–17

Placement of spinal cord stimulation system. *A*, Making a 5- to 7-cm longitudinal incision. *B*, Disconnecting the stylet from the lead. *C*, Exposing the lead beyond the tip of the needle. *D*, Slipping the Tuohy needle off the lead body. *E*, Suturing the lead anchor. *F*, Guiding the tool subcutaneously along the tunneling route and pulling the assembly through the passing straw. *G*, Suturing the wide end of the extension connector. *H*, Stimulator used after electrodes are in place to confirm the area of stimulation prior to starting the pocket. *I*, Checking incision length. *J*, Inserting the extension connector pins into the connector block. *K*, Tightening each set's screw on the connector block. *L*, Inserting the stimulator (implantable pulse generator [IPG]) into the pocket with the lettered side facing the skin. *M*, IPG buried subcutaneously and the incision closed in a standard fashion.

local anesthetic infiltration (Fig. 43–17). Patients must be alert and responsive enough to report on stimulation coverage. Therefore, general anesthesia is contraindicated and appropriate and judicious sedation may be employed by the anesthesiologist. Entry into the epidural space, using the manufacturer's supplied modified Tuohy needle, is facilitated by a slightly paraspinal approach. It is important to keep the angle of entry as shallow as possible, to more easily advance the lead cephalad. With a shallower angle, steering of the lead is easier because of the mechanical advantage it affords.

Fluoroscopy combined with the standard loss-of-resistance technique increases the chance of atraumatic entry into the epidural space. Real-time imaging can often guide placement of the lead through resistance in the epidural space, along the way to final placement. A single lead should be placed slightly ipsilateral to the painful side and as close as possible to the physiologic midline for bilateral pain coverage. Coverage of the painful region with stimulation paresthesia determines the final lead placement. A dual lead may be necessary for better coverage in the same side or for bilateral coverage of the extremity. Various electrode placements are illustrated in the Figure 43–18.

IMMEDIATE POSTIMPLANT CHANGES

The ideal stimulation pattern—and resulting pain relief—are often lost within the first few weeks after implantation. Periodic reprogramming then becomes essential. As the fibrous tissue invests the lead electrodes, resistance to delivery of the electrical impulses increases. The result is the need to substantially increase the amplitude over time. This should be expected, and the patient made aware that it is a normal occurrence. This maturation process can often require reprogramming of the electrode array, pulse width,

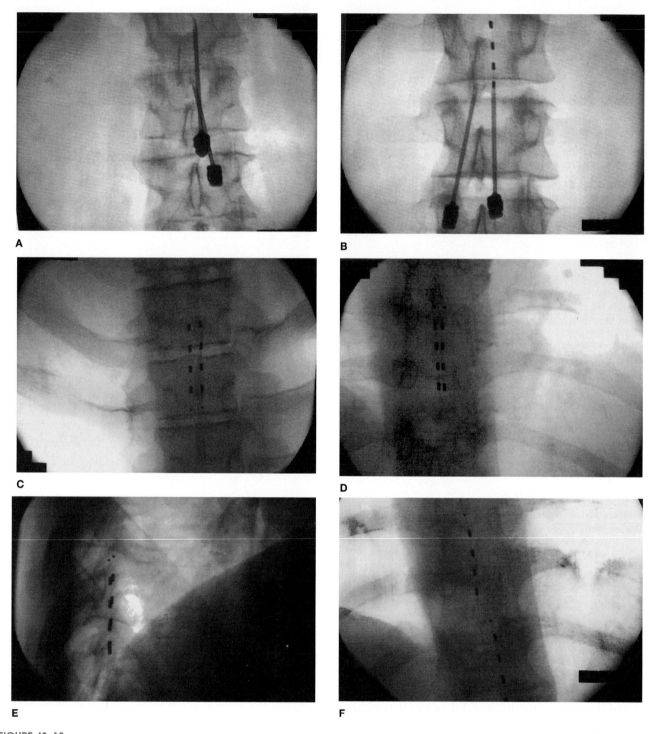

FIGURE 43–18

A, When two electrodes are needed, the Tuohy needles could be entered at two different levels, as shown. *B,* Another way of inserting Tuohy needle at the same level. *C,* This radiograph shows dual leads off of midline. *D,* Anteroposterior view in the radiograph shows dual leads close to the midline. *E,* Lateral view of two leads in place. *F,* When a larger area needs to be stimulated, the leads can be placed one over the other, as shown.

and frequency. The three-dimensional space surrounding the lead can be altered by the natural process of healing in a manner that renders the stimulator system ineffective, despite a successful trial.

Migration of the lead after maturation is much less likely, but it still occurs with relative frequency. "Electrical repositioning" of the electrode array recovers

the optimal stimulation pattern. Multiplication of the other particles improves the comfort of the stimulator signal, which is a matter of individual patient preference.

At our institution, routine clinic visits for stimulator reprogramming are scheduled approximately every 3 to 6 months after the optimal stimulation programs are initiated. This is essential in patients with simulator systems that do not provide multiple patient-controlled programs. By varying the programs from time to time, accommodation can be avoided. *Accommodation* describes the phenomenon by which the body comes to "ignore" a steady, unvarying electrical stimulus over time. Patients who leave their stimulator systems on continuously develop accommodation much more rapidly, and this stimulation becomes ineffective, if not actually painful, over the long term. Most patients do best in a ""cycling" mode; for example, 1 minute on, 1 minute off. This cycling mode also serves to prolong pulse generator battery life by relying on the "carry-over" analgesic effect experienced by most SCS patients. This carry-over effect can last seconds to hours.

TISSUE CHANGES AFTER 4 WEEKS

Once the patient has passed the 4th postoperative week, the system can be said to have matured. The body has now formed a fibrous capsule around the various components of the implant, which is less likely to migrate or produce any of the complications mentioned in the previous section. Several potential difficulties still lie in wait for the unsuspecting physician implanter.

SACRAL NERVE STIMULATION

Anatomy

The sacrum is a large, triangular bone situated below L5 (Fig. 43–19). Its apex articulates with the coccyx. Its anterior surface is concave. Anteriorly, four transverse ridges cross its median part. The portions of the bone between the ridges are the bodies of the sacrum. There are four anterior sacral foramina through which the sacral nerves exit and lateral sacral arteries enter. The posterior surface of the sacrum is convex. There are rudimentary spinous processes from the first three or four sacral segments in the midline. The laminae unite to form the sacral groove. The sacral hiatus is formed by the failure of the laminae of S5 to unite posteriorly. The tubercles that represent remnants of the inferior articular processes are known as the *sacral cornua*; they are connected inferiorly to the coccygeal cornua. Laterally, one can identify four dorsal sacral foramina. They transmit the posterior divisions of the sacral nerves. The sacrum may have many variations. The bodies of S1 and S2 may fail to unite or the sacral canal may remain open throughout its length.

Indications

- Voiding disorders
  - Urinary incontinence
  - Urinary retention
  - Voiding dysfunction
- Chronic pelvic pain
  - Interstitial cystitis
  - Pudendal neuralgia
  - Vulvodynia

Contraindications

- Local infection
- Any infection involving the bladder or the pelvis
- Coagulopathy

Preparation of the patient

PHYSICAL EXAMINATION

Examine for superficial infection in the surgical area and for distorted anatomy that may affect performance of the procedure.

LABORATORY

- Complete blood count with platelets
- Prothrombin time, partial thromboplastion time
- Platelet function test or bleeding times
- Urinalysis
- Magnetic resonance imaging (optional) for canal size

PREOPERATIVE MEDICATION

For preoperative medication, use the standard American Society of Anesthesiologists' recommendations for conscious sedation.

Procedures

TRIAL SACRAL STIMULATION

Patients must undergo acute percutaneous electrical stimulation of the ventral ramus at the level of the third (S3), and possibly S2 and S4 sacral foramina, to establish functional integrity of the sacral nerves, to locate the nerves that can elicit beneficial responses, and to confirm that nerve stimulation elicits contractions of the appropriate muscle groups. The search for the S3 foramen can be done either with anatomic palpation or fluoroscopy (Fig. 43–20).

If adequate responses are obtained during the acute testing, then test stimulation needs to be conducted for several days (not to exceed 7 days). Stimulation is achieved by replacing the stimulation needle with a temporary screening lead placed through the needle and connected to the same external screener that is used during the test phase. The amplitude of stimulation and "on/off" are controlled by the patient.

The patient controls the amplitude of the stimulation so that it is sensate but painless. Patients are informed that the sensation can change according to their positioning (sitting, standing, lying) and movements. Continuous stimulation is used (day and night, 10 Hz, 210 milliseconds), and patients must be educated to manage power according to the severity of symptoms and feelings. They have to report all modifications of stimulation parameters on the voiding diary.

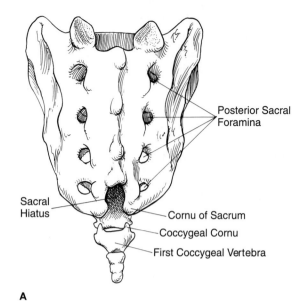

Posterior Sacral
Foramina

Sacral
Hiatus

Cornu of Sacrum

Coccygeal Cornu

First Coccygeal Vertebra

A

FIGURE 43–19

A, Anatomy of the sacrum. *B*, Anterior view of the sacrum with the anterior primary rami exiting. Note the presence of the coccygeal nerve. *C*, Lateral view of the sacrum shows both the anterior and posterior primary rami of the sacral nerves exiting their respective foramina.

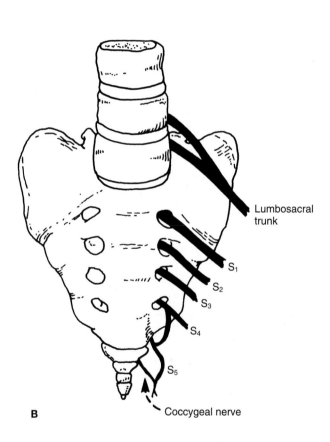

Lumbosacral
trunk

S₁

S₂

S₃

S₄

S₅

B   Coccygeal nerve

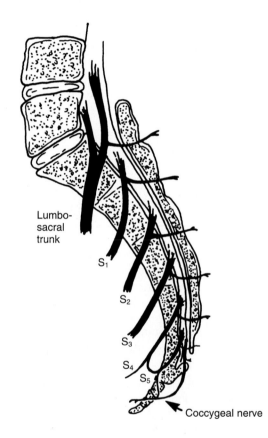

Lumbo-
sacral
trunk

S₁

S₂

S₃

S₄

S₅

Coccygeal nerve

C

PERMANENT SACRAL STIMULATION

Sacral nerve root stimulation is performed under light sedation, using local infiltration. Patients are positioned prone on a radiolucent table. Electrodes are placed percutaneously in the epidural space under fluoroscopic guidance at the appropriate level as determined by patient paresthesia. The lumbar and sacral nerve roots are approached in a caudal direction (retrograde approach). In this approach, a Tuohy-type needle is inserted into the skin at a level superior

rather than inferior to the interlaminar space and advanced in a caudal rather than a cranial direction. To reach sacral nerve roots, it is imperative to insert the needle in the same direction that the nerve root travels within the epidural nerve root sleeve. Therefore, the needle has to be placed in a paramedial fashion and advanced caudally into the epidural space. Once the epidural space is penetrated, the electrode will then follow the path of the needle and continue to advance toward the targeted nerve root (Fig. 43–21). The experts

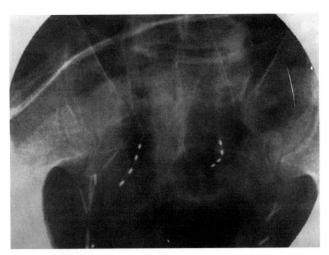

FIGURE 43–20

Anteroposterior view of electrodes through S3 foramina bilaterally for trial-testing of the area of stimulation and analgesia.

in this technique (Quattrode or Octrode) recommend multielectrode systems. Initial positioning is according to the anatomically predicted locations appropriate for the patient's pain. The exact position of the physiologic target varies and can be determined only intraoperatively by communicating with the patient about the location of the perceived paresthesias as different neural targets are stimulated. The perceptual threshold is defined as the stimulation amplitude at which level the patient first perceives the paresthesias. The discomfort threshold is the amplitude at which the paresthesias become uncomfortable. In all patients, criteria for a successful trial includes a greater than 50% reduction in pain level, a reduced consumption of pain medications, and an increase in activities of daily living. If the patient had a successful trial, then permanent sacral electrodes are implanted.

Complications

- Epidural hematoma
- Spinal headache
- Infection
- Lead migration
- Seroma or stitch abscess
- Wound dehiscence

Helpful Hints

If the patient has had pervious scar formation that makes it difficult to pass the electrode, the physician may put a curve at one end of the guidewire to use as a tool for opening the space. Alternatively, a tunneling catheter with a soft spring tip and a small syringe, such as the Tun-L-Kath, can be used to open the space using 1 mL of saline. When the space is opened, the lead can be advanced.

EFFICACY OF SPINAL CORD STIMULATION

There are numerous retrospective studies that tout the efficacy of SCS. These studies or reports usually lump together patients who have various pain syndromes of different kinds. The substance of many of these studies suggests that, for many such syndromes, efficacy is approximately 60% and relief lasts about 2 years. After 2 years, for whatever reasons, in some patients efficacy seems to fall off. SCS is effective not only for neuropathic pain of appendicular and axial origin but also for complex regional pain syndrome, peripheral vascular disease, and the pain of intractable angina.

The most comprehensive published study is the one by North and associates,[23] in which patients with up to 18 years' follow-up were subjected to an extensive questionnaire.

If one considers only the most stringently analyzed series, good to excellent results are reported in 40% to 60% of the implanted patients.[23–27] In these published series, the percentage of patients with no or minimal results varied between 30% and 60%. Other less rigorous general series in the literature claim good to excellent results, ranging from 47% to 66%, and failure

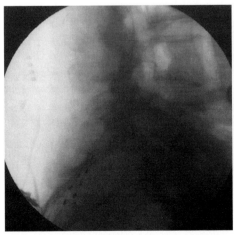

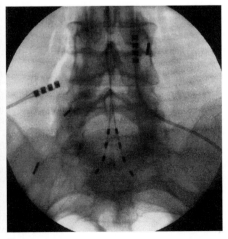

A   B

FIGURE 43–21

A, Radiographic imaging (anteroposterior view) of lumbosacral area that shows retrograde placement of electrodes toward sacral nerve roots. B, Radiographic imaging (lateral view) of the lumbosacral area that shows retrograde placement of electrodes in the caudal canal.

▽ TABLE 43–2 Most Relevant Published General Series on Spinal Cord Stimulation for Chronic Pain Management

Primary Author	Publication Year (Time Span of Implants)	Type of Study[¶]	Number of Implanted Patients	Average Follow-Up (Years)	Extended Trial Screening	Results (%) None/Poor	Results (%) Fair	Results (%) Good/Excellent
Barolat—Group A[31],[*]	1998 (1985–1992)	3	102	3.8	No	51	15	34[#]
Barolat—Group B[32],[†]	1998 (1985–1992)	3	80	3.8	Equivalent to yes	37.5	11.5	51[#]
Burchiel[32]	1996 (1990–1992)	Retrospective	70	1	Yes	22	43	35
Devulder[33]	1991 (1982–1990)	1	69	At least 2	Yes	30	11	59
Koeze[25]	1987	3	26	22	No	30	20	50
Kumar[28]	1991 (1980–1989)		94	3.4	Yes	44	Not applicable	56
Kupers[34]	1994	3	70	3.5	Yes	27	21	52
Ohnmeiss[26]	1996	Retrospective	40	2	No	30	44	26
Meglio[35]	1989 (1979–1986)							
Nielson[36]	1975 (1969–1973)	2	130	[‡]	Yes	39	12	49
North[23]	1991 (1971–1990)	3	171	7	Yes	37	11	52
Racz[37]	1989 (1984–1986)	2	26	1.8	No	21	18	61
Ray[38]	1982 (1976–1982)	1	78	1.8	Yes	23	20	57
Siegfried[39]	1982 (1972–1980)	1	89	4	Yes	39	24	37
Simpson[29]	1991	2	60	2.3	24 Yes; 26 No	20	33	47
Spiegelmann[27]	1991 (1987–1989)	3	30	1	Yes	36	4	60

[*] All implanted patients.
[†] Implanted patients, excluding the ones who never experienced any pain relief (equivalent to patients in published series with trial screening who passed the trial and underwent implantation).
[‡] In 32% of patients <1 year, in 45% of patients > 1 < 2 years, in 24% of patients > 2 years.
[§] Patients who rated their pain relief at the survey between 25% and 49%.
[#] Patients who rated their pain relief at the survey 50% or better.
[¶] The key to the type of study is the following:
1, Detailed data; 2, Detailed data + Methodology of data collection clearly specified; 3, Detailed data + Methodology of data collection clearly specified + survey by disinterested third party.

rates ranging between 20% and 39%.[28, 29] Limiting success to only reports of good/excellent relief, however, would not do justice to an average of 20% of implanted patients who still use the stimulator with moderate pain relief. See Table 43–2 for studies on SCS by various groups.

The psychological preparation of the patient for the procedure seemed to have a substantial impact on the results. The authors believe that this is due in part to the elimination of patients who have frank psychopathology. In a larger percentage, however, the better results are to be explained by the fact that patients who underwent psychological counseling came to the surgical implantation better prepared mentally and with a more realistic approach. One feels that administering psychological testing is just as important as providing extensive psychological support before, during, and following the implantation procedure. Therefore, continuing psychological screening as an integral part of SCS implantation program is appropriate.[30]

Percutaneous implantation neurostimulator electrode/epidural 63650; revision/removal of implanted spinal neurostimulator pulse generator or receiver 63688; revision/removal supina neurostimulator electrode 63660; placement of spinal neurostimulator pulse generator/receiver 63685

REFERENCES

1. Shealy CN, Mortimer JT, Reswick J: Electrical inhibition of pain by stimulation of the dorsal column: Preliminary clinical reports. Anesth Analg 46:489–491, 1967.
2. Foreman RD, Beall JE, Applebaum AE, et al: Effects of dorsal column stimulation on primate spinothalamic tract neurons. J Neurophysiol 39:534–546, 1976.
3. Handwerker HO, Iggo A, Zimmerman M: Segmental and supraspinal actions on dorsal horn neurons responding to noxious and non-noxious skin stimuli. Pain 1:147–165, 1975.
4. Feldman RA: Patterned response of lamina V cells: Cutaneous and dorsal funicular stimulation. Physiol Behav 15:79–84, 1975.
5. Stanton-Hicks M: Lumbar sympathetic nerve block and neurolysis. In Waldman S (ed): Interventional Pain Management, 2nd ed. Philadelphia, WB Saunders, 2001, pp 485–492.

6. Picaza J, Hunter S, Cannon B: Pain suppression by peripheral nerve stimulation. Appl Neurophysiol 40:223–239, 1977/1978.
7. Ebraheim NA, Biyani A, Brown JA: Anatomic considerations of halo pin placement. Am J Orthop 25:754–756, 1996.
8. Weiner R, Reed K: Peripheral neurostimulation for control of intractable occipital neuralgia. Neuromodulation 3:217–221, 1999.
9. Oakley JC, Weiner RL: Spinal cord stimulation for complex regional pain syndrome: A prospective study of 19 patients at two centers. Neuromodulation 2:47–51, 1999.
10. Bennett DS, Alo KM, Oakley J, Feler CA: Spinal cord stimulation for complex regional pain syndrome (RSD): A retrospective multicenter experience from 1995–1998 of 101 patients. Neuromodulation 3:202–210, 1999.
11. Broseta J, Roldan P, Gonzalez-Darder J, et al: Chronic epidural dorsal column stimulation in the treatment of causalgia pain. Appl Neurophysiol 45:190–194, 1982.
12. Barolat G, Schwartzman R, Woo R: Epidural spinal cord stimulation in the management of reflex sympathetic dystrophy. Stereotact Funct Neurosurg 53:29–39, 1989.
13. Stanton-Hicks M: Spinal cord stimulation for the management of complex regional pain syndromes. Neuromodulation 2:193–202, 1999.
14. Mannheimer C, Augustinsson LE, Carlsson CA, et al: Epidural spinal electrical stimulation in severe angina pectoris. Br Heart J 59:56–61, 1988.
15. Augustinsson LE: Spinal cord stimulation in severe angina pectoris: Surgical technique, intraoperative physiology, complications, and side effects. Pace 12:693–694, 1989.
16. Murphy DF, Giles KE: Dorsal column stimulation for pain relief from intractable angina pectoris. Pain 28:365–368, 1987.
17. deJongste MJL, Hatvast RWM, Ruiters MHJ, ter Horst GJ: Spinal cord stimulation and the induction of *c-fos* and heat shock protein 72 in the central nervous system of rats. Neuromodulation 1:73–85, 1998.
18. Kobaina FJ, Dominguez M, Diaz M, et al: Spinal cord stimulation for relief of chronic pain in vasospastic disorders of the upper limbs. Neurosurgery 24:63–67, 1989.
19. Augustinsson LE, Holm J, Carl A, et al: Epidural electrical stimulation in severe limb ischemia: Evidences of pain relief, increased blood flow, and a possible limb-saving effect. Ann Surg 202:104–111, 1985.
20. Jacobs MJ, Jorning PJ, Joshi SR, et al: Spinal cord electrical stimulation improves microvascular blood flow in severe limb ischaemia. Ann Surg 207:179–183, 1988.
21. Groth KE: Spinal cord stimulation for the treatment of peripheral vascular disease. Adv Pain Res Ther 9:861–870, 1985.
22. Claeys LGY: Spinal cord stimulation and chronic critical limb ischemia. Neuromodulation 2:1, 1999.
23. North RB, Kidd DH, Zahurak M, et al: Spinal cord stimulation for chronic, intractable pain: Experience over two decades. Neurosurgery 32:384–395, 1993.
24. Matsui T, Asano T, Takakura K, et al: Beneficial effects of cervical spinal cord stimulation (cSCS) on patients with impaired consciousness: A preliminary report. Pace 12:718–725, 1989.
25. Koeze TH, Williams AC, Reiman S: Spinal cord stimulation and the relief of chronic pain. J Neurol Neurosurg Psychiatry 50:1424–1429, 1987.
26. Ohnmeiss D, Rashbaum R, Bogdanffy M: Prospective outcome evaluation of spinal cord stimulation in patients with intractable leg pain. Spine 21:1344–1350, 1996.
27. Spiegelmann R, Friedman WA: Spinal cord stimulation: A contemporary series. Neurosurgery 28:65–70, 1991.
28. Kumar K, Nath R, Wyant GM: Treatment of chronic pain by epidural spinal cord stimulation: A 10-year experience. J Neurosurg 75:402–407, 1991.
29. Simpson BA: Spinal cord stimulation in 60 cases of intractable pain. J Neurol Neurosurg Psychiatry 54:196–199, 1991.
30. Daniel M, Long C, Hutcherson M, Hunter S: Psychological factors and outcome of electrode implantation for chronic pain. Neurosurgery 17:773–777, 1985.
31. Barolat G, Katchik B, He J: Long-term outcome of spinal cord stimulation for chronic pain management. Neuromodulation 1:19–30, 1998.
32. Burchiel KJ, Anderson VC, Brown FD, et al: Prospective multicenter study of spinal cord stimulation for relief of chronic back and extremity pain. Spine 21:2786–2794, 1996.
33. Devulder J, Vermeulen H, DeColvenaer L, et al: Spinal cord stimulation in chronic pain: Evaluation of results, complications, and technical considerations in 69 patients. Clin J Pain 7:21–28, 1991.
34. Kupers RC, Van den Oever R, Van Houdenhove B, et al: Spinal cord stimulation in Belgium: A nationwide survey on the incidence, indications, and therapeutic efficacy by the health insurer. Pain 56:211–216, 1994.
35. Meglio M, Cioni B, Rossi GF: Spinal cord stimulation in management of chronic pain: A 9-year experience. J Neurosurg 12:519–524, 1989.
36. Nielson KD, Adams J, Hosobuchi Y: Experience with dorsal column stimulation for relief of chronic pain, 1968–1973. Surg Neurol 4:148–152, 1975.
37. Racz GB, McCarron RF, Talboys P: Percutaneous dorsal column stimulator for chronic pain control. Spine 14:1–4, 1989.
38. Ray CD, Burton CV, Lifson A: Neurostimulation of a large clinical practice. Appl Neurophysiol 45:160–166, 1982.
39. Siegfried J, Lazorthes Y: Long-term follow-up of dorsal column stimulation for chronic pain syndrome after multiple lumbar operations. Appl Neurophysiol 45:201–204, 1982.

Intrathecal Implantations

HISTORY

In 1979, Wang and colleagues[1] reported that the use of morphine for cancer-related pain at doses of 0.5 to 1 mg resulted in excellent pain relief for 8 to 30 hours. Yaksh[2] documented the physiologic basis of the pain relief produced by the intraspinal administration of opioids as the modulation of inhibitory mechanisms occurring at the spinal cord.

Opioids produce a profound inhibition of the evoked discharge of spinal nociceptive neurons, resulting in a significant elevation of the pain threshold in animals.[3] At analgesic doses, spinal opioids, unlike local anesthetic agents, have no effect on the response to light touch, autonomic outflow, or voluntary motor function. The analgesic functions of intraspinally administered opioids are dose dependent and stereospecific. Opioids have a highly regular structure-activity relationship and are antagonized in a dose-dependent fashion by naloxone. This highly regular pharmacology suggests an effect mediated by receptors that are located in the spinal cord. Opiate-binding studies revealed high levels of binding in the substantia gelatinosa, where the bulk of the small primary afferent fibers terminate. The local action of morphine in the substantia gelatinosa inhibits the discharge of nociceptive neurons, thereby inhibiting the transmission of pain.[3, 4]

Although percutaneous externalized epidural or even intrathecal catheter placement is feasible for short-term treatment, vulnerability to infection and economic considerations preclude serious considerations for long-term use (>3 months).[5, 6]

Coombs,[7] Poletti,[8] and their coworkers initially described the use of an implanted reservoir that, on repeated compression, delivered a bolus of medication into the epidural space. Percutaneous injection of an implanted infusion port connected to a spinal catheter was also described.[9] Theoretical and practical objections to bolus dosing arose when primate studies indicated that tolerance to the opioids developed more rapidly when they were delivered in this manner.[10] These techniques also required sufficient personnel to obtain and administer the medication, primarily morphine, on an outpatient basis. Infusion ports could be connected to external pumps, which avoided the risk of rapid tolerance but resulted in the patient's discomfort and increased risk of infection.[11]

ANATOMY

Usual lumbar anatomy knowledge is required for intrathecal catheter placement. In addition, one must be aware of the anatomic structures related to performance of a chronic intrathecal infusion of sterile, preservative-free morphine sulfate or other analgesics (such as hydromorphone, clonidine, and local anesthetics). Chronic intrathecal infusion of baclofen injection is accomplished for severe spasticity of spinal or cerebral origin.

INDICATIONS

In general, intraspinal pain therapy using implantable drug administration systems has been reserved for patients whose condition is considered chronic. This technique is not indicated for acute pain syndromes. Chronicity may be defined in terms of time (e.g., pain lasting longer than 3 or 4 months that is inadequately relieved by standard medical management.)[12] Chronicity may also be defined in terms of pain present more than 1 month beyond what a normal healing process would be expected to take.

With regard to cancer-related pain, although the disease is progressive, if the pain is expected to last beyond 3 months, it can be thought of as chronic. The indication for use of implantable drug administration systems then includes the treatment of chronic pain of both cancer-related and non–cancer-related varieties.

Inclusion Criteria
- Pain type and generator appropriate
- Demonstrated opioid responsivity
- No untreated psychopathology that might predispose to an unsuccessful outcome
- Successful completion of a screening trial

Exclusion Criteria
Absolute
- Aplastic anemia
- Systemic infection
- Known allergies to the materials in the implant
- Known allergies to the intended medications
- Active intravenous drug abuse
- Psychosis or dementia

Relative
- Emaciated patient
- Ongoing anticoagulation therapy
- Child before fusion of the epiphyses
- Occult infection possible
- Recovering drug addict
- Opioid nonresponsivity (other drugs may be considered)
- Lack of social or family support
- Socioeconomic problems
- Lack of access to medical care

EQUIPMENT

- Implantable intrathecal infusion pump
- Connecting tubing
- Intrathecal catheter (if separate)
- Appropriate surgical instruments for implantation

DRUGS

- Local anesthetics for infiltration
- Drug to be used for intrathecal infusion

PREPARATION OF THE PATIENT

LABORATORY

- Complete blood count with platelets
- Prothrombin time, partial thromboplastin time
- Platelet function studies and bleeding time

PREOPERATIVE MEDICATION

For preoperative medication, use the standard American Society of Anesthesiologists' (ASA) recommendations for conscious sedation.

MONITORING

Use the standard ASA-recommended monitoring protocol.

PROCEDURES

Implantation may take place with the patient under general or local anesthesia with monitoring. Local anesthesia is often preferred in an outpatient setting because it lends itself to rapid recovery after the procedure. When general anesthesia is chosen, the use of muscle relaxants is frequently deferred until after the catheter is threaded into the intrathecal space. The steps are as follows:

1. Before the implantation, spend some time with the patient to decide on the side and location of the pump. About the only area amenable to the implantation of these generally large devices is the right or left lower quadrant of the abdomen. The anatomic constraints tend to be the iliac crest, the symphysis pubis, the ilioinguinal ligament, and the costal margin. These structures should not touch the pump when the patient is in the seated position. The task is easier with more obese patients and can be difficult with cachectic cancer patients.
2. Position the patient in the lateral decubitus position on the operating table with the side of implantation upward. At this stage, C-arm fluoroscopy may be necessary if a new intrathecal catheter is to be placed (Fig. 44–1).
3. Position the instrument to permit an anteroposterior view, allowing easy lumbar puncture and identification of the catheter tip level (Fig. 44–2).
4. Implant the catheter through a paramedian approach after making a 5- to 8-cm incision in the skin down to the lumbar fascia (Fig. 44–3).
5. Document a good flow of cerebrospinal fluid (CSF), and clamp the catheter to the drape to prevent CSF loss.
6. Pack the incision with an antibiotic-soaked sponge.
7. If the existing catheter is to be used as the permanent delivery catheter, as in the screening technique, place the patient on the operating table in the decubitus position, with the implantation side upward and the exiting screening extension catheter downward. Preparation and draping for implantation then proceeds as usual.
8. Reopen the previous back incision, and disconnect the disposable extension catheter from the permanent intrathecal catheter. Have the circulating nurse pull it out from under the patient.

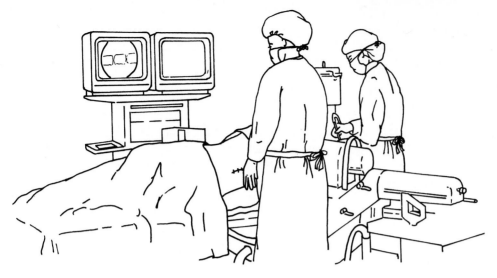

FIGURE 44–1

Preparing and draping the patient.

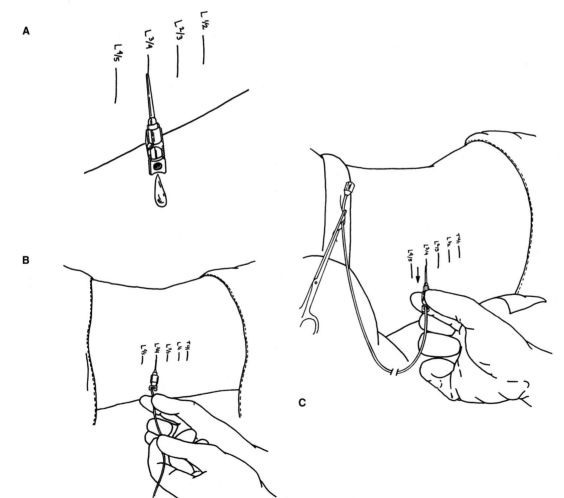

FIGURE 44–2

A, Observing the backflow. B, Inserting the distal catheter section. C, Withdrawing the needle slightly to minimize leakage.

A

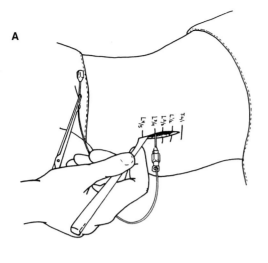

B

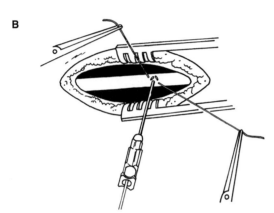

FIGURE 44–3

A, Making a small vertical incision to expose the supraspinous ligament. *B*, Placing pursestring sutures around the catheter.

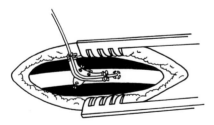

FIGURE 44–5

Inserting the catheter into an anchor and securing it with ligatures.

A

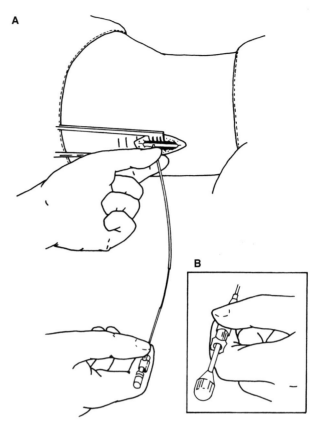

B

FIGURE 44–4

A, Removing the introducer needle. *B*, Withdrawing the needle and guidewire.

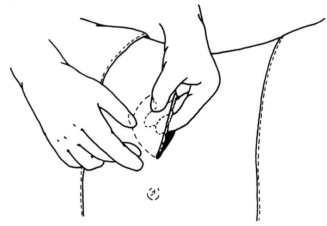

FIGURE 44–6

Forming a pump pocket.

9. Clamp the intrathecal catheter to prevent CSF loss. The rest of the implantation proceeds in the usual manner (Figs. 44–4 and 44–5).

10. Turning attention to the lower quadrant of the abdomen, make a 10-cm incision down the underlying subcutaneous fat layer. Fashion a subcutaneous pocket large enough to admit the particular pump being used. Generally, if all four fingers can be admitted to the meta-carpophalangeal joints in the pocket, it is large enough (Fig. 44–6).

11. Undermine the upper side of the incision roughly the width of the pump or about 2.5 cm to allow closure without tension. The eccentric location of the pocket allows the pump to be placed in such a fashion that the refill port is clear of the incisional scar and easier to locate. An ideal pocket is one that allows the pump to

be placed in such a fashion that the refill port is clear of the incisional scar and easier to locate. Another aim is to have a pocket that allows placement of the pump without struggle but is tight enough to aid in preventing pump rotation. The depth of the pocket below the skin is critical for programmable pumps. A depth greater than 2.5 cm may not allow reliable telemetry.

12. In fashioning the pocket, maintain meticulous hemostasis to avoid postoperative hematoma formation. At this point, pack the pocket with an antibiotic-soaked sponge.

13. Next, tunnel the catheter connecting the intrathecal catheter to the pump (the extension catheter) from the pump pocket to the back incision using a malleable tunneling device. Shunt tunneling tools may also be used, and the tunneling system provided with the programmable pump works well. Because most constant-flow-rate pumps come with the extension catheter connected to the pump at the factory, the catheter must be attached to the programmable pump (Fig. 44–7).

14. Make a connection between the extension catheter and the intrathecal catheter using a male-to-male tubing connector (usually provided with the catheter selected). This connector may be made of titanium or a plastic material.

15. Cover this construct with some type of anchoring device, which is secured to the connector with 2-0 nonabsorbable braided tie, and anchor the construct to the underlying muscle fascia in a figure-of-8 fashion. Do not skip the anchoring; without it, the intrathecal catheter will migrate, usually coiling itself under the skin (Fig. 44–8).

16. Connect the extension catheter to the previously prepared programmable pump, and secure it to the pump with a 2-0 braided tie. Pumps with a previously attached catheter must be placed into the pocket at the time of catheter tunneling.

17. Place the programmable pump into the subcutaneous pocket. The SynchroMed pump in its polyester (Dacron) pouch may be placed without need for further suturing. Pumps without this pouch may have anchoring loops manufactured around the pump circumference. The use of these structures is problematic. Place a nonabsorbable stitch into a tissue that does not necrose rapidly, as do fat and muscle. Use at least two stitches to prevent rotation; three may be necessary to prevent flipping. A dermal or fascial stitch is usually required, and there is a risk that the anchor will be painful. If this technique is used, place the stitches into the pocket

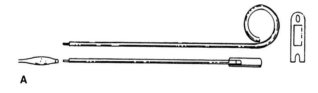

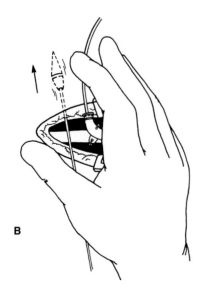

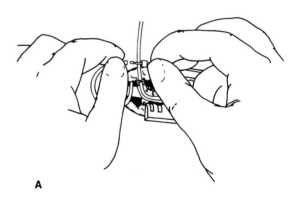

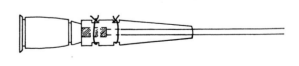

FIGURE 44–7

A, Assembling the tunneling tool or preparing the catheter passer. *B,* Creating a subcutaneous tunnel.

FIGURE 44–8

A, Inserting a metal tubing connector into the proximal catheter section. *B,* Suturing a sleeve onto the connector.

first, then through the pump suture loops. Place the pump into the pocket, and tie the sutures. If the pocket is carefully fashioned, even a pump lacking a Dacron pouch may be placed without suturing, especially in thin patients (Fig. 44–9A).

18. Carefully close the incisions. An interrupted, inverted layer of 2-0 absorbable suture in the abdomen and 3-0 absorbable suture in the back is sufficient. Then appose the skin edges with Steri-Strips. If tension is a problem, use surgical staples to reinforce the closure (Fig. 44–9B).

19. The intrathecal pump is programmed prior to connection to the intrathecal catheter with a continuous mode and single bolus. The bolus setting serves to clear the intrathecal tubing and infuse the drug to the tip of the catheter. By having the catheter filled with drug, potential drug-related adverse effects could be monitored in a hospital environment. This is done by bolusing the catheter with 0.4 mL of infusion drug over an hour (Fig. 44–10).

COMPLICATIONS

SURGICAL PROBLEMS

In the perioperative period, bleeding with subsequent development of a pocket hematoma is perhaps the most troublesome and preventable problem. Meticulous attention to hemostasis during pump pocket formation prevents this situation. Prevention is aided by placing an abdominal binder, such as a 6-inch elastic wrap around the abdomen and lightly compressing the fresh pump pocket for 24 to 48 hours. This compression dressing helps avoid accumulation of blood or fluid in the pocket.

The possibility of epidural and intrathecal hemorrhage with the obvious risk of neurologic injury is frequently mentioned. This complication, unfortunately, is likely to be unnoticeable at the time of catheter implantation. Preoperatively, care should be taken to discontinue nonsteroidal anti-inflammatory drugs and reverse any anticoagulation. Signs of a developing hematoma are usually a sudden increase in focal back pain associated with tenderness, progressing numbness, or weakness in the lower extremities, and loss of bowel or bladder control resulting in either retention (constipation) or incontinence. This clinical presentation warrants immediate imaging studies with magnetic resonance imaging (MRI) or computed tomography (CT) myelography and emergent neurosurgical intervention if there is neurologic deterioration.

With implantable devices, one of the most feared complications is that of wound infection. Prophylactic antibiotics have been controversial, but a consensus seems to have developed for using some preoperative antibiosis. One method is to use a cephalosporin intravenously 1 hour before surgery with subsequent antibiosis. Some clinics use daily prophylaxis while an externalized screening electrode trial is performed. Intraoperatively, antibiotic irrigation may be used. Attention on the part of surgical personnel to handling all parts with care and avoiding unnecessary contact with any, even prepared, skin may cut down on contamination.

Although not all wound infections require removal of the device, general experience with foreign bodies implanted in the body, such as CSF shunts, spinal instrumentation, and prosthetic devices, indicates that all but superficial infections require system removal.[13] Implantable pumps contain an internal filter that guards against direct contamination resulting in meningitis. However, with infection tracking along the intrathecal catheter, either an epidural abscess or meningitis may result.

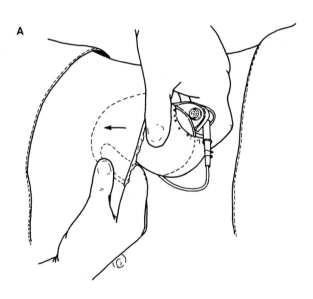

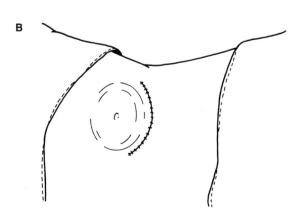

FIGURE 44–9

A, Inserting a pump into the pocket. *B,* Closing the pocket and spinal incisions.

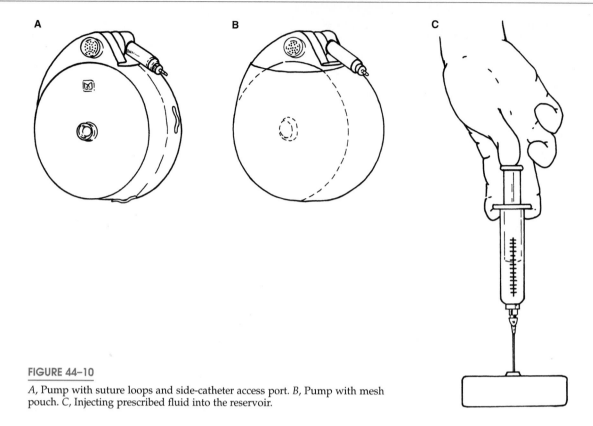

FIGURE 44–10

A, Pump with suture loops and side-catheter access port. *B,* Pump with mesh pouch. *C,* Injecting prescribed fluid into the reservoir.

Neurologic injury is a definite possibility whenever the CSF space is entered. Needle placement, even when guided fluoroscopically, is essentially "blind" with respect to intraspinal neural structures. Potential injury to the nerve roots can occur and, to some extent, can be mitigated by performing the catheter placement using local anesthesia. The patient under local anesthesia will report a radiating electric shock–like or burning sensation in the distribution of the involved nerve root. The needle should be immediately withdrawn and placement at a different level should be considered.

With catheter placement, the spinal cord is at risk. Catheters that are spring wound or have stiffening wired internally must not be forced through the spinal canal because the tip may be buried in an intramedullary position. Penetration of the spinal cord often results in the production of dysesthesias or a burning, stinging pain below the lesion that is not nondermatomal and may not result in noticeable neurologic signs immediately. Intramedullary infusion of drug may result in progressive signs of a spinal cord lesion, and this should be immediately evaluated with MRI or CT myelography and dealt with appropriately by the neurosurgeon.

CSF leaks are a natural consequence of placing catheters in the subarachnoid space. The opening created in the dura mater by the introducing needle is larger than the entering catheter, predisposing to some potential leakage. The dura mater has a moderate amount of elasticity, which probably explains why the incidence of leaks is not higher. If the particular technique used seems

to result in a relatively high incidence of spinal headache or CSF collection under the skin, a blood patch injecting 10 to 20 mL of autologous venous blood one level above the catheter entry point or at the entry point under fluoroscopic control (to avoid shearing the intrathecal catheter) may treat this problem effectively.

DEVICE-RELATED PROBLEMS

The most frequently reported complications with implantable pump systems involve some failure in the catheter system. Pump complications are quite rare. Early reports contained many catheter-related complications.[14, 15] With the development of more thick-walled and reinforced catheters, new anchoring techniques, and paraspinous approaches to placement, this problem seems to have decreased.[16]

Catheter tip obstruction can be a problem and may require revision of the catheter. This problem is usually suspected when the expected and measured residual volumes vary by more than 20%. A complete evaluation of the catheter must be performed if obstruction, kinking, or separation is suspected. This evaluation is made more important by the increasing reports of sterile granulomatous masses forming at the tip of the catheter. These masses may cause obstruction but most commonly produce increasing pain and a progressive neurologic deficit.[17]

Evaluation of a catheter problem includes some type of imaging. Simple radiography with a soft tissue technique can demonstrate breakage or suggest a kink, migration, or disconnection from the extension or pump catheter. The evaluation of suspected obstruction related to an intraspinal problem or catheter leakage requires the use of the injection side port, if present. Injection of non-ionic contrast material confirms obstruction and often shows the point of leakage. The risk with this technique is that delivery of a large bolus of medication directly into the subarachnoid space will lead to significant overdosage. When this procedure is performed, preparation for management of an overdose should be made. An attempt to aspirate the catheter should take place before injecting the contrast material to avoid this problem. In the absence of a side port, the evaluation of catheter problems is more difficult. A radioisotope may be injected into an emptied pump, and if the system is programmable, a bolus is programmed; if it is nonprogramable, an appropriate time must elapse and the catheter is scanned.

Treatment of catheter problems usually requires removal and replacement of the catheter. Occasionally, a disconnected catheter may simply be reconnected, usually with local anesthesia. Demonstration of a granulomatous mass may require neurosurgical intervention to resect the lesion.

Pump-related complications common to nonprogrammable and programmable systems include overfilling of the pump, failure of the self-sealing septum at the refill port, and movement of the pump in the pocket. Overfilling can result in overpressurization with delivery of an unpredictable amount of drug, failure of the system, or activation of the reservoir valve preventing infusion with a programmable pump. Nonprogrammable pumps may show a slight decline in drug delivery as they approach their refill time. The decline is most likely due to a decrease in the pressure of gas against the bellows as the Freon reaches the maximum volume it has to occupy. This behavior should be anticipated and may require a slight shortening of the refill time if it is troublesome to the patient.

Programmable pumps have an additional set of potential problems because of the internal modules and mechanical components necessary with this type of device. Battery failure, pump rotor failure, and failure of the telemetry or electronic modules may occur. The battery lifetime of the pumps has been quite acceptable and is generally in the range of 3 to 5 years. Battery depletion requires surgical removal of the existing pump and replacement with a new pump. Pump rotor stalls may be confirmed by taking a radiograph of the pump showing the rotor, programming a bolus dose, and repeating the radiograph 15 minutes later. The pump rotor should have turned 90 degrees if the rotor is functioning. A stalled rotor requires pump replacement. Failure of the electronic or telemetry module results in inability of the pump to receive a change in programming. The pump will, however, continue to function as a nonprogrammable pump at its last prescription infusion rate. The decision to replace the pump is based on the need to make programming changes.

Movement of the pump in the pocket may result in dislodgment of the catheters (extension or intrathecal, or both). The pump may rotate in the pocket, resulting in a coiling of the catheter much like that of a fishing reel, or it may flip in the pocket, resulting in a progressive winding of the catheter. Revision of the pump and possibly the catheters may be necessary if catheter movement is occurring. A flipped pump is usually noticed by the patient but may be noted and verified in the clinic at the time of attempted refill. Revision of the pump is probably necessary and often requires anchoring the pump.

HELPFUL HINTS

An important concern is the patient's current opioid use and how to manage it at the time of screening. Eliminating opioids before screening any cause unwarranted discomfort to the patient and may add to the expense of the trial.[18] A complete conversion from systemic opioid to intraspinal opioid may result in an abstinence syndrome. Therefore, a clinical protocol during the screening trial is necessary to prevent withdrawal effects. One such protocol, suggested by Krames,[16] involves converting 50% of the pretrial oral dose to an intrathecal equivalent dose and withdrawing the remaining oral dose by 20% per day, converting it to an equianalgesic intrathecal dose. The dose may then be increased to effecting intrathecally while systemic medication is decreased.

For the tunneled catheter period, the patient is usually kept in the hospital for a 3-day period, although some clinicians are beginning to use outpatient trials of 1 week or longer. The length of trial may be an important consideration. Presumably, the longer the trial proceeds, the less likely it is that a placebo response will account for the outcome. It is fair to say that most clinicians feel that a longer screening trial predisposes to a more successful outcome.

If the screening trial is successful, the patient generally reports at least 50% pain relief as measured by some standard self-reports to no intolerable side effects. The patient then proceeds to implantation of the chosen drug administration system.

EFFICACY

Although most patients with chronic non–cancer-related and cancer-related pain are adequately managed with oral analgesic medications, electrostimulation, or behavioral techniques, studies indicate that only about half of the patients so treated with back pain or neuropathic pain achieve good reduction of pain, and a full 21% are unresponsive to opioid therapy.[19, 20] Long-term results are even less satisfactory, with only 16.7% reporting adequate relief.[21]

CANCER-RELATED PAIN

Early studies of cancer-related pain demonstrated that intrathecal administration of opioids was much more effective than other routes of administration.[9, 22-25] The most common early use of intrathecal infusion of morphine was for cancer-related pain.

In a retrospective, multicenter study of the use of intraspinal morphine for all types of pain, 32.7% of the patients analyzed had cancer-related pain.[22] The average length of treatment in the study was 14.6 months (range, 8 to 94 months). Patients with cancer-related pain were treated with higher initial doses and escalated to a stable level more rapidly than those with non–cancer-related pain. The most frequently used drug was morphine. In the population with cancer-related pain, 13.6% had somatic pain, 25.4% neuropathic pain, 16.9% visceral pain, and 44.1% a mixed pain presentation. The long-term stability of dosing in the population with cancer-related pain has also been documented elsewhere.[26]

Cancer pain of all types remains an excellent indication for the use of intrathecal opioids, especially with a programmable pump, which can aid in matching pain relief to progression of disease. It is probable that about 5% to 10% of the population with cancer pain are candidates for an implantable pump system according to the selection criteria noted previously.

NON–CANCER-RELATED PAIN

The use of intrathecal opioids for non–cancer-related pain has increased despite a lack of prospective studies. The most definitive data supporting such an increase in use are those provided by the survey of physicians in the United States by Paice and colleagues[22] for cancer-related pain and including non–cancer-related pain and by the retrospective study of Winkelmuller and Winkelmuller from Europe.[19]

In the American study, two thirds of the patients had non–cancer-related pain. The most common condition was failed back syndrome (42.4%). Other pain syndromes treated included complex regional pain syndrome (5.6%), postherpetic neuralgia (5.1%), and peripheral nerve injury (3.7%). The most common screening technique was continuous epidural infusion (35.3%), followed by bolus intrathecal injection (33.7%). Psychological screening was used for 77.6%. Morphine was the most commonly infused drug (95.5%), but a wide variety of medications were used. Doses for neuropathic pain tended to be higher at 6 months than for somatic or vis-

ceral pain. A local anesthetic (bupivacaine) was used as an adjuvant to morphine in 19.8%. These patients had a linear increase in dose over time, eventually reaching stable levels by 1 year at 9.2 mg per 24 hours. By physician report, 52.4% of the patients had excellent pain relief, 42.9% good relief, and 4.8% poor relief, testifying to the considerable efficacy of this technique.[22]

Specific outcome measures employed by Paice and colleagues[22] included activities of daily living (ADL), employment, percentage of pain relief, a global pain relief score incorporating intensity and pain medication changes, and activity levels. ADL were 82% improved. Patients with visceral pain showed the greatest improvement in ADL. Twenty-four of the patients with non–cancer-related pain returned to work.

In a long-term follow-up of 120 patients with non–cancer-related pain in Europe with a mean of 3.4 years (range, 0.5 to 5.7 years), 73 patients had mixed neuropathic and nociceptive pain because of multiple back surgeries and 34 had conditions such as postherpetic neuralgia, stump and phantom limb pain, and various peripheral nerve injuries.[20] Six months after implantation, the average pain intensity score was 30.5. At the conclusion of follow-up, the score was 39.2. The best initial response was seen in the group with nociceptive pain, which had a 77% initial reduction in pain intensity and declined to 48% at last follow-up. Groups with deafferentation and neuropathic pain benefited from therapy and over the long term showed the best results, with 68% and 62% pain reduction as measured by visual analog scale, respectively.

Although these results for a population of patient unresponsive to more conventional methods are impressive, prospective studies comparing this therapy with alternative therapies would establish intrathecal infusion of medication as a treatment of choice in a more rigorous fashion. The current acceptance in clinical practice empirically validates the technique but also makes prospective and certainly randomized studies difficult to implement.

Infusion programmable pump 32362; implantation, revision, or repositioning of intrathecal or epidural catheter or implantable reservoir/infusion pump 62350; removal of reservoir or pump previously implanted for intrathecal or epidural infusion 62365; removal of previously implanted intrathecal or epidural catheter 62350

REFERENCES

1. Wang JK, Nauss LA, Thomas JE: Pain relief by intrathecally applied morphine in man. Anesthesiology 50:149–150, 1979.
2. Yaksh TL: Spinal opiate anesthesia: Characteristics and principles of action. Pain 11:293–346, 1981.
3. Yaksh TL, Rudy TA: Analgesia mediated by a direct spinal action of narcotics. Science 192:1357–1358, 1976.
4. Yaksh TL, Rudy TA: Narcotic analgesics: CNS sites and mechanisms of action as revealed by direct intracerebral injection techniques. Pain 4:299–359, 1978.

5. Bedder MD, Burchiel K, Larson SA: Cost analysis of two implantable narcotic delivery systems. J Pain Symptom Manage 6:368–373, 1991.

6. DuPen IL, Williams AR: Management of patients receiving combined epidural morphine and bupivacaine for the treatment of cancer pain. J Pain Symptom Manage 27:15–127, 1992.

7. Coombs DW, Saunders RL, Baylor MS, et al: Relief of continuous chronic pain by intraspinal narcotics infusion via an implanted reservoir. JAMA 250:2336–2339, 1983.

8. Poletti CE, Cohen AM, Todd DP, et al: Cancer pain relieved by long-term epidural morphine with permanent indwelling systems for self-administration. J Neurosurg 55:581–584, 1981.

9. Brazenor GA: Long-term intrathecal administration of morphine: A comparison of bolus injection via reservoir with continuous infusion by implanted pump. Neurosurgery 21:484–491, 1987.

10. Muller H, Lueben V, Zierski J, Hempleman G: Long-term spinal opiate treatment. Acta Anaesthesiol Belg 39:83–86, 1988.

11. Akahoski MP, Furuike-McLaughlin T, Enriquez NC: Patient-controlled analgesia via intrathecal catheter in outpatient oncology patients. J Intravenous Nurs 11:289–292, 1988.

12. Krames ES, Olson K: Clinical realities and economic considerations: Patient selection in intrathecal therapy. J Pain Symptom manage 14(Suppl):S3–S13, 1997.

13. Blount JP, Campbell JA, Haines SJ: Complications in ventricular cerebrospinal fluid shunting. Neurosurg Clin North Am 4:633–656, 1993.

14. Coffey RJ, Cahill D, Steers W, et al: Intrathecal baclofen for intractable spasticity of spinal origin: Results of a long-term multicenter study. J Neurosurg 78:226–232, 1993.

15. Penn RD, York MM, Paice JA: Catheter systems for intrathecal drug delivery. J Neurosurg 78:226–232, 1993.

16. Krames ES: Intrathecal infusion therapies for intractable pain: Patient management guidelines. J Pain Symptom Manage 8:36–46, 1993.

17. Krames ES: Intraspinal opioid therapy for chronic nonmalignant pain: Current practice and clinical guidelines. J Pain Symptom Manage 11:333–352, 1996.

18. Turner JA, Loeser JD: The importance of placebo effects in pain treatment and research. JAMA 221:1609–1614, 1994.

19. Winkelmuller M, Winkelmuller W: Long-term effect of continuous intrathecal opioid treatment in chronic pain of nonmalignant etiology. J Neurosurg 85:485–467, 1996.

20. Zenz M, Strumpf M, Tryba M: Long-term oral opioid therapy in patients with chronic nonmalignant pain. J Pain Symptom Manage 7:69–77, 1992.

21. Schulzech S, Gleim M, Maier C: Morphintabletten bei chronischen nicht-tumorbedingten Schmerzen. Welche Faktoren beeinflussen Erfolg oder Misserfolg einer Langzeittherapie. Anaesthesist 42:545–556, 1993.

22. Paice JA, Penn RD, Shott S: Intraspinal morphine for chronic pain: A retrospective multicenter study. J Pain Symptom Manage 11:71–80, 1996.

23. DeCastro J, Meynadier J, Zenz M: Regional Opioid Analgesia. Dordrecht, Kluwer Academic, 1991, pp 393–425.

24. Eriksen K, Bigler D, Jensen NH, et al: Langtidsbehandling med morfin intratekalt ved svaere cancers mertetilstande. Ugeskr Laeger 151:2365–2366, 1989.

25. Motsch J, Belser W, Ismaily AJ, et al: Kontinuierliche intrathekale Opiattherapie mit tragbaren Medikamentenpumpen bei Karzinomschmerzen. Anasth Intensivther Notfallmed 23:271–275, 1988.

26. Schultheiss R, Schramm J, Neidhardt J: Dose changes in long-term and median-term intrathecal morphine therapy of cancer pain. Neurosurgery 31:664–670, 1992.

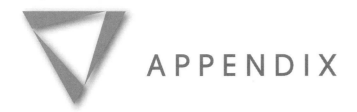

APPENDIX

SPECIAL EQUIPMENT NEEDED FOR PROCEDURES

EQUIPMENT FOR RADIOFREQUENCY

- Figure A–1. Radiofrequency machine
- Figure A–2. SMK radiofrequency 10-cm needles with 2-mm tip
- Figure A–3. RF radiofrequency 10-cm needles with 5-mm tip
- Figure A–4. Tew radiofrequency 10-cm needles with 10-mm tip
- Figure A–5. RFK small radiofrequency 10-cm needles with 15-mm tip
- Figure A–6. Intravenous catheter, 16 gauge, and intravenous catheter, 14 gauge
- Figure A–7. Radiofrequency 15-cm needles with 15-mm tip
- Figure A–8. SM straight radiofrequency needle with 5-mm tip, and SM straight radiofrequency needle with 10-mm tip

This radiofrequency equipment is applicable to the following chapters: 6 to 12, 17, 20 to 22, 26 to 29, 35, and 36.

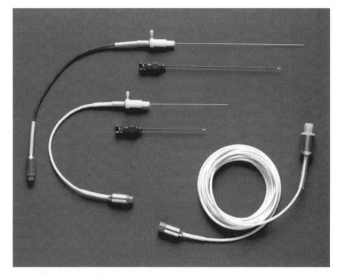

FIGURE A–2

SMK radiofrequency 10-cm needles with 2-mm tip.

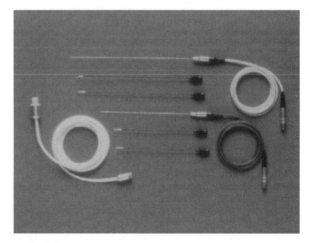

FIGURE A–3

RF radiofrequency 10-cm needles with 5-mm tip. (Courtesy of Radionics, Division of Tyco Healthcare, Burlington, Massachusetts.)

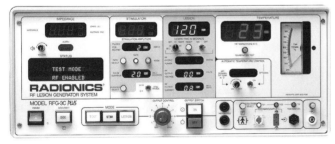

FIGURE A–1

Radiofrequency machine faceplate (Radionics).

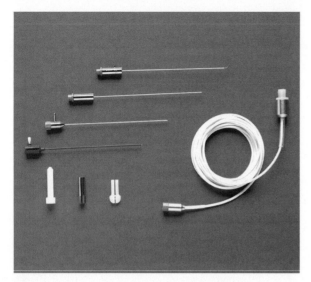

FIGURE A–4
Tew radiofrequency 10-cm needles with 10-mm tip.

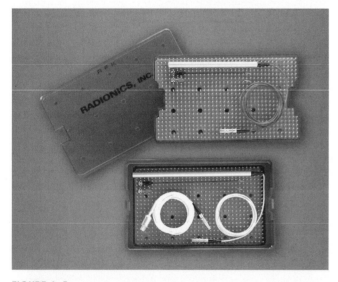

FIGURE A–5
RFK small radiofrequency 10-cm needles with 15-mm tip.

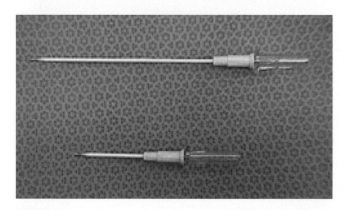

FIGURE A–6
Intravenous catheter with 16 gauge, and intravenous catheter with 14 gauge.

EQUIPMENT FOR BALLOON NEUROLYSIS

- Figure A–9. Fogarty catheter 4 French

This radiofrequency equipment is applicable to Chapter 6.

EQUIPMENT FOR CRYONEUROLYSIS

- Figure A–10. Cryoneurolysis machine and cable
- Figure A–11. Cryo probe set with probe 12g, 14g, 16g, 18g

This equipment is applicable to Chapters 10 and 19.

EQUIPMENT FOR EPIDURAL TECHNIQUE

- Figure A–12. Tuohy epidural needle
- Figure A–13. LOR (loss of resistance) syringe

This radiofrequency equipment is applicable to Chapters 16 and 24.

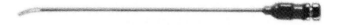

FIGURE A–7
Radiofrequency 15-cm needles with 15-mm tip (curved blunt).

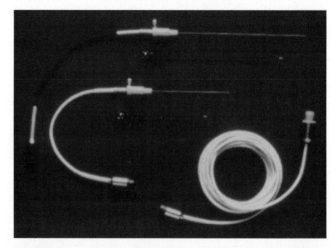

FIGURE A–8
SM straight radiofrequency needle with 5-mm tip, and SM straight radiofrequency needle with 10-mm tip. (Courtesy of Radionics, Division of Tyco Healthcare, Burlington, Massachusetts.)

FIGURE A–9
Fogarty catheter 4 French for trigeminal balloon neuroplasty.

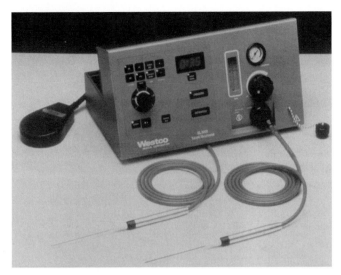

FIGURE A-10

Cryoneurolysis machine and cable. (Courtesy of Westco Medical Corporation, Dahlgren, Virginia.)

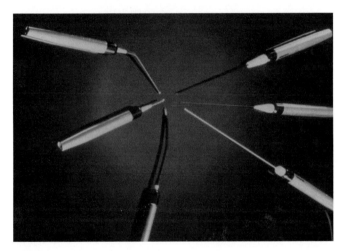

FIGURE A-11

Cryo probe set with probe 12g, 14g, 16g, 18g. (Courtesy of Westco Medical Corporation, Dahlgren, Virginia.)

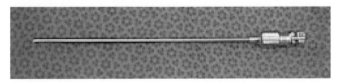

FIGURE A-12

Tuohy epidural needle.

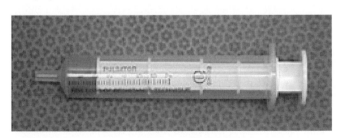

FIGURE A-13

LOR (loss of resistance) syringe for epidural procedure.

EQUIPMENT FOR PROVOCATIVE DISCOGRAPHY

- Figure A–14. Chiba needle
- Radiofrequency needle

This radiofrequency equipment is applicable to Chapters 17 and 31.

EQUIPMENT FOR PRESSURE MONITORING SYSTEM FOR DISCOGRAPHY

- Figure A–15. Discography monitoring equipment

This equipment is applicable to Chapter 31.

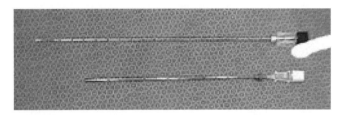

FIGURE A-14

Chiba needles to be used for discography.

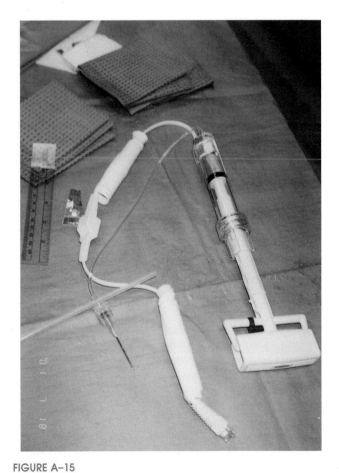

FIGURE A-15

Discography monitoring equipment includes the screw-type syringe with integrated pressure monitoring.

EQUIPMENT FOR CONTINUOUS INFUSION OF PERIPHERAL NERVES

- Figure A–16. RK epidural needle, 16 gauge
- Figure A–17. Tun-L-XL epidural catheter
- Figure A–18. BD Longdwel catheter with needle

This equipment is applicable to Chapters 18 and 39.

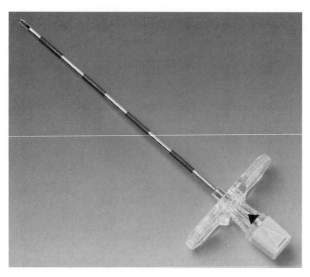

FIGURE A–16

RK epidural needle 16 gauge from Epimed, Inc. This needle is designed to minimize the potential to shear epidural catheters.

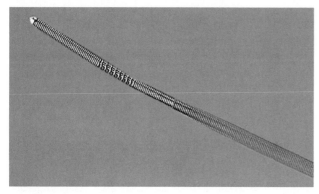

FIGURE A–17

Tun-L-XL epidural catheter from Epimed, Inc. This springwire, reinforced catheter with a "soft" tip helps attenuate the potential for neural tissue damage.

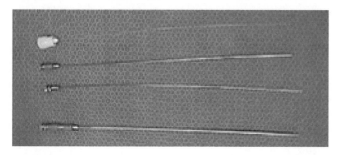

FIGURE A–18

BD Longdwel catheter with needle. A catheter-over-needle system for peripheral nerve continuous infusions.

EQUIPMENT FOR INTRADISCAL ELECTROTHERMAL COAGULATION

- Figure A–19. Oratek electrothermal coagulation machine
- Figure A–20. Spina-Cath

This equipment is applicable to Chapter 32.

EQUIPMENT FOR VERTEBROPLASTY

- Figure A–21. No. II gauge bone biopsy needle
- Figure A–22. Mixing bowl and ladle
- Figure A–23. Disposable PMMA injection

This equipment is applicable to Chapter 33.

EQUIPMENT FOR AUGMENTATION

- Figure A–24. IPG and ANS—Genesis
- Figure A–25. Medtronic
- Figure A–26. Programming equipment
- Figure A–27. Electrodes

This equipment is applicable to Chapter 43.

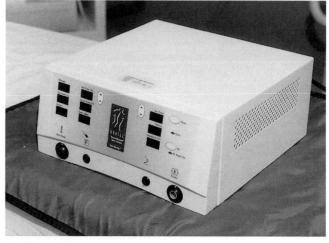

FIGURE A–19

Oratec electrothermal coagulation machine. This is the base unit for intradiscal electrothermal coagulation (IDET).

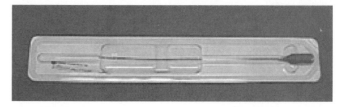

FIGURE A–20

Spine-Cath. An intradiscal catheter inserted into the disc for IDET lesioning.

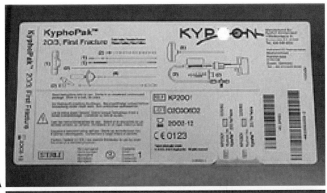

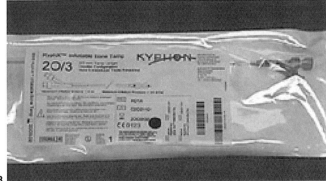

FIGURE A–21

No. 11 gauge bone biopsy needle for injection of bone cement. This needle is used for vertebroplasty and kyphoplasty.

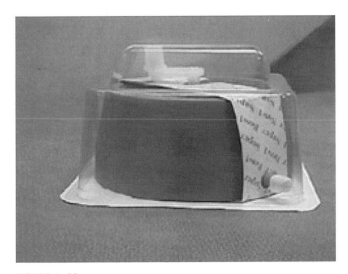

FIGURE A–22

Bowl and ladle for mixing injectable bone cement in vertebroplasty.

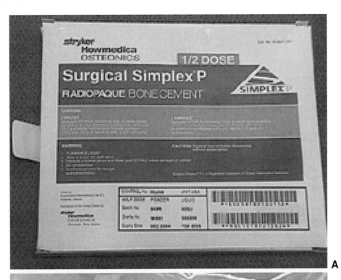

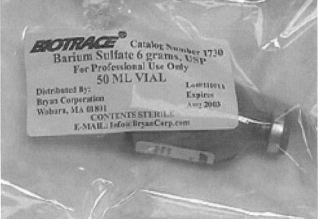

FIGURE A–23

Disposable PMMA injection kit. *A,* Bone cement ingredients. *B,* Radiopaque barium sulfate additive to bone cement.

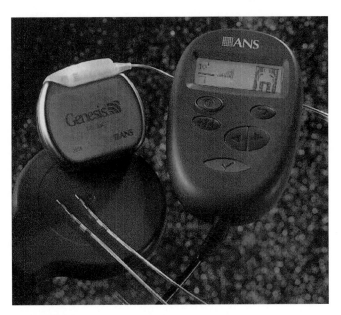

FIGURE A–24

ANS—Genesis IPG (implantable pulse generator) on the left; patient programmer on the right; two percutaneous quadripolar electrodes in the foreground.

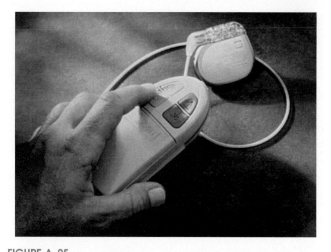

FIGURE A–25

Medtronic Itrel 3 implantable pulse generator (IPG) battery is in the background; the patient's controller is in the foreground.

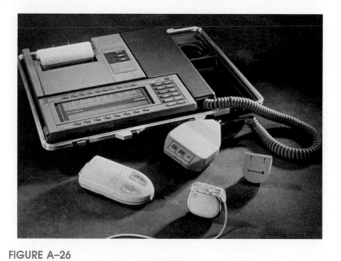

FIGURE A–26

Medtronic programmer for the physician for the implantable pulse generator used in dorsal column stimulation. Patient's programmer, IPG, and magnet are in the foreground.

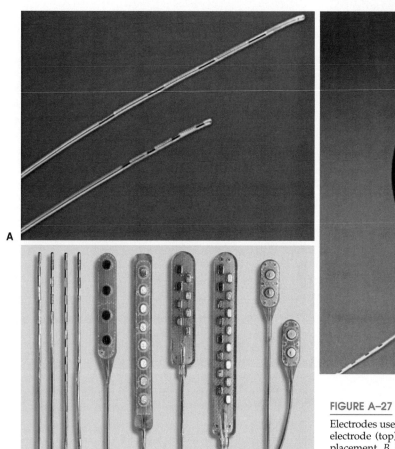

A

B

C

FIGURE A–27

Electrodes used in column stimulation. *A*, Medtronic Pisces Quad Plus electrode (top) and Pisces Quad electrode (bottom) for percutaneous placement. *B*, Medtronic Pisces Quad electrode. *C*, Percutaneous and laminotomy electrodes from ANS.

EQUIPMENT FOR INTRATHECAL PUMP

- Figure A–28. Programmable pump with catheter
- Figure A–29. Fixed rate pump with catheter

This equipment is applicable to Chapter 44.

EQUIPMENT FOR EPIDUROSCOPY

- Figure A–30. Epiduroscope with neuroplasty catheters and introducers

This equipment is applicable to Chapter 42.

EQUIPMENT FOR RADIOGRAPHIC IMAGING

- Figure A–31. A typical fluoroscopy C-arm

This equipment is used for all radiographic imaging in this book.

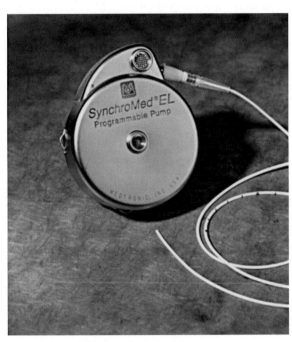

FIGURE A–28

Programmable pump with catheter.

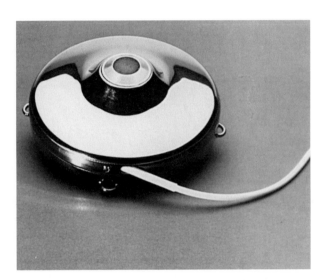

FIGURE A–29

Fixed-rate pump with catheter.

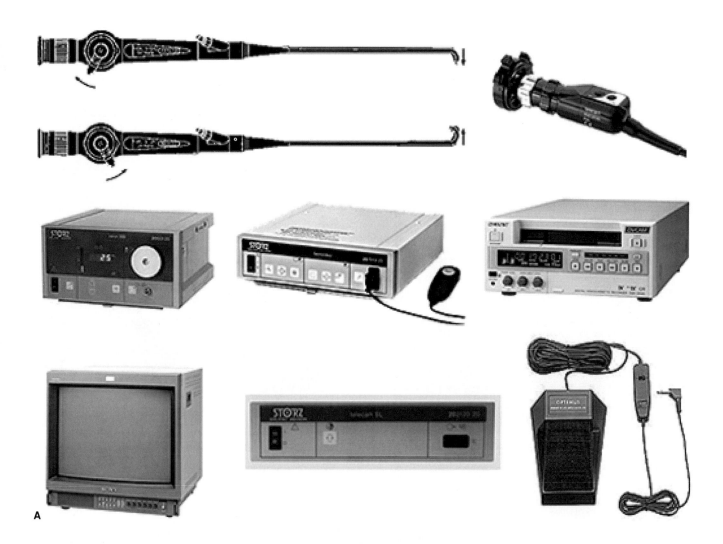

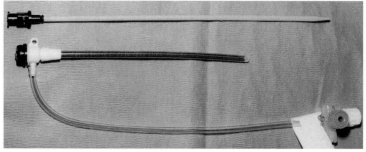

FIGURE A–30

Epiduroscope with catheters and introducers. *A,* The various components of the epiduroscopy system. *B,* Dilator (top) and introducer cannula (bottom).

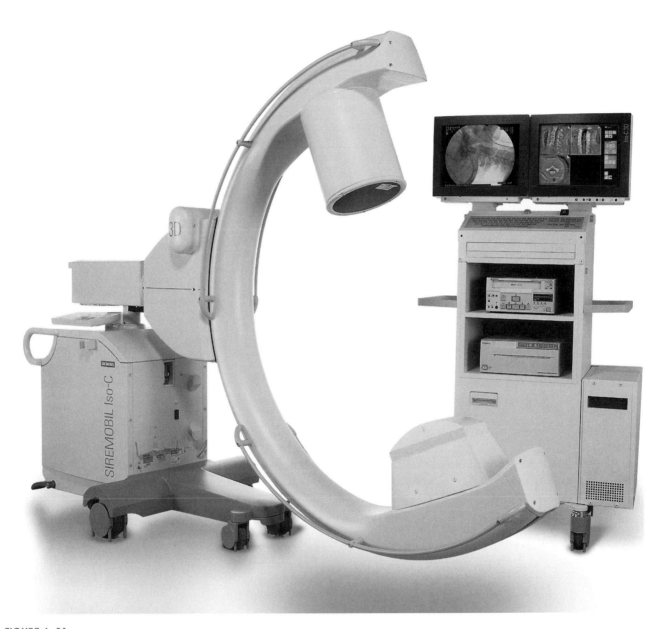

FIGURE A–31

A typical fluoroscopy C-arm. (Courtesy of Siemens.)

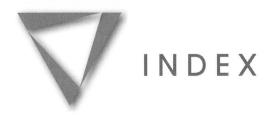

INDEX

Note: Page numbers followed by f refer to figures and those followed by t refer to tables.

A

A fibers, transmission role of, 24, 282
Abdominal pain syndromes
  lower thoracic blocks for. *See* Celiac
    ganglion block; Splanchnic nerve
    blocks.
  upper thoracic blocks for. *See* Intercostal
    nerve block.
Abdominal viscera, innervation of
  celiac plexus, 164–165, 165
  intercostal, 117–118, 118f
  splanchnic, 158, 158f
Abscess, epidural, with thoracic discogram,
  152
Absorbed dose, of radiation, 9
AC (alternating current), in radiography
  physics, 2, 3, 6
Accessory nerve nuclei, compromise with
  upper cervical conditions, 81–82, 81f
Accommodation, of electrical stimulus, 297
Adhesions, perineural, epiduroscopic lysis
  of, 274, 279
Air acceptance test, for epidural nerve
  blocks, 103
Air-core transformer, physics of, 3
Alcohol injection, for neurolysis. *See* Ethyl
  alcohol.
Alcoholic neuritis, from ethyl alcohol, 23
Alternating current (AC), in radiography
  physics, 2, 3, 6
Amide local anesthetics
  metabolism of, 15–16, 16f
  pharmacology of specific, 18–19, 18f
Ammonium salts, as neurolytic agent, 26
Amperage, in radiography physics, 2, 3, 5
Amplitude, in electromagnetic radiation, 2, 2f
Analgesia. *See specific anatomical block.*
Anatomy. *See specific block or procedure.*
Anesthesia dolorosa, with glossopharyngeal
  nerve block, 59
Anesthetics
  dermatomal, 24
  epidural, 2-chloroprocaine as, 17–18
  local. *See* Local anesthetics.
  regional, 19, 24
Angstrom, in electromagnetic radiation, 2, 2f
Annulus fibrosus, of intervertebral discs,
  207–208, 207f
  in intradiscal electrothermal coagulation,
    208, 210, 210f
  lumbar, 197–198, 197f, 200
  thoracic, 61, 152
Anode, of x-ray tube, 6f, 7
  electrical energy conversion in, 2
  electron interaction with, 1f, 2–3
Anterior approach, to celiac ganglion block,
  164, 170–173, 172f
  advantages of, 164, 170–171

Anterior approach *(Continued)*
  CT or ultrasonographic guidance for, 164,
    171–172, 172f
  disadvantages of, 171
  important precautions for, 172–173
Antiarrhythmic agents, local anesthetics as,
  18, 19
Antibiotics
  for decompressive neuroplasty, 261
  for discograms, 108, 150
    lumbar provocative, 199–200, 206
  for intradiscal electrothermal coagulation,
    208–209, 211
  for intrathecal implants, 307
  for skin damage, 68, 136, 200, 232
  for vertebroplasty, 216, 219
Aortic plexus, anatomy of, 231–232, 231f
Arrhythmias, secondary to nerve blocks, 59,
  71, 74
Articular processes, of thoracic and lumbar
  vertebrae, 213f, 214
Aspiration test, mandatory
  for cervical epidural nerve block, 104
  for trigeminal ganglion block and
    neurolysis, 40, 47
  with suprascapular nerve block, 130
Ataxia
  with atlantoaxial joint block, 89
  with atlanto-occipital joint block, 85
Atlantoaxial joint block, 86–90
  anatomy for, 86–87, 86f–87f
  complications of, 89–90
  contraindications to, 87–88
  drugs for, 88
  efficacy of, 90
  equipment for, 88
  helpful hints for, 90
  history of, 86
  indications for, 87
  patient preparation for, 88
  positioning for, 88, 88f–89f
  procedural technique for, 88–89, 89f
    contrast injection and interpretation, 89,
      90f
    drug injection, 89
Atlantodental joint. *See* Atlantoaxial joint
  block.
Atlanto-occipital joint block, 81–85
  anatomy for, 81–82, 81f
  complications of, 85
  contraindications to, 82
  drugs for, 82
  efficacy of, 85
  equipment, 82
  helpful hints for, 85
  history of, 81
  indications for, 82
  patient preparation for, 82

Atlanto-occipital joint block *(Continued)*
  positioning for, 82, 83f
  postprocedure monitoring of, 85
  procedural technique for, 82–85
    contrast injection and interpretation,
      84–85, 84f
    hyalgan injection, 85
    needle entry, 83–84, 83f–84f
Atomic structure, in radiography physics, 1,
  1f
Attenuation coefficient, of x-ray beam, 9–10
Augmentation techniques
  for spinal cord, 282–300
    contraindications to, 283
    drugs for, 283
    efficacy of, 299–300, 300t
    equipment for, 283
    for cervical spinal cord, 285–290
    for occipital nerve, 283–285
    for sacral nerve, 297–299
    for thoracolumbar spinal cord, 290–297
    history of, 282, 282t
    indications for, 283
  for vertebral body. *See* Vertebroplasty.
Autotransformer, physics of, 4
Axillary approach, to brachial plexus block
  helpful hints for, 116
  history of, 111
  technique for, 114–115, 115f
Axillary artery, in brachial plexus block,
  114–115

B

Balloon compression. *See* Percutaneous
  balloon decompression.
Barium sulfate powder, for vertebroplasty,
  215
Blind techniques, for piriformis muscle
  injection, 252–253, 253f
Blood patch, for cerebrospinal fluid leaks,
  308
Blunt-tip needle
  for lumbar sleeve and dorsal root block,
    154, 156
  for lumbar sympathetic block, 177, 180
Bodies, of thoracic and lumbar vertebrae,
  213–214, 213f
  in vertebroplasty, 218, 218f–219f, 219
Botulinum toxin, for muscle injections
  piriformis, 252
  psoas and quadratus lumborum, 222, 225
Brachial plexus block, 111–116
  Chassaignac's tubercle in, 111, 113
  complications of, 113, 114, 115
  drugs for, 112
  efficacy of, 112, 116
  equipment for, 111